Springer Series in Cognitive Development

Series Editor
Charles J. Brainerd

Springer Series in Cognitive Development

Series Editor: Charles J. Brainerd

Wolfgang Schneider   Michael Pressley

Memory Development
Between 2 and 20

With 17 Illustrations

Springer-Verlag
New York Berlin Heidelberg
London Paris Tokyo

Wolfgang Schneider
Max-Planck-Institut für Psychologische Forschung
Munich, West Germany

Michael Pressley
Department of Psychology
University of Western Ontario
London, Ontario
Canada N6A 5C2

Series Editor
Charles J. Brainerd
Program in Educational Psychology
University of Arizona
Tuscon, Arizona 85715 USA

Library of Congress Cataloging-in-Publication Data
Schneider, Wolfgang, 1953–
  Memory development between 2 and 20.
  (Springer series in cognitive development)
  Bibliography: p.
  Includes index.
  1. Memory in children.   2. Memory in youth.
I. Pressley, Michael.   II. Title.   III. Title: Memory
development between two and twenty.   IV. Series.
BF723.M4S35   1988   155.4'13   88-15981

Printed on acid-free paper.

Typeset by Publishers Service, Bozeman, Montana
Printed and bound by Edwards Brothers, Inc., Ann Arbor, Michigan
Printed in the United States of America.

9 8 7 6 5 4 3 2 1

ISBN 0-387-96742-7 Springer-Verlag New York Berlin Heidelberg
ISBN 3-540-96742-7 Springer-Verlag Berlin Heidelberg New York

Dedicated to our wives, Elisabeth and Donna, and to our children, Christof, Felix, and Timothy

Series Preface

For some time now, the study of cognitive development has been far and away the most active discipline within developmental psychology. Although there would be much disagreement as to the exact proportion of papers published in developmental journals that could be considered cognitive, 50% seems like a conservative estimate. Hence, a series of scholarly books devoted to work in cognitive development is especially appropriate at this time

The *Springer Series in Cognitive Development* contains two basic types of books, namely, edited collections of original chapters by several authors, and original volumes written by one author or a small group of authors. The flagship for the Springer Series is a serial publication of the "advances" type, carrying the subtitle *Progress in Cognitive Development Research*. Each volume in the *Progress* sequence is strongly thematic, in that it is limited to some well-defined domain of cognitive-developmental research (e.g., logical and mathematical development, development of learning). All *Progress* volumes will be edited collections. Editors of such collections, upon consulting with the Series Editor, may elect to have their books published either as contributions to the *Progress* sequence or as separate volumes. All books written by one author or a small group of authors are being published as separate volumes within the series.

A fairly broad definition of cognitive development is being used in the selection of books for this series. The classic topics of concept development, children's thinking and reasoning, the development of learning, language development, and memory development will, of course, be included. So, however, will newer areas such as social-cognitive development, educational applications, formal modeling, and philosophical implications of cognitive-developmental theory. Although it is anticipated that most books in the series will be empirical in orientation, theoretical and philosophical works are also welcome. With books of the latter sort, heterogeneity of theoretical perspective is encouraged, and no attempt will be made to foster some specific theoretical perspective at the expense of others (e.g., Piagetian versus behavioral or behavioral versus information processing).

C.J. Brainerd

Preface

We first met in May 1982 at the University of Notre Dame. MP was a visiting professor and WS was touring the United States as part of a leave from the Max Planck Institute to Stanford. At the time of the meeting, we had both been researching memory development for some time and had been thinking about metamemory in particular. It was apparent immediately that we shared many of the same points of view. We both had a no-nonsense, "what-do-the-data-say" attitude about the study of memory development. MP was particularly impressed by WS's thorough analysis of metamemory, one eventually published as Schneider (1985c).

We met again from time to time at conferences. In the summer of 1984, MP came to the Max Planck Institute, a visit reciprocated by WS to the University of Western Ontario in the spring of 1985. At that time we were working on the good strategy user model (along with John Borkowski). The result was an integrative framework for thinking about memory functioning, one that included cognitive, metacognitive, and noncognitive components. The latest version is taken up in Chapters 6 and 7 of this volume.

The summer of 1986 brought MP back to Munich, as WS was finishing his habilitation. It was clear that we were once again thinking about many of the same issues, and once again, the differences in our thinking were much smaller than the similarities. There seemed to be good reason to think about putting our common thoughts into a book. WS suggested parts of his habilitation as a starting point; MP agreed. This volume is the result of many rewritings and reworkings from that point of departure. We especially tried to focus on the main themes and methods in memory development. We felt it important, however, to take positions on some of the more controversial issues of the day. We debated long and hard about some of the perspectives offered here, but in the end believe that our conclusions are eminently defensible in light of the available data. We also went well beyond the habilitation, especially in developing our theory of good strategy use in light of the extensive memory development data base.

This book is intended for a number of audiences. First of all, it is meant as a coherent introduction to memory development for students and professionals who have little background in either cognitive or developmental psychology. We tried to write a good book for advanced undergraduate and first- and second-year graduate courses. It is also a volume for our peers, however, in that we do try to provide clear stances on many of the major issues of the day. We worked hard to separate the "wheat from the chaff" and, thus, have identified the literature that we hope our peers will consider seriously as they plan future research. There was no hesitation to indicate gaps in the literature, thus hoping that some of the senior scientific community might be stimulated by our discussion and consider filling in those gaps. For student readers, these gaps might provide many thesis and dissertation opportunities.

This volume will be updated with a second edition in a few years. Most of the revision will follow from new work that will appear in the literature, but some of it will involve rethinking the work already conducted. Please do not hesitate to let us know if you believe that some data and/or interpretations not presented in this volume should be considered for the revision.

There are a lot of people who deserve thanks for their contributions to our work. Both of us agree that John Flavell has influenced our thinking enormously. WS has visited Stanford several times in the 1980s; John was MP's advisor during his early graduate school years. Flavell's influence is apparent throughout this volume. Our mutual friend and frequent coauthor John Borkowski also deserves thanks. He continuously challenges us to think about memory differently than we would have otherwise. Many of these ideas were developed in part in the South Dining Hall on the campus of the University of Notre Dame. WS acknowledges the support of his colleagues and staff at the Max Planck Institute. He is particularly grateful to Franz Weinert, who first stimulated his interest in memory development about a decade ago and has provided continuous support since then. WS's ideas about the memory-metamemory relationship have been expanded by his discussions with Marcus Hasselhorn, Joachim Körkel, Beth Kurtz, Beate Sodian, Gerhard Strube, Monika Knopf, and Michael Waldmann. MP bounced many of these ideas off his graduate students, including Barbara L. Snyder, Teresa Cariglia-Bull, Eileen Wood, and Patricia Devolder. Bill Rohwer of Berkeley and Joel Levin have provided continuous feedback for 15 years about MP's work on elaboration, some of which is summarized in Chapter 7.

We hope that we wrote a book that summarizes the field well in a fashion that is interesting. Let us know what you think.

Munich, FRG   Wolfgang Schneider

London, Ontario, Canada   Michael Pressley

Contents

1. A Brief History of Memory Development Research

The aim of this book is to give an integrative introduction to theory and research on memory development from early childhood to early adulthood. Research on memory development has been stimulated by a shift in both experimental and developmental psychology away from behaviorist theories toward cognitive theories, a shift that emphasizes information processing considerations. The discovery of Piaget by American developmental psychology (Bruner, 1964; Flavell, 1963) also encouraged the cognitive "Zeitgeist" in developmental psychology (Ornstein, 1978a). A "Symposium on Memory Development," which posed the question, "What actually develops?" (Flavell, 1971) was an additional stimulant.

While in 1965 the key word "memory" was not used in the index of *Child Development Abstracts and Bibliography* (as noted by Kail & Hagen, 1977a), every issue of that outlet now includes abstracts for a number of studies of memory. It would have been much easier to summarize this field even a decade ago (Wimmer, 1976) with most of the important research programs covered comprehensively in a single edited volume (Kail & Hagen, 1977a). Since then, there has been a dramatic increase in the amount of research and the approaches taken by memory development researchers. For instance, although Flavell and Wellman (1977) summarized most of the existing metamemory research in a single chapter, Forrest-Pressley, MacKinnon, and Waller (1985a, 1985b) published two entire volumes about metacognition research programs, with much of the research focussing on metamemory.

Students and scholars not specializing in memory development could easily be overwhelmed by the quantity and diversity of this literature. Thus, a main purpose in writing a book about the highlights of memory development is to make accessible the most important ideas and research in this area. In doing so, we focus on what we view as the main components of the memory system including short-term memory structures, memory strategies, metamemory, and the nonstrategic knowledge base. Separate chapters are dedicated to these main components, with interactions between components considered at appropriate places (e.g., strategy development as it relates to development of the nonstrategic knowledge base and to meta-memory). The book concludes with chapters that focus on how the components function interactively and the challenge of improving memory through instructional development of components and their interactions. Before turning to recent research on memory development, however, we provide some history in this chapter.

1885–1935

Investigations of Immediate Memory

Most of the developmental memory studies at the turn of the century were concerned with the memory span, that is, with immediate memory. Given the interest of German psychologists in memory in general, it should not be surprising that much of the memory development research at that time was conducted in Germany. Ebbinghaus himself was concerned with memory-span capacity at different age levels, with particular interest in identifying the developmental memory-span curves for various types of materials (Ebbinghaus, 1885, 1887, 1902). Thus, many studies were conducted in which children were exposed to meaningless syllables, single-syllable words, or numbers with recall required immediately after one presentation. For instance, Ebbinghaus found that learners between 18 and 20 years of age were able to recall about 1½ more syllables or words than 8- to 10-year-old learners. It was also determined early that meaning played a significant role in determining the amount recalled (Netschajeff, 1902). For instance, whether nonsense words were one or two syllables in length had little impact on span. On the other hand, Binet and Henri (1894a, 1894b) found that preschoolers exhibited substantially better memory for sentences with many words (e.g., 38 words in length) than for short lists (e.g., seven items) of meaningless words. As a rule, the core verbal units that suggested meaning were remembered best.

Frequently, experimental investigations were commissioned for the purpose of answering particular practical questions, for instance, what the effects of intensive practice (five hours) was on the mental alertness of students. Often a number of different age groups were tapped in these investigations, making it possible to construct descriptive curves of memory-span development.

Other investigations were prompted by theoretical issues. In two studies in particular (Lobsien, 1902a; Netschajeff, 1900), 9- to 18-year-olds were administered a series of memory tasks, including immediate memory span for multidigit numbers and for serial word lists. The words on these lists included terms that described sensations (cool, hot), described sounds (music, bell) or referred to abstract concepts (cause, justice). In addition, memory for actual sounds and objects was tested. For all types of items, memory-span performance increased with age, with better memory for objects and labels describing sensations than for sounds and abstract concepts. Lobsien's analyses of the exact recall sequences yielded another important result—that memory of items in order develops later than simple free recall of list items. At all age levels, however, fewer items were produced in the correct serial order than were recalled overall.

Meumann (1907a) and Offner (1924) regarded both Lobsien's (1902a) and Netschajeff's (1900) investigations as particularly valuable in that they highlighted the existence of several memory functions that did not develop in parallel. Thus, the same 9-year-old children who could produce about 30% of a list of nonsense syllables were more successful when the trial consisted of numerical series of the same length (about 60% recall) or meaningful word lists (about 70%) (e.g., Jacobs, 1887; Lobsien, 1902a; Pohlmann, 1906). These findings, moreover, were consistent with earlier studies conducted by Kirkpatrick (1894) and Lobsien (1911a). In Kirkpatrick's study, schoolchildren were able to recall seven out of 10 meaningful words on average, regardless of whether the words were read or heard. In contrast, the subjects in Lobsien's experiment (aged 7 to 15 years) recalled only 2.3 out of 10 nonsense words on average.

A number of studies of immediate memory span were made using the "word-pair method" developed by Ranschburg (1901), the forerunner of the paired-associate learning technique. On each trial a series of word pairs were presented with subjects instructed to repeat each pair several times. At testing, the experimenter read the first pair member with subjects required to recall its pairmate. Nagy (1930) conducted experiments with this technique. His participants were 700 schoolchildren between the ages of 7 and 19. There were four different lists, each composed of 12 word pairs. Lists differed systematically in terms of the abstractness/concreteness dimension. Nagy found that abstract word pairs were harder to remember than concrete ones.

Investigations of Long-Term Memory and Forgetting

One of the first investigations of children's retention and forgetting of verbal materials (Vertes, 1913, 1931) used the word-pair method. Vertes was interested in the interval between learning and testing as a determinant of recall in children 6 to 18 years of age. The test for immediate retention was followed by two delayed tests at intervals of one day and one week. That more than 80% of the material was recalled on the immediate memory test suggests that the concrete words on the list were easy to memorize, particularly for the older children. After an interval of one day, the rate of forgetting was about 8% in the 6- to 13-year-old sample and no more than 3% in the 13- to 18-year-old group. After one week the results were astonishing for children older than 10 years of age. They actually remembered more than they had on the previous tests. Younger children (especially 6-year-olds) performed worse after a week than they had after 24 hours.

How do these findings compare with classic forgetting curves (e.g., Ebbinghaus, 1885)? Ebbinghaus conceived of forgetting as a quantitative fading of memory and a nonlinear function of passage of time. This relationship could be expressed as (retention/forgetting) $= k/(\log \text{time})^c$ with k and c referring to constants. In everyday language, this function specified that the rate of forgetting is greater shortly after learning than it is later. Vertes results clearly did not conform to this principle, with Vertes offering three potential explanations. One was that the word-pair method was not the same approach that Ebbinghaus used to study retention and forgetting. The second was that there was already a substantial literature suggesting that forgetting did not occur as specified by Ebbinghaus' formula. The third explanation was that forgetting might be different for children than for adults.

Vertes third hypothesis is by far the most important one in this context. Vertes was aware of the comprehensive analyses of retention and forgetting in children and adults that had been made by Radossawljewitsch (1907). Radossawljewitsch's study was stimulated by criticisms of Ebbinghaus' experimental method. In particular, Meumann, Radossawljewitsch's advisor, doubted Ebbinghaus' findings because neither he nor his collaborators were able to replicate them, and because they did not accord with the experiences of everyday life and work.

Radossawljewitsch's subjects were 16 students between 20 and 40 years of age and 11 children (aged 7 to 13). The participants learned nonsense syllables and meaningful materials (poems) and were tested on immediate memory and relearning after lapses of 5 minutes, 20 minutes, 1 hour, 8 hours, and subsequently after 2, 6, 14, 30, and 60 days. Compared to adults, children needed a very large number of repetitions to learn a series for the first time, but the children forgot less of the material that was learned and their rate of forgetting seemed less than that of adults. These differences were most salient at long retention intervals (30 to 60 days). The rate of forgetting of meaningful material in both age groups was similar to the forgetting rate for nonsense syllables, but "savings" (i.e., reduction in time to relearn the material completely) were generally greater for meaningful material.

Although the slopes of the forgetting curves were different for children and adults, the most important finding was the forgetting curves obtained for the two groups did not correspond to the curve obtained by Ebbinghaus. Although the curves were in accord with the assumption that forgetting is a decelerating function of time, they differed from the curve obtained by Ebbinghaus in that forgetting did not take place as rapidly. In particular, the children's rate of forgetting was slower than the rate reported by Ebbinghaus. The discrepancy between the two sets of data was very great—Ebbinghaus forgot more information in one hour than adults in Radossawljewitsch's study forgot in eight hours. Finkenbinder (1913) conducted research aimed at reconciling the discrepancy between the outcomes in the experiments conducted by Ebbinghaus and Radossawljewitsch. Although there is no need to consider Finkenbinder's methods or results in detail, one of his main conclusions is important. He argued that the rapid rate of forgetting by Ebbinghaus was probably due to the relatively rapid rate of self-presentation in that study.

Studies of General Memory Development

A study by Brunswik, Goldscheider, and Pilek (1932) differed from earlier investigations in that the goal was to provide a general description of memory in school-age children. In addition, the issues addressed in this study were derived directly from a truly developmental theory, Charlotte and Karl Bühler's doctrine of phases and stages. The study was also unique compared to previous research in that statistical significance tests were used. Brunswik et al.'s (1932) experiments focused on verbal memory of children 6 to 18 years of age. For the younger students in the study, nonsense syllables, one-syllable words, and numbers were used as the learning materials and only immediate retention was tested. The tests for older students involved short-term and long-term memory for poems, memory of Bühler's paired concepts (e.g., rabbit and fir tree-Easter and Christmas), as well as "Mars number tasks," another pair-associate test involving combinations of numbers and nonsense syllables.

Six- to 13-year-olds required more practice to learn nonsense syllables than words or numbers. This difference was particularly marked for the youngest children. With increasing age, the number of repetitions to learn these types of materials declined. The findings for the older students, however, were not equally clearcut. While the typical age trend was obtained with the Mars numbers (i.e., olders learned more easily), no age differences were reported for the two tasks involving more meaningful materials (poems and paired concepts). For the paired-concepts task, this was probably due to marked ceiling effects. That was not the case for poems, however.

Although no exact figures were reported for delayed recall, the results with meaningful learning materials were generally similar to the findings reported by Vertes (1913, 1931)—higher scores were obtained after one week than had been obtained at immediate recall. As in Vertes' work, the rate of forgetting was greater for the older subjects compared to the younger ones.

In addition to the tests of verbal memory, Brunswik et al. (1932) included nonverbal tests of memory span. The "School of Balls" test involved nine exercises with a ball, with subjects required to repeat these in correct sequence. Recall and recognition of nine geometric figures as well as serial recall of nine different colored patterns was also required. Meaningful memory span was assessed by recalling a picture story (Christmas eve), learning 24 pairs of real objects, and remembering instructions in correct sequential order (i.e., following instructions to tidy up the classroom).

The major findings on the span tasks were that memory for meaningless materials peaked by about age 12, whereas the maximum span for Gestalt memory configurations and meaningful elements continued to develop into adolescence. Given the different developmental patterns, Brunswik et al. (1932) concluded that there must be different memory functions. Their view was that the rote-associative memory system was dominant early in development and was eventually replaced by higher functions, a view that was generally consistent with the Bühlers' theories of development.

In their efforts to make their findings congruent with the Bühlers' perspectives, Brunwik et al. (1932) interpreted their complex data too uniformly, however. The alert reader will have noticed already that the conclusion that rote-associative processes predominate in young children is inconsistent with the data on the verbal

learning tasks; the younger children required more practice to learn nonsense syllables than meaningful words, with continuous improvement in the learn of nonsense
syllables up until age 18, even though ceiling effects were obtained with meaningful
material much earlier in development. In addition, other scientists have failed to
find support for the position that children can skillfully learn nonmeaningful
material by rote before they can master more meaningful materials (e.g., Fechner,
1965; Weinert, 1962). For instance, Weinert found that 6-year-olds learned word
pairs composed of familiar words much more easily than they learned pairs consisting of meaningless, unfamiliar syllables.

Notwithstanding its shortcomings, the study by Brunswik et al. (1932) is a valuable contribution to memory development. The use of more precise methods and various learning materials gave rise to more specific hypotheses concerning age
differences in memory development. The disparate growth curves obtained for
different memory functions were consistent with the data in previous studies (e.g.,
Netschajeff, 1900, 1902; Offner, 1924). The graphical representation of the general
development of immediate memory is particularly interesting in light of the assumptions of the day about the course of memory development. Their curve was based on
scores from about 700 students and represented an aggregation across all measures
included in the study, using a special standardization procedure (see Fig. 1.1). The
outcomes recorded in Fig. 1.1 correspond closely to those reported by Nagy (1930)
and Vertes (1913, 1931) who found linear and steep rises in performance from 6 to
11 years of age. Brunswik et al.'s results are also consistent with other reports that
there is a plateau in performance during pre- and early adolescence (e.g., Bourdon,
1894; Lobsien, 1911a, 1911b; Nagy, 1930; Pohlmann, 1906). On the other hand,
the findings of Brunswik et al. differ substantially from the results obtained by
Ebbinghaus who concluded that the period from ages 13 to 15 was characterized
by a major increase in memory performance. From the slope of Brunswik et al.'s
curve, it seems likely that maximum performance had not yet been obtained by age
18. This aspect of the data was consistent with Meumann's (1907a) and Pohlmann's
(1906) results, indicating that immediate retention for verbal materials continues
to increase up to the age of 25, and only then is there an enduring plateau in performance. Finally, the findings of Brunswik et al. (1932) concerning long-term
memory for meaningless material are also supportive of Meumann's and Radossawljewitsch's earlier results. The retention of older children and adolescents appears
even lower than that of younger children. The results of Brunswik et al. were also
consistent with the apparently paradoxic outcomes in Vertes, indicating improvements in performance after long time intervals.

Individual Differences in Memory Development

The majority of the early studies attached great importance to the identification of
interindividual differences in memory development. At the time these studies were
conducted, demonstrations that adults produced superior recall than children were
by no means trivial, for there were hypotheses that children would learn some types
of material (e.g., nonsense syllables; Meumann, 1907a) better than adults would. In

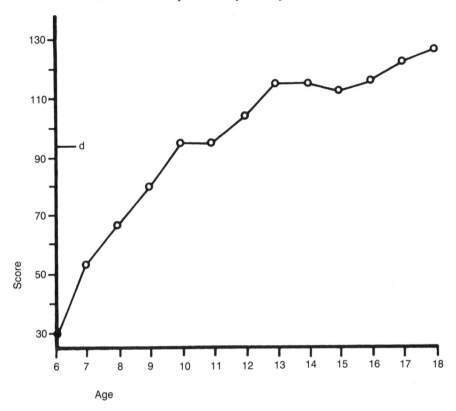

FIGURE 1.1. Memory development in children and adolescents. Data from Brunswik et al. (1932).

addition, there was a great deal of concern with sex differences. Many of the opponents of coeducation sought to win the cause of separate education by arguing that girls had inferior intellectual aptitudes. Since women were portrayed as not being able to keep up with men, coeducation was considered a "sin against nature" by some (Braunshausen, 1914, p. 95f). The early studies also dealt extensively with the possibilities that there were memory types and that there are important relationships between memory and intelligence.

SEX DIFFERENCES

Although Bolton (1892) assumed that girls were in general superior to boys, Ebbinghaus (1897), Lobsien (1911a), and Nagy (1930) all reported higher performance levels for boys in younger populations (9 to 12 years of age), while girls did better in older age groups. In general, Bolton's findings were consistent with the bulk of the data, however (e.g., Brunswik et al., 1932; Kesselring, 1911; Netschjeff, 1900; Pohlmann, 1906; Vertes, 1913, 1931), although in most cases the differences in favor of girls were small. One of the greatest difficulties in interpreting this entire literature is that any minor difference was interpreted as important, however. The study by Brunswik et al. (1932) was an exception in this respect since it included significance tests to evaluate mean differences. A comparison of sex differences across several memory tasks revealed that the differences were relatively weak, especially compared to the age differences found for the same tasks.

Memory Types

Research on memory types in children was inspired on the one hand by the everyday observation that memory for figures, melodies, stories, and other materials can vary enormously within the same person, and on the other hand by mnemonists whose proficiency seem clearly confined to one modality (Braunshausen, 1914; Offner, 1924). Classifying students into groups of acoustic-auditory, optic-visual, tactile-motor, or mixed-memory types seemed directly relevant to the design of instruction in school. There was also an interest in determining whether there is an optimal combination of visual and auditory instruction (Kemsies, 1900, 1901; Kirkpatrick, 1894).

A particularly prominent study at the turn of the century was by Netschajeff (1900) who asked students about their learning habits and classified them as visual, auditory, or motor-memory types on the basis of their responses during these interviews. It should be noted that Netschajeff was fully aware of the methodological problems arising in any such classification. For example, it was difficult to find clearcut memory types, with only about 10% of the sample classified unequivocally. In addition, the individual differences that were detected proved not to be stable (Meumann, 1907a; Pohlmann, 1906; Radossawljewitsch, 1907). Despite the difficulties, Braunshausen (1914) and Offner (1924) still regarded knowledge about memory types as potentially important in terms of practical consequences for instruction. However, use of memory types in planning instruction was never implemented extensively, although there are even contemporary attempts to show instruction to accommodate memory types (see Cronbach & Snow, 1977).

Relationships Between Intelligence and Memory

An informal observation of the day was that bright students did not always have good memories. This issue was investigated empirically by cross-classifying subjects in terms of relative academic achievement and relative memory performance. In a study of memory span, Bolton (1892) and Ebbinghaus (1897) found evidence in support of the everyday observation. The correlations between academic achievement and memory span were low. Others, however, found more striking relationships between simple memory performance and achievement (e.g., Binet, 1909; Bourdon, 1894; Meumann, 1912; Pohlmann, 1906; Winch, 1906). Meumann's and Binet's studies were particularly noteworthy in that academic ability was not inferred from school achievement, but was instead measured using psychometric and experimental techniques. Not surprisingly, the more meaningful and complex the to-be-memorized materials, the greater the correlation between memory and intelligence (Brunswik et al., 1932; Vertes, 1913, 1931). When all of the data were considered, the relationship between intelligence and memory performance proved positive, although the correlations were not particularly high in many cases. This finding seems to be in line with Bolton's (1892) conclusion:

Intellectual acuteness, while more often accompanied by a good memory span and great power of concentrated and prolonged attention, is not necessarily accompanied by them (p. 379).

SUMMARY

In the first three decades following Ebbinghaus' classic work, a great number of studies of children's memory were undertaken using methods closely related to the paradigms of general memory research. Much of this research was conducted in Germany. The large number of replication studies make clear that early research on memory development was systematic and programmatic. Interest focused more on performance than on process. The major conclusions that could be drawn from the data available by the mid-1930s can be summarized briefly:

1. In general, memory performance (e.g., immediate recall) improves over the school years and continues increasing until about the age of 25.
2. A particularly steep, linear increase in levels of performance can be observed between the ages of 7 and 11, with a plateau between the ages of 13 to 16.
3. The slope of the age curve differs depending on the type of memory function investigated and the type of learning material used.
4. A sharp distinction must be made between the development of immediate and long-term retention. Contrary to the findings for immediate recall, long-term retention seemed better for younger children and declined with increasing age.
5. Regardless of the age group or task studied, sex differences were small.
6. On average, there were positive correlations between memory performance and intellectual aptitude.

When these early studies are examined today, a number of deficiencies in them are apparent. For one, very few tasks were studied, and thus, it should not be surprising that the shape of the learning curve cited in summary point 3 would not prove to be general across the many memory tasks considered by contemporary workers. There were few control groups and frequent confoundings in these studies. For instance, these early investigators did not recognize the many problems associated with evaluating retention when the amount of time required to learn material varies dramatically between groups, as it did between children and adults (e.g., Underwood, 1964). Contemporary recognition of this methodological difficulty makes obvious one factor that may have accounted for children's retention seeming to be better than adults' retention in these early studies. Finally, there were few inferential statistical analyses in these studies. Despite these reservations, we emphasize how impressive it is that generally replicable findings emerged from this work. These pioneers made a lot of important progress.

1936–1965

The state of German research on memory development from 1935 to 1965 can be described easily. No important empirical studies of memory development were published in Germany between 1933 and 1961. The great progress made by German researchers in the early 20th century came to a halt as the winds of war gathered and exploded over Europe. Theoretical perspectives that predominated in the immediate postwar period (i.e., Gestaltist, phenomenological) did not encourage analytic research on memory or memory development.

American Research

The situation was much different in America. Learning theories were popular, including ones that encouraged research on verbal learning. The major issues outlined by Ebbinghaus' classical study (e.g., serial position effects, massed vs. spaced practice, meaningfulness, interference) remained as part of this tradition until well into the 1950s. The verbal learning theorists were not particularly interested in developmental issues, however, since their primary concern was identification of general laws (see Keppel, 1964; Goulet, 1968; McGeoch & Irion, 1952; Munn, 1954; Weinert, 1964). In this sense, conclusions by contemporary authors (Brainerd & Pressley, 1985a; Kail & Strauss, 1984) that there was a dearth of research on memory development prior to 1965 applies to American developmental psychology between 1936 and 1965.

Developmental learning research during this period was most often conducted in simple learning paradigms, with studies of classical and instrumental conditioning and discrimination learning. The few studies of verbal learning that were conducted were concerned with list learning (free recall), serial learning, and paired-associate learning (Spiker, 1960). Studies of free recall and serial learning were natural extensions of the earlier research on memory span, since memory-span tasks consisted of free and serial recall of progressively longer lists. Paired-associate learning allowed the possibility of independent manipulation of stimulus and response characteristics. The task was easily adaptable with children, and it was possible to gain insights into the processes that children were using to mediate their paired-associate learning (Goulet, 1968; Spiker, 1960). Unfortunately, however, most of the verbal learning studies with children were descriptive, with studies often conducted at a single age level. Research on children's verbal learning was rarely programmatic, with single-shot studies common. The brief review of verbal learning issues that were studied from 1936 to 1965 is meant only to provide examples of the kind of American research that was being conducted during the era and is limited only to examples that provided an analysis of age trends and examined hypotheses of age by learning process interactions.

PAIRED-ASSOCIATE LEARNING

Developmental processes were typically studied within the three basic paired-associate transfer paradigms (i.e., A-B, A-C; A-B, C-B; A-B, A-Br). In each of these three paradigms, subjects learned two paired-associate lists. The first list was designated A-B, and the second was defined by its similarity to the first. The A-B, A-C paradigm involved identical stimuli on the two lists, but unrelated responses. The A-B, C-B paradigm involved lists with identical responses but different stimuli. The A-B, A-Br paradigm involved identical stimuli and responses except that the stimuli and responses were paired differently on the two lists. The interference theory (e.g., Postman, 1961) that motivated use of these transfer paradigms assumed that the similarity of the successive tasks typically produced negative transfer. For instance, learning of the second list was assumed to be harder than learning of the first list from this theoretical perspective. Subsequent recall of either list when two lists were learned was hypothesized to be harder than recall if only one list had been learned.

The substantial role played by verbal associative strength of stimuli to responses as a determinant of learning rate was demonstrated in studies by Castaneda, Fahel, and Odom (1961) and Wicklund, Palermo, and Jenkins (1965). Linear, positive relationships were produced in these studies between the verbal associative strengths of to-be-learned pairs and the speed of children's learning. This observation suggested a developmental hypothesis, derived from interference theory. Since verbal-associative strength is largely determined by the relationship of the to-be-learned materials to the knowledge base, and since the knowledge base should be richer for older compared to younger children, meaningful A-B and A-C associations should be stronger for older compared to younger children. Thus, there is the possibility of greater interference with older compared to younger children.

This hypothesis was tested in a study by Kopenaal, Krull, and Katz (1964) for preschool, kindergarten, and third-grade children. All children learned two consecutive paired-associate lists following the A-B, A-C paradigm. After 24 hours subjects in the retroactive inhibition conditions recalled the first list. These retroactive inhibition conditions tapped whether learning a subsequent list interfered with recall of the first list. Subjects in the proactive inhibition conditions recalled the second paired-associate list. These conditions tapped whether learning the first list interfered with retention of the second list. The outcomes were consistent with the developmental hypothesis that was derived from interference theory. The third-grade children showed significant retroactive and proactive inhibition; the kindergarten subjects only experienced significant retroactive interference; preschoolers evidenced no interference (all comparisons relative to control conditions in which subjects learned only one list).

FREE RECALL

The studies by Bousfield and his associates (Bousfield, 1953; Bousfield, Cohen, & Whitmarsh, 1958) on free recall of word lists stimulated many studies with college students, with a number of variables systematically manipulated including interitem associative strength, meaningfulness, and list length. Only a few developmental studies of free recall were conducted during this period, however. An important one was the classic study by Bousfield, Esterson, and Whitmarsh (1958). They compared the degree of associative clustering in free recall of third-grade, fourth-grade, and college students. The theoretical rationale of the study was derived from Heinz

Werner's (1948, pp. 234-243) assumption that organizational principles change during development. According to Werner, perceptual-sensory ordering is initially dominant but is replaced later by a tendency to organize conceptually. Thus, the word lists used by Bousfield et al. (1958) could be classified either on the basis of perceptual categories (color) or conceptual categories (meaning). An important aspect of this study was that it included measures of clustering presumed to tap processing more directly than simply the amount of material recalled. The most important finding was that both recall and clustering on the basis of categoric information correlated positively with age. Contrary to expectations, color clustering was low in all age groups.

Laurence (1966) used Tulving's (1962a) measure of subjective organization. Subjective organization is the tendency to recall unrelated list items in a constant order from one trial to the next. To test the validity of Tulving's hypothesis that recall varies positively with subjective organization, Laurence included college students as well as elderly adults and children between 5 and 10 years of age. The subjects were presented a free recall task involving 16 unrelated pictures. There were striking differences in the subjective organization levels of children and adults. Young adults learned more quickly than either children or the elderly. The elderly learned faster than 5- to 8-year-old children, but at about the same rate as 10-year-olds. In contrast to the simple recall differences between the younger and older adults, however, there were negligible differences in subjective organization between these two groups of adults. Despite the comparable recall levels for the elderly and the 10-year-olds, the elderly had higher subjective organization scores. In addition, high correlations between subjective organization and recall for both adult samples and the 8-year-old and 10-year-old children, but not for the younger participants, creates problems for Tulving's hypothesis. Thus, across the life span, subjective organization and recall appear to manifest different developmental trends. The data provided by Laurence were not consistent with the simple cause-and-effect relationship proposed by Tulving.

SUMMARY

Developmental changes were not central concerns of North American verbal learning researchers. In an important review of children's learning research during this period, Keppel (1964) emphasized the striking correspondence between college student data and results in the few investigations conducted with children. Our point of view is that this was nothing more than an attempt (and a lame one at that) to legitimitize verbal learning researchers' lack of interest in developmental issues. Goulet's (1968) subsequent review of verbal learning in children is especially noteworthy for critically examining the presumed correspondence between the child and adult data. As the studies of free recall and paired-associate learning that were covered here make evident, it cannot be assumed that the processes that mediate verbal learning at different age levels are qualitatively identical. The experiments by Koppenaal et al. (1964) and Bousfield et al. (1958) stand out for having proposed developmental functions and for producing data substantiating important ontogenetic differences.

The majority of the developmental studies of verbal learning that were undertaken were conducted at the end of the 1950s or at the start of the 1960s. We note that these studies anticipated a great deal of work on children's paired-associate and list learning that was conducted after 1965. Traditional verbal learning techniques played an important role in the major advances in developmental memory research during the 1970s and 1980s.

Soviet Research

Soviet researchers were particularly interested in the development of meaningful memory (i.e., memory mediated by prior knowledge) compared to rote, "mechanical" learning. A prototypical example of Soviet thinking is provided by Smirnov's (1948, cited by Smirnov, 1973) analysis of rote versus logical memorizing at different age levels. In particular, Meumann had asserted that logical memory begins to predominate at about 13 or 14 years of age, and thus, differences in learning that favor meaningful material over nonsense material should increase with age. Smirnov evaluated this claim by examining studies that used nonsense syllables as indicators of rote learning and meaningful word materials to tap logical memory, a methodological approach that was generally consistent with European thinking in the first half of this century (Brunswik et al., 1932; Lobsien, 1911a; Pohlmann, 1906). Meumann's proposal that the advantage of memorizing meaningful material versus nonsense material should steadily increase with increasing age was not substantiated by Smirnov's review. In fact, the efficiency of memorizing nonsense material increased more rapidly with age than did the efficiency of learning meaningful material. The superiority of "logical" over rote memory (i.e., memory of meaningful materials over nonmeaningful materials) was more pronounced in elementary school children than it was in adolescents. Concerning this apparently paradoxical result, Smirnov argued that in the older children, rote memorizing without consideration of meaning is only rarely found. With age, children have a greater ability to give meaning to meaningless material, and thus, they transform what could be a mechanical and rote process (i.e., learning of nonsense materials) into a meaningful one. A great deal of modern data support this latter conclusion (e.g., development of uninstructed use of elaboration, Chapter 6).

The increasing relevance of conscious, independent, and goal-oriented memory activity as the causal origin of memory development was emphasized by a number of Soviets in the 1930s (see reviews by Leontjev, 1977; Meacham, 1977; Smirnov & Zinchenko, 1969). Two major concerns can be distinguished in the empirical studies. One was the study of *involuntary memory*, which was not regarded as an independent, goal-directed operation. Involuntary memorizing occurs when the ultimate goal of the subject is not memory, but something else, often comprehension in the Soviet studies. In such cases, memory is involuntary in that it is a byproduct of comprehension. The second focus was *voluntary memory*, which is a product of activities that are driven by a goal to remember. The Soviets assumed that superior forms of memory develop on the basis of the transition from natural and involuntary memorizing to subject-controlled and voluntary memory involving the use of mediating processes and cues (Leontjev, 1931, cited by Leontjev, 1977).

INVOLUNTARY MEMORY

As Zinchenko (1967) pointed out, the practical significance of involuntary memory in people's everyday lives had been underestimated by many. Early research projects on involuntary remembering were undertaken at the end of the 1930s and at the start of the 1940s, concentrating primarily on the effects that active intellectual participation had on memory performance (see Smirnov, 1948; Zinchenko, 1939, cited by Zinchenko, 1967). A study by Zinchenko (1939, cited by Smirnov & Zinchenko, 1969), one that produced a striking set of results, can be used to illustrate research on involuntary memory. Illustrations of various objects depicted on 15 pieces of cardboard were presented to schoolchildren and adults. A two-digit number was recorded in the right-hand corner of each piece of cardboard. Subjects in one experimental condition were asked to categorize the picture objects. In the second experimental condition subjects were asked to arrange the cardboard pieces in sequence on the basis of the numbers. Immediately following completion of the task, subjects in both conditions were unexpectedly instructed to describe and list the items. The findings were clearcut. The adults who had been asked to categorize the materials recalled many more pictured objects than numbers. The second group (who has sequenced the cards) recalled many more numbers than pictures. The pattern of results was similar with children. From these findings, Zinchenko concluded that active intellectual participation determines what is remembered.

VOLUNTARY MEMORY

A nice example of research on voluntary memory was provided by Istomina (1948; cited in Istomina, 1977), who sought to determine when and under what conditions voluntary memorizing and voluntary recall first emerge. This classical study is often cited in the Soviet literature under the rubric of "motivation and memory," since it involved a comparative analysis of the memory performance of preschoolers (aged 3 to 7) in an exciting game situation versus a typical laboratory task. Under laboratory conditions the experimenter read five words to children and asked them to recall the list after a short delay. During the game the children were asked to go on an errand to a store and buy five items for the kindergarten. As indicated in Table 1.1, the children's memory performance was much better given the shopping task.

Istomina assumed that the systematic recall differences favoring the game over the laboratory task were due to different motivational incentives for the children. Remembering presumably was an intrinsically important goal and had real meaning for the children in the game situation, especially in comparison to the laboratory situation. Consequently, they probably showed greater interest in the task.

One of the earliest studies on the use of retrieval cues following voluntary memorizing activities was conducted by Leontjev (1928; cited by Leontjev, 1977) with normal and mentally retarded children between 9 and 14 years of age. In one condition, 15 words were presented with subsequent recall required. A second condition differed in that pictures could be selected from a larger group of pictures for

TABLE 1.1. Mean number of items recalled by preschoolers and kindergarteners as a function of age and activity (Lab vs. Game).*

Age (yr)	Activity	
	Lab	Game
3–4	0.6	1
4–5	1.5	3
5–6	2.0	3.2
6–7	2.3	3.8

*Reconstructed after Istomina (1977, pp. 109, 111).

use as retrieval cues. Normal grade-school children's recall increased enormously in the retrieval cue condition. For the handicapped children, however, the effect of retrieval cues was much smaller, and in some cases, even negative. The use of retrieval cues seemed to make the task too complicated for the retarded children. Leontjev obtained results similar to the grade-school retarded data when a group of preschool children participated in the same task. Preschoolers did not benefit from the opportunity to select and use retrieval cues.

Children's learning from text was examined in a large number of studies of voluntary memory. This research was stimulated both by theoretical concerns about the development of organizational processes that could be applied to text and to the pragmatic possibility of providing guidelines for educators. For instance, Korman (1944, 1945; cited by Yendovitskaya, 1971) studied preschool children's memory for connected material (fairy tales). Korman was impressed by the children's ability to recall the main events of the stories correctly. Although he noted that the children frequently departed from the original sequence of events, the deviations were often logically consistent with the story. The recall differences found between groups of 4- to 5-year-olds and 6-year-olds were primarily quantitative. The younger children recalled the skeleton of the story, whereas the older children gave a more detailed and precise recall of the fairy tale.

A more systematic study with preschool children was reported by Smirnov (1948; cited by Smirnov, 1973), who was particularly interested in the impact of text structure on children's recall. Second, fourth, and sixth graders were presented two texts, with sentences arranged in a coherent fashion or randomly. After two attempts at recalling the two texts, subjects were instructed to break up the texts into pieces of information that went together (done from memory). For random texts, this was a difficult mental reconstruction of the text. The most important finding was that the youngest subjects (second graders) were not able to reorganize the text. Only a small percentage of fourth and sixth graders were able to break up the text into meaningful elements, and these successes were usually obtained when subjects were reading the coherent text. Although most of the children could identify that random texts were harder to break up than coherent texts, they were not consciously aware of the structural differences between the texts. It was interesting that children often recalled a considerable number of coherent transitions between topics in random stories when asked to recall the story freely, even though they had trouble rearranging the random story elements, a finding consistent with recent data (reviewed in Chapters 5 and 6). Given this obvious divergence between conscious and unconscious processes, Smirnov concluded that meaningful grouping processes first proceed in an unconscious way before becoming conscious activities.

In another experiment conducted by Smirnov (1948; cited by Smirnov, 1973) with second, fourth, and sixth graders, the goal was to determine which cognitive processes influence encoding and intentional memorizing of text. There were large individual differences for each age group, which were particularly pronounced for the youngest group. Only a few of the most capable second graders evidenced a process like self-checking, which was observed more frequently in older children. Selective repetition of material also increased with age. In general, there were age-related increases in text recall that were presumably due to the use of increasingly complex and flexible coding strategies.

Correlation Between Voluntary and Involuntary Memory

Leontjev tested hypotheses derived from Vygotsky's (1978) cultural-historical theory of mental development. In particular, Leontjev conducted studies to determine whether there were qualitative shifts in children's memory with development. He particularly believed that there were important shifts between preschool and the early grade-school years.

In Leontjev's first series of experiments on involuntary memorization, the to-be-learned materials (nonsense syllables and meaningful words) were given to subjects without instructions to memorize or to use cues. The subsequent instruction to recall the materials was therefore unexpected. In the second series of experiments using the same material, an explicit memorizing instruction was given (i.e., these were studies of voluntary memorization). The most important finding was that preschoolers' memory performance hardly differed across these experiments. On the other hand, children in the early grade-school years profited considerably from the introduction of memory cues and achieved higher levels of performance under voluntary memory instructions. Subsequent comparisons of voluntary memorization with and without external memory cues (pictures) produced greater memory performance for older school children and adults when no cues were provided. Leontjev (1931, cited by Smirnov, 1973) interpreted these findings as consistent with the Soviet theory that older children use internal memory cues more efficiently than external memory cues.

Similar experiments were undertaken by Zinchenko (1939, cited by Zinchenko, 1967; Smirnov, 1973). In one of his studies, picture recall performances of pre-school children, schoolchildren, and adults were compared under conditions of involuntary versus voluntary memorization. Voluntary memory was again tested with and without external memory cues. For the preschool children, involuntary memorization instructions produced better recall than voluntary memory directions. The higher involuntary memorizing scores obtained by Zinchenko's preschoolers as compared to Leontjev's subjects are probably attributable to the mnemonic orientation given in Zinchenko's experiments. Zinchenko's directions elicited a goal-directed activity (classification of picture materials), on the basis of which the meaning of the item would be deduced. For the younger grade-school children, voluntary memorization by use of external cues yielded the highest recall scores, whereas for older children and adults, recall was approximately equal across voluntary and involuntary procedures.

The experiments subsequently conducted by Smirnov (1948, cited by Smirnov, 1973) were designed to test the generalizability of Zinchenko's findings, since Zinchenko had limited himself to only one type of activity, namely, the classification of pictures. Smirnov also included words and sentences as test material. The subjects were second and fourth graders and college students. The design of the experiment was rather complex. In both involuntary and voluntary memorizing conditions, intensity of processing was varied. For instance, writing words dictated by the experimenter or finding spelling errors in sentences were regarded as less intensive intellectual activities than combining words in a meaningful way to evaluating the meanings of sentences.

The efficiency of involuntary memorizing was higher the more intensive the intellectual processing with the learning material. This result is consistent with Zinchenko's findings, according to which, under specific conditions, involuntary memory may be superior to voluntary memory. Depth of processing and the level of intellectual activity connected with it are the most important conditions affecting the efficiency of involuntary memorization. With increasing age, the effectiveness of involuntary memorizing decreases relative to voluntary memorization, that is, the number of cases where voluntary memorizing proves more efficient than involuntary memorizing increase.

The relationship between voluntary and involuntary memory in developmental processes was also analyzed in correlational studies undertaken by Istomina (1977), Samokhvacova (1962, 1965; cited by Smirnov & Zinchenko, 1969), and Barkhatova (1964; cited by Smirnov & Zinchenko, 1969) with preschoolers, schoolchildren, and adults. The correlational coefficients obtained varied considerably with the age of subjects and the type of task used. Aggregated across tasks, the mean correlation between involuntary and voluntary memory was 0.80 for the 3- to 4-year-olds, but only 0.45 for the 5- to 6-year-olds. Mean correlations decreased steadily up until grade 8 (0.40 in grade 2; 0.21 in grade 5; and 0.09 in grade 8), but increased again up to 0.26 for college students. The interindividual differences were explained in the sense that the younger preschool children more frequently behaved the same way when given involuntary and voluntary memorization instructions. Older children's memory behaviors differed considerably when given voluntary instructions compared to involuntary directions, with more memorizing activity and higher performance when voluntary memorizing instructions were provided.

RELATIONSHIP BETWEEN VISUAL AND VERBAL-LOGICAL MEMORIES

According to Blonskii (1935), four distinct forms of memory (motor, emotional, visual, and verbal) constitute the ontogenetic stages of memory. Blonskii considered most important the hypothesis that visual memory develops before verbal memory.

Particularly relevant to this theory were studies comparing recall of pictures and verbal material, especially ones conducted by Farapanova (1953, 1958; cited in Smirnov, 1973). In her experiments, the subjects (second, fifth, and seventh graders as well as college students) were asked to memorize different types of materials. On the first trial subjects were given pictures of objects that could easily be named by children; on the second trial they were provided verbal materials that could be visualized (i.e., names of concrete objects); on the third trial subjects were provided pictorial materials that were difficult to label (i.e., pictures of various types of fish and mushrooms); and on the fourth trial, abstract verbal materials were provided. The central hypothesis was that visual and verbal memory would always be involved in memorization, but that the role they played would differ depending on materials. The most important result was that at all age levels, the memorization of easily named pictures was best; the recall of visualizable words was also high, but not as good. Much poorer recall was obtained for hard-to-name pictures and hard-to-visualize words. The second graders remembered hard-to-label pictures better, while the older schoolchildren and the adults did better with abstract words. Recall of both visual and verbal material increased with age, but recognition and recall scores increased faster with age for words than for pictures. As a result, the difference between recall of pictures and words tended to diminish with increasing age.

A very similar experimental procedure was used by Kornienko (1955; cited in Smirnov, 1973) with preschool children. In a series of trials, subjects were asked to memorize and recall a number of toys, the same number of familiar words, and the names of trees and shrubs that were unfamiliar to children. The results were compatible with the ones obtained by Farapanova. At all age levels (younger, middle, and older preschoolers), the highest recall and recognition scores were obtained for the toys. Memory for familiar words ranked second.

Maltseva (1948, 1958; cited in Smirnov, 1973) adopted a different approach to the problem of comparing visual and verbal memory. In her studies, visual and verbal stimuli were used as retrieval cues for encoding and recalling text materials, with second, fourth, and sixth graders as well as college students serving as subjects. All subjects performed better with visual cues. Consistent with the other results, older subjects benefited relatively more from verbal cues, however. That is, recall differences due to the use of visual versus verbal cues decreased with increasing age.

Taken together, the findings from various studies are similar. The role of the verbal system increased with age in all of these experiments. There was a gradual reduction in the dominance of the visual system observable from the preschool through the grade-school years. Nonetheless, even in adults, visual material was better recalled than abstract material. Soviet researchers assumed that optimal recall occurs when the visual and verbal systems function together.

SUMMARY

Relative to western researchers of the day, Soviet scientists emphasized more the development and evaluation of particular theoretical positions (see Meacham, 1977, for an extensive overview). The Soviets believed that qualitatively distinct memory processes and learning activities are prevalent at different age levels. The support for this position was provided principally by studies of involuntary and voluntary memorization.

A number of conclusions followed from this data base:

1. Three- to 4-year-olds generally did not show intentional memory behaviors when instructions to remember were provided. That these children were not very active when attempting to memorize was apparent in a number of analyses. More optimistically, preschoolers' memories could be improved by manipulations that increased their meaningful processing of material.
2. The first signs of goal-directed activities in the memorization of objects, pictures, and words were observed among 5-year-olds. They appear to set goals about what they want to remember and try to achieve these memory goals. Unfortunately, they usually did not possess means by which to accomplish most memory goals.
3. Six- to 7-year-olds more frequently possessed methods that facilitated the recall of objects and pictures. Nonetheless, the repertoire of memorizing methods was observed to be limited to simple repetition. Conscious reorganization strategies were rarely observed.
4. Additional improvements in performance were noted between the second- and fifth-grade levels, with development greater during this period than during the fifth- to seventh-grade interval (Smirnov & Zinchenko, 1969).

There are many problems in appraising the Soviet literature, however. In general, western reviewers in the 1980s must rely on secondary sources, for the primary sources are either not available at all or not readily accessible. These secondary sources are often incomplete with respect to designs, procedures, and results. Even more disheartening, when primary sources are located and translated, they, too, are often vague about how studies were conducted and analyzed, given a different emphasis in the Soviet Union on the importance of the methods and results sections compared to the discussion section in scientific articles. (Reading any issue of *Soviet Psychology* makes this point obvious.)

When westerners can peruse the methods of important experiments (e.g., Istomina, 1977), it is clear that Soviet experimental studies are not as well controlled as American studies, with this conclusion especially compelling for studies conducted before 1960. For instance, "practice" controls in Istomina (1977) did not really control for practice! (See Smirnov, 1973, for a description of these procedures.) At least one other confounding is apparent as well. The experimenter repeated the names of the objects several times in the game situation, but only once in the lab task. Istomina's (1977) findings and conclusions must, therefore, be viewed with caution, especially since western researchers have had difficulty replicating that memory is better in a natural game-like situation compared to in the laboratory. Neither Weissberg and Paris (1986) nor Schneider and Brun (1987) could reproduce Istomina's finding.

More optimistically, other Soviet outcomes have been duplicated by western researchers using contemporary methodologies. Consistent with Smirnov (1973), Murphy and Brown (1975) found that preschoolers' involuntary memorization of

picture lists that were meaningfully processed (i.e., categorizing items as pleasant
or unpleasant) was greater than their voluntary memorization of materials. Christie
and Schumacher (1975) replicated Korman's study (cited by Yendovitskaya, 1971).
Young children were able to produce essential text information (i.e., the logical,
core sequence of a story) but did not recall the details of the main events. Replications such as these suggest that a concise, fair assessment is that Soviet scholars
were doing important work on memory development during the middle third of
this century.

The Modern Era

Most of the rest of this book is concerned with research conducted since 1965. The
modern conception of memory is in terms of interacting components, with memory
development a product of developing components in ever more complex interactions. For simplicity of organization, we consider each important part of memory in
Chapters 2 through 5. Some interactions between these components are taken up in
Chapters 2 through 5 as appropriate, although much of the discussion of interactions
between components is deferred until Chapters 6 and 7. In those chapters we detail
a complete model of competent memory that we refer to as the Good Strategy User
Model.

Most of the research that is taken up in the subsequent chapters was carried out
in the west. Although Genevan and Soviet influences were important stimulants for
some studies that are reviewed, the most influential theoretical perspective by far
is the general information processing approach. Thus, the four chapters on components of memory development are about components that are common to most information processing models of performance.

For readers who are not familiar with information processing, a few simple
distinctions should help as advance organizers for Chapters 2 through 5. Many
information-processing models divide memory into short-term and long-term components (e.g., Atkinson & Shiffrin, 1968). Information that is in short-term memory
is currently in consciousness. Thus, when a person reads a story, they may be aware
at any given instant of the exact wording of the last sentence read and a few other
pieces of recently encountered information. Perhaps one or two points covered a
while back in the text are activated as well—maybe because they were associated
with information that was processed recently. Only a limited amount of information
can be consciously processed at any one time—that is, short-term capacity is
limited. (Whether there are developmental changes in this short-term capacity is
taken up in Chapter 2.) If nothing is done with information held in short-term
memory, it is usually forgotten quickly. (Short-term memory is short-term in that
what is there usually does not stay there for long!) In contrast to short-term memory
is a long-term store that contains virtually everything that the person knows. Particularly relevant here, this long-term store contains knowledge of procedures (i.e.,
strategies) that can operate on information in short-term storage. The development
of strategy use is taken up in Chapter 3. In addition to knowing procedures, people

know many others things—concepts, associations between concepts, hierarchic classifications of concepts, schemas, etc. This nonstrategic knowledge (world knowledge) often has direct effects on the memorability of newly encountered content, as well as profound influences on whether strategies operate efficiently or can operate at all. This knowledge base as a determinant of children's memory and memory development is considered in particular in Chapter 4. Whether strategic procedures are used correctly depends on knowing when and where to use particular procedures, a form of metacognition (i.e., knowledge about thinking). Metacognitive knowledge is also stored in long-term memory, with the metacognition (metamemory in particular) the topic of Chapter 5. In relegating strategies, nonstrategic knowledge, and metamemory to long-term memory, we emphasize that when these components are activated, they operate in consciousness, and thus, short-term capacity determines their use in part. This interaction between short-term memory and long-term components is just one of many interactions that will be considered in the chapters that follow, but it is a very important one. Thus, we devote a chapter to short-term capacity before moving on to consideration of long-term components.

2. Capacity

This chapter examines an extremely simple hypothesis about the development of memory—perhaps memory improves with development because children's "capacity" to remember increases, with capacity at least partially determined by neurological development. We explore the capacity question first because it is important to understand the nature of capacity and its development, since all strategies, metacognition, and world knowledge that is used by the child must operate within the constraints posed by capacity. A second reason for dealing with studies of capacity early in the book is that research on this topic is directly related to the earliest studies that examined memory development, the work on memory span conducted at the turn of the century and reviewed briefly in the last chapter.

Before beginning this discussion, readers are forewarned that summarizing research on the capacity hypothesis is not easy, a fact that becomes obvious by reading the reviews of short-term capacity that have been provided by others (Dempster, 1981, 1985; Hasselhorn, 1986; Weinert, 1979). The greatest source of confusion is the fact that various models of short-term memory have been formulated. These range from a rather passive system, as proposed by Atkinson and Shiffrin (1968) and described by Brown and DeLoache (1978) as a "container" model, to an extremely active "working memory" system with several components in interaction, including both central processing and peripheral mechanisms such as subvocal rehearsal (e.g., Baddeley, 1981, 1986). As described by Case and his colleagues (e.g., Case, 1978; Case & Kurland, 1980; Case, Kurland, & Goldberg, 1982), short-term memory and working memory differ in that the former involves only storage and reproduction of information but the latter includes the capacity to transform information being held in the short-term system (also, Dempster, 1985). The current trend is more to focus on the active, multicomponent short-term processing that is captured by the working memory construct.

Dempster (1985) reviewed in detail potential sources of development for short-term capacity. Important candidate explanations included the possibility that there is an increase with development in the maximum number of representations from long-term memory that can be activated or reactivated simultaneously and that the speed of information activation and deactivation increases. One important hypothesis is whether apparent age-correlated increases in representational activation capacity are due to changes in strategy or to other changes including the possibility that there are more neurologically determined "slots" (Miller, 1956) with development. Following Dempster (1985), we take the position that structural changes can only be assumed (i.e., developmental increases in the number of storage slots), if age differences cannot be reduced to differences in nonstructural strategic or nonstrategic characteristics.

Potential Determinants of Performance on Memory-Span Tests

Memory-span tasks are structured simply and provide reliable data. Subjects are usually presented sequences of stimuli at a constant speed (e.g., one item per second). Short sequences (e.g., three items) are used first, with subsequent presentations increased by one item at a time until the subject can no longer produce the entire sequence. Even Ebbinghaus (e.g., 1897; 1902; 1905) realized that developmental improvement on these tasks was determined in part by the type of material being memorized, with the slopes of developmental memory-span curves varying as a function of item type (see Figure 2.1). That performance on memory-span tasks is materials dependent was an early stimulus for the hypothesis that strategic operations might be mediating developmental differences in apparent memory span.

Strategies and Skills

REHEARSAL

Strategic mediation of memory-span performance seemed likely for digit span, for which marked developmental improvement occurs. Age differences were hypothesized to be due to developmental increases in spontaneous use of rehearsal. This hypothesis was assessed by analyzing developmental memory-span data for "primacy effects." The assumption was that use of rehearsal provides greater encoding opportunities for material presented early in a list compared to later material, and hence, greater memory of first compared to later material would suggest the operation of rehearsal (e.g., Atkinson & Shiffrin, 1968; Waugh & Norman, 1965). Although researchers were able to find primacy effects in children's digit-span data, they generally did not obtain developmental differences in the presence of primacy effects (e.g., Harris & Burke, 1972; Huttenlocher & Burke, 1976). Thus, this research tactic failed to yield support for the position that develop-

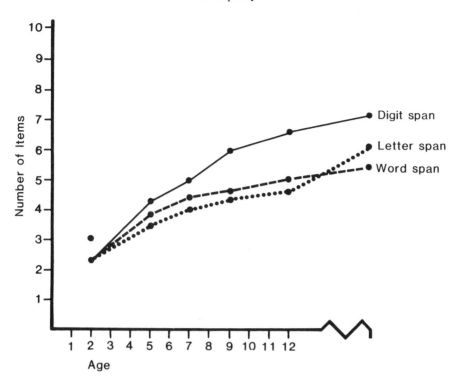

FIGURE 2.1. Developmental differences in digit span, letter span, and word span (constructed from Dempster, 1981, Figs. 1, 2, and 3). Copyright 1981 and used by permission.

mental improvements in memory-span performance are due to developmental shifts in the use of rehearsal.

Frank and Rabinovitch (1974) tried another tactic. They studied "running memory span" in 7- to 11-year-olds. "Supraspan" lists were presented with subjects required to recall as many items as possible from the end of the list. They reasoned that since the end of long lists cannot be anticipated, active repetition would be suppressed. If the rehearsal hypothesis were true, then developmental differences apparent with normal digit span should not materialize with running digit span. That performance did increase some between 7 and 9 years of age for running digit span suggested that, at the very least, more than just rehearsal mediated the developmental changes in digit-span performance.

This sample of data makes obvious that rehearsal alone could not account for between-age digit-span differences. See Dempster (1981, 1985) for additional commentary.

GROUPING

Another strategy hypothesis was that active grouping and regrouping of to-be-learned materials mediated developmental differences in span performance. This hypothesis followed from the observation that adults spontaneously group items given a span task and that adults generally remember more items on lists that contain temporal or rhythmic groupings (Dempster, 1981, reviewed the relevant literature).

The studies of the developmental grouping hypothesis are restricted to experiments about temporal grouping by the experimenter. Unfortunately, the effects of such grouping were not entirely predictable. For instance, Rohwer and Dempster (1977) predicted that age differences in memory span with temporal grouping should increase since older children would be more likely to take advantage of the experimenter-provided groupings. Alternatively, Huttenlocher and Burke (1976) hypothesized that young children would be less likely to group items spontaneously and thus, would benefit from the experimental intervention (see also Engle & Marshall, 1983; Samuel, 1978). All authors contributing to this literature, however, predicted interactions between age and grouping variables.

The tests of the grouping hypotheses were plagued with methodological difficulties, not the least of which were ceiling effects for older subjects (who were often provided lists barely longer than their memory spans) and floor effects for the younger subjects (who were provided lists far longer than their spans). When the predicted age by grouping interactions were obtained (Frank & Rabinovitch, 1974; Huttenlocher & Burke, 1976), ceiling and/or floor effects were present in the data. When data were consistently mid-range, there was little evidence of developmental interaction (Engle & Marshall, 1983; Harris & Burke, 1972; McCarver, 1972; Samuel, 1978). There is little support for the grouping hypothesis.

CHUNKING

Miller (1956) introduced the "magic" number "7 (+ or − 2)" as the maximum number of chunks of verbal information that could be held in short-term memory. The magic in this approach was that although capacity in terms of chunks was invariant, individual differences in short-term memory capacity (e.g., Simon, 1974) could be explained in terms of different-size chunks. Simon reviewed a number of tests of his hypothesis and concluded:

The psychological reality of the chunk has been fairly well demonstrated, and the chunk capacity of short-term memory has been shown to be in the range of five to seven. Fixation of information in long-term memory has been shown to take about 5 to 10 seconds per chunk (1974, p. 487).

From this perspective, age differences in memory span are presumed to be due to larger and larger information sequences being encoded as chunks with increasing age. With larger chunks, the amount of information that can be stored and processed simultaneously increases proportionately. In contrast to repetition and temporal grouping procedures, the degree of chunking that is possible depends on the amount of previous knowledge about the respective stimuli; thus, it is a knowledge-specific strategy (Chi, 1978).

Dempster (1978) compared the short-term memory performances of 7-, 9-, and 12-year-old children who were presented various materials (numbers, consonants, words, nonsense syllables). The systematic variation of letter sequences was of special importance to the "chunking" hypothesis. The comparison of memory for consonant sequences that cannot be recoded easily and memory for generally known consonant-vowel sequences was compared. Age differences in memory span were in fact very dependent on material type (see also Chi, 1976). Only minimal age differences were found for consonant sequences that could easily be integrated, whereas relatively marked developmental differences were obtained for consonant-vowel sequences. In short, developmental differences were obtained for the task that could be mediated by chunking, but not for the one that did not require chunking.

Unfortunately, Burtis (1982) failed to obtain data that complemented Dempster's (1978) finding. Burtis presented 10- to 14-year-olds with easy-to-recode, somewhat difficult-to-recode, and difficult-to-recode consonant sequences. Regardless of age, Burtis' subjects seemed to chunk all of these materials, undermining the conclusion that chunking alone could account for age-correlated increases in recall of consonants.

Although it is difficult to explain the discrepant findings in these two studies, in neither piece of research were students' prior familiarity with the consonant sequences determined directly. A study carried out by Chi (1978) did control this factor with more complex materials. She compared the abilities of chess experts and novices in memorizing chess board positions. Most fascinating from a developmental perspective, the children were the experts in this study and the adults the novices. Although the children performed more poorly than the adults on a digit-span task, the results were reversed for recall of the chess positions. Chunking was implicated in the post-experiment interviews, with child experts indicating that they viewed the whole chessboard as the unit of learning. The children who knew a lot about chess were in a better position to create chunks than were the less knowledgeable adults. Chi's (1978) study made clear that chunking can play an important role in mediating some types of memory performance differences. Whether it plays a similar role in mediating performance on memory-span tasks that include numbers, words, or letters as stimuli, is still unclear. Again, see Dempster (1981), who takes this issue up in greater detail.

ITEM SEQUENCING

Some researchers (e.g., Chi, 1977; Dempster, 1981; Huttenlocher & Burke, 1978) suggested that age differences in memory span may be due in part to the requirement that materials on memory-span lists be reproduced in order. They believed that this ordering requirement would especially penalize very young subjects since very young children are not familiar with the sequential ordering of ordinal numbers.

In support of this hypothesis, Chi (1977) reported 100% improvement in recall performance by 5-year-olds when the order of items was not considered. Case et al. (1982) ignored ordering of information in their study of children's short-term memory, and obtained higher "memory span" values than are obtained when correct serial ordering is required (cf., Flavell, Friedrichs, & Hoyt, 1970; Yussen & Levy, 1975). Thus, although the data base is not extensive at this point, there is some support for the hypothesis that sequential ordering skill may be part of the cause of age differences in memory span.

Speed of Information Processing

Although there is little compelling evidence for the hypothesis that strategic varia-bles are causally connected to age-related changes in memory span, there remains the question of whether nonstrategic factors might account for developmental increases in span performance. One of these is the speed of information processing (Dempster, 1985).

There is no doubt that speed of processing generally increases with age during childhood. For instance, the rate of item identification (i.e., the time necessary to recognize or name to-be-remembered items) decreases with age. Chi (1977) com-pared recognition time for faces in 5-year-old children and adults and discovered that the time needed by the children was much greater than the time needed by adults. Both groups needed more time to name the faces, although the difference favoring adults over children remained on the naming task. Spring and Capps (1974) produced complementary results for 7- to 14-year-olds. See Keating and Bobbitt (1978) for similar developmental results on another task.

There are also clearcut data indicating that rate of item identification is correlated with memory-span performance. In Chi (1977) the differences in memory span per-formance between kindergarten children and adults were reduced drastically when the time of picture presentation was reduced by half for adults, and thus, the effects of processing speed were diminished. Case et al. (1982) discovered a monotone and almost linear relationship ($r = -.74$) for children from 3 to 6 years of age between reaction time rate and memory span. Case et al.'s correlation was significant, even when the effect of age was removed statistically ($r = -.35$). Nicolson (1981) reported a similarly high correlation. In short, it seems as if the relationship between rate of processing and memory span is very pronounced both between and within age groups. Individuals who process rapidly have relatively large memory spans.

Case et al. (1982) also tested whether there was a causal relationship between speed of activation and memory-span performance. This was tested by constructing to-be-recalled lists that were composed of materials that were named at the same rate by children and adults. Case et al. reasoned that if memory span is dependent on speed of naming, then span differences between children and adults should be eliminated with materials that are processed at the same rate by both groups. On the other hand, if span increases are mediated by other factors, then memory-span per-formance should be better for adults than children, even with materials processed at the same speed. Case et al. in fact found that with speed of processing equated, children and adults had comparable memory spans. Nicolson (1981) reached a simi-lar conclusion with a sample of 8- to 12-year-old children, reporting no age-related memory-span differences when reading speed was equated across age levels. It seems likely that speed of item identification is an important determinant of memory span and developmental differences in speed can at least partially explain correlated span differences.

Summary

The exact determinants of individual differences in memory-span performance are not known at this time. In our judgment there is good reason to continue research on the chunking, speed of processing, and serial-ordering factors that were reviewed here. We particularly believe that there is a great deal of room for additional true experiments in this area. For instance, if the chunking hypothesis is correct, then teaching children who do not chunk to chunk should increase their functional memory spans. Manipulations that increase the rate of item identification should also have a positive effect on memory-span performance. Thus, perhaps serial lists could be constructed from materials that were initially unfamiliar to subjects. If some subjects were given familiarity training to the point that their recognition of particular items was very rapid and others were not given such training, it would be expected that prefamiliarized subjects would have greater memory spans for lists composed of the familiar materials than would subjects not provided familiarization training. A lot more work could and should be done on the memory-span problem. Because only brief coverage of this problem was provided here, we strongly suggest that readers who are interested in these issues read the reviews provided by Dempster (1981, 1985).

Are There Really Development Changes in Memory Span?

Answering this question requires a brief overview of one particular developmental theory, Pascual-Leone's (e.g., 1970) theory of constructive operators. It has prompted a number of studies on the development of memory capacity. The theory is a new interpretation of Piaget's structural model of intellectual development (see also Ewert & Schumann, 1983). The central claims of the theory are stated in terms of the Piagetian concept of schema. Pascual-Leone divides schema into three components. There are figurative schema, which are roughly equivalent to the "chunks" reviewed earlier in this chapter; there are operative schema, which can be interpreted as rules or strategies; and there are executive schema, which are essentially task solution plans. The activation of particular figurative or operative schema is orchestrated by executive schema.

Pascual-Leone believes that a quantitatively specifiable parameter can be used to explain many of the qualitative phenomena described by Piaget. This is "central computing space" or "mental space" (abbreviated M-space). M-space is the maximum number of schema that a person can activate and/or coordinate simultaneously. Particularly critical to developmental psychology, Pascual-Leone hypothesizes that there is a linear increase from 3 to 16 years of age in this mental capacity. Capacity is hypothesized to increase by one schema every two years. At every age level, a constant "a" is added to this maximum number of schema. This constant stands for the additional storage space needed for the executive schema that is coordinating the activation of the other "k" schema. Hence, total capacity at any given age is equal to a + k, with k varying between 1 and 7 and equal approximately to (age − 2)/2.

Designing tasks that permit assessment of the k component is not easy. Pretraining of the task is necessary so that the child has the necessary executive skills to carry out the task. The task must involve some mental transformations so that he or she is tapping the many aspects of short-term capacity that are presumably represented by k. In addition, it is important to suppress strategies like chunking. That is, the size of each chunk must be known by the experimenter in order to determine k, and that is very difficult if subjects are recoding materials into larger chunks.

Pascual-Leone (1970) relied heavily on one particular task to provide a measure of M-space, the "compound visual stimulus information" task (CVSI). This task requires children between 5 and 11 years of age to react motorically by clapping or raising their hands in response to various visual stimuli (e.g., a square, the color red). After subjects master stimulus-action pairings (e.g., a square calls for clapping, red calls for raising hands), the critical measurements are taken. Combination stimuli are presented (e.g., a red square) and subjects are required to make every response that would be appropriate for such a stimulus (i.e., both clap and raise hands). The compound stimuli vary in complexity. The results obtained by Pascual-Leone were perfectly consistent with his model in that the complexity of stimuli that subjects could respond to increased with age. For instance, 5-year-olds could perform correctly for compound stimuli made up of two stimuli-action sequences, whereas 11-year-olds could respond correctly to compounds requiring five stimulus-action sequences. A number of other studies have also provided data consistent with Pascual-Leone's assumption that there are age-correlated increases in M-space (e.g., Burtis, 1982; Case, 1972; Case & Serlin, 1979; Ewert & Schumann, 1983; Globerson, 1983).

Nonetheless, there are a number of objections that can be raised against the conclusion that mental capacity increases with age. First of all, from a theoretical perspective, it is somewhat disturbing that the amount of space allocated to executive action is considered constant across childhood (i.e., equal to the invariant parameter "a" at all age levels). Just the fact that mental processes are executed more rapidly with increasing age (as reviewed briefly earlier in this chapter) would suggest that the functional capacity used by executive schema might change. In particular, with increasing age and increasing speed, it might be expected that the amount of space required for the executive actions would decrease. In addition, the assumption that stimulus-action pairings are equal to one same-sized chunk at all age levels poses difficulties. The speed of recognition and execution of these pairings should also increase with age, and thus, reduce the amount of capacity required to attend to and execute a single pairing. In short, speed of information processing was not taken into account by Pascual-Leone (1970). More recent data suggest that speed of information processing may better account for developmental shifts in complex tasks than do other factors (e.g., Case et al., 1982).

In addition, there are disturbing problems with the data that are reported in support of Pascual-Leone's theory. First of all, different measurement methods produce differ age norms (e.g., compare Pascual-Leone, 1970, with Globerson, 1983). Sometimes the same methods produce different age norms (e.g., compare Case, 1972, with Globerson, 1983). Sometimes there are obvious alternative explanations of the developments that are reported. For example, consider when numerical material is used in a transformation task such as the "digit placement task" used by Case (1972) and Globerson (1983). Subjects are presented numerical series where, except for the last item, the numbers increase. The subject's task is to put the last number in the correct position in the series. There is the obvious possibility that developmental improvement on the task is mediated by improvement with age in numerical ordering skills rather than simply changes in M-space as assumed by investigators in the Pascual-Leone tradition.

In addition, all of this is complicated by the fact that there were procedure by age confoundings. For instance, the number of reactions required in Pascual-Leone's M-space tests were systematically confounded with age (i.e., younger children were given fewer stimulus-action pairings to learn and produce in reaction to compound stimuli). See Trabasso and Foellinger (1978) and Trabasso (1978) for a thorough review of the problems in Pascual-Leone's research as well as Pascual-Leone's responses (Pascual-Leone, 1978; Pascual-Leone & Sparkman, 1980).

What has emerged from the investigations of memory span that have been conducted as part of the evaluation of Pascual-Leone's theory is a revision of the theory. Case et al. (1982; Case, 1985) have provided the leadership in this effort, proposing that there are developmental increases in *functional* capacity due to more efficient processing of stimuli (e.g., faster recognition and speed of processing). Particularly critical to Case's position is the argument that the amount of space required to operate on stimuli functionally decreases with increasing age given more efficient operation of the executive actions. This, in turn, frees up more space for storage of material and accounts largely for the increases in memory-span performance that are observed.

Summary

Several general conclusion emerge from the data considered in this chapter. There is no reason to assume that age-correlated performance increases in memory span should be interpreted as enlargement of some biologically determined capacity. Developmental increases in memory-span performance, however, are probably not due to use of strategies alone, which was another popular hypothesis. In fact, only one strategy, chunking, seems worthy of additional investigation as a potential contributor to memory-span improvements. Factors that likely contribute to developmental increases in span include developmental increases in speed of information processing and automatic item sequencing. In particular, more efficient execution of operations "frees up" more space for storage (Case et al., 1982).

We note as well that intraindividual differences only were considered in this chapter, and thus, all of these conclusions are relevant only to *intraindividual* differences in memory span performance. That is, they are explanations about how the same person can perform differently on memory span tests at one developmental level compared to another developmental level. As such, they cannot serve as explanations of *interindividual* differences in memory-span performance, which may very well be determined by biologically mediated differences in capacity or other factors (e.g., biologically mediated differences in speed of processing).

This research on memory span is important because it has been revealing about the "hardware" that the developing child possesses. As the discussion turns to strategies, metacognition, and the knowledge base as determinants of developmental improvements in memory performance, it is important to remember that although the actual capacity of the child's biological endowment may not change, the functional capacity does because of more efficient and speedier processing. Increases in speed of basic processes presumably contribute to more efficient execution of strategies and more rapid identification and use of metacognition and world knowledge. With increasing age, use of strategies and their coordination with relevant metacognition and world knowledge should be more certain. Thus, much of the development that is documented in the rest of this book is probably highly dependent on the development of more efficient, basic processing (i.e., better and quicker use of the biologically determined capacity that is available).

3. Development of Encoding and Retrieval Strategies

The influence of neobehaviorism in American experimental research decreased markedly during the 1960s as the limits of the stimulus-response frameworks became more and more evident. Many experimental findings could not be explained using conventional S-R terminology (e.g., Kail & Strauss, 1984), which was based on the premise of a passive organism. This made it necessary to give up the "black-box" approach that characterized much of American learning (including verbal learning) research in favor of a model of a cognitively active organism (Hagen, Jongeward, & Kail, 1975).

American research on cognitive development was influenced at this time by a number of factors. One of these was the growing awareness of Piaget's theory. A differentiation was made by the Genevans between the development of intentional recall and the development of the operations that determine intelligence and memory. Memory was viewed as highly dependent on these general operations which changed dramatically with development (Piaget & Inhelder, 1973). Most relevant here, the Piagetians believed that qualitative changes in memory would follow from these shifts, since memory was viewed as completely dependent on operational intelligence. This motivated studies aimed at identifying qualitative shifts in memory during development.

The empirical studies on memory conducted by Piaget and Inhelder were concerned mainly with testing two hypotheses that followed from their theory: (1) They believed that children's memory performance depends on their basic understanding of the task as determined by their level of cognitive development. Thus, identical stimuli are processed differently and in turn remembered differently by different age groups. (2) If it is true that children's cognitive processes reorganize themselves over long periods of time, then the memory for a specific event should also be affected in that the memory trace itself should change over time, and at least in some cases, be improved as the child matures (Liben, 1977, 1982; Naus & Halasz, 1979). Although Piaget and Inhelder reported positive support for both hypotheses, numerous American attempts at replication were less successful (Liben, 1977), especially for the claim that there is long-term improvement in memory performance (see also Weinert & Knopf, 1983). The decline in interest in the Piagetian theory of memory was in part due to these failures, although many developmentalists continued to believe that there were qualitative changes in memory over the course of childhood.

A second influence on developmental reseachers was a major insight gained from Soviet research – that it was important to differentiate voluntary from involuntary (i.e., intentional from incidental) memory (see Chapter 1). The Soviet perspectives on intentional and incidental learning were similar to those of Piaget and his associates. Both groups believed that most of children's memories and knowledge of the world were built up through incidental processing that occurs as part of the continual interactions with the world (Brown, 1975). Involuntary memory was viewed as a byproduct of the use of information in specific situations and determined in part by how information is processed and used (Smirnov & Zinchenko, 1969; Yendovitskaya, 1971). Thus, if a child tries to figure out the meaning of a stimulus, meaningful properties of the object will be remembered; if the child focusses on physical aspects of a stimulus, physical attributes are encoded. Many studies have confirmed Soviet hypotheses about the influence of incidental memory processes on memory in preschoolers and school children (e.g., Geis & Hall, 1976, 1978; Ghatala, 1984; Ghatala & Levin, 1981, 1982; Levin & Ghatala, 1982; Owings & Baumeister, 1979; Sophian & Hagen, 1978). Nonetheless, much of the Soviet research was embedded in dialectical models (e.g., Riegel, 1974, 1975) that were not nearly as appealing to North American developmentalists (nor as available or comprehensible to them; e.g., Wozniak, 1972, 1975) as the models of human information processing that predominated in adult cognitive psychology in the late 1960s and early 1970s. Thus, the Soviet position had limited impact.

The "cognitive turn" in North American experimental psychology made popular some old concepts that had almost been forgotten. So it was, for example, that the differentiation made by William James (1890) between "primary" and "secondary" memory was the basis of Waugh and Norman's (1965) specification of the first contemporary model of memory. Primary memory was postulated as a limited capacity store, with rehearsal as the only means of preventing forgetting and permitting transfer of information to the permanent, secondary memory. A short time later, Atkinson and Shiffrin (1968, 1971) presented a greatly expanded version of this model, which can be considered the most popular of the multistore conceptions (see Hagen, Jongeward, & Kail, 1975). Analogous to computer programming languages, the model differentiates between invariant structural elements ("hardware") and control processes that can be modified ("software"). In Atkinson and Shiffrin's model, the structural components are the sensory registers, long- and short-term memories. Information passes through the sensory registers into the short-term memory, which holds in consciousness both inputs from the sensory registers and activated information from long-term memory. The limited capacity of short term

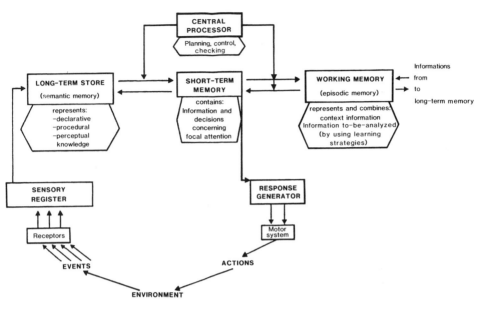

FIGURE 3.1. A general model representing memory structures and processes (modified after Wippich, 1984).

memory can be extended by control processes such as rehearsal, which also increases the probability that this information will reach the unlimited capacity long-term memory.

Although this model was at first well received by developmentalists, its use in developmental explanations was reduced considerably by an alternative proposal by Craik and his associates (Craik & Jacoby, 1975; Craik & Lockhart, 1972; Jacoby & Craik, 1979). Craik et al.'s levels of processing approach criticized the computer model as a useful metaphor for adult cognition. It replaced the notion of a multistore model with a conception that defines the "depth" or level of processing of incoming information. The role of subject-controlled memory processes and semantic memory was clearly more important in this model than in the multistore concept. The resistance of the memory trace to forgetting is viewed as a function of the "processing depth." While shallow processing is associated with attending more to physical features of a stimulus, deeper processing involves more complete and meaningful processing. Given the similarity of this position and Soviet theories of incidental memory being determined by activities that the learner engages in, it is not surprising that developmentalists were attracted to Craik's thinking.

Nonetheless, depth-of-processing models did not completely replace multi-store models (Lachman & Lachman, 1979). New structural models of thinking arose, ones that included central processing and storage as well as levels-of-processing components (Bower, 1975, 1978; Kintsch, 1975 Raaijmakers & Shiffrin, 1980, 1981). A version of such a model is presented in Figure 3.1. Combined structural and depth-of-processing models are compatible with much more of the available data than simpler alternatives (e.g., Bower & Hilgard, 1981). Virtually all of the developmental data reviewed in this chapter are compatible with this type of combined model.

The pioneering work of John Flavell and his associates (e.g., Flavell, 1970; Flavell, Beach, & Chinsky, 1966; Keeney, Cannizzo, & Flavell, 1967; Moely, Olson, Halwes, & Flavell, 1969) especially stimulated research on information processing in children. Their early research was concerned with children's use of verbal mediators in storage and recall of verbal information. Flavell and colleagues particularly focused on conscious and intentional memory activities, although Flavell (e.g., 1970) always recognized the importance of incidental learning to the development of children's knowledge. Consistent with a distinction made by Maccoby (1964), Flavell's group studied two potential difficulties in particularly great detail. One possibility was that young children do not produce mediators that can effectively promote learning (i.e., they have a production deficiency). Alternatively, children might produce mediators when learning, but the mediators would fail to facilitate performance as they do for older children and adults (i.e., the children would have a mediational deficiency; Reese, 1962).

The usefulness of the distinction between production and mediational deficiencies was apparent in Keeney et al. (1967). First, it was determined that some first-grade children used a verbal-rehearsal strategy during list learning, whereas other first-grade children failed to do so. Memory was clearly better for the children who produced the rehearsal strategy. When the production-deficient children were taught the rehearsal strategy, their memory improved dramatically, however. Thus, the children who failed to use the strategy spontaneously had a production deficiency, but not a mediational deficiency. Moely et al. (1969) also demonstrated a production deficiency in grade-school children. In this case, kindergarten, first-, and third-grade children failed to use a sorting-clustering strategy when learning lists of potentially categorizable pictures (see p. 53, this volume). Again, it proved possible to teach the strategy to these children. As in Keeney et al., there were consistent correlations between use of the sorting-clustering strategy and memory performance.

The conclusion that was reached following these early experiments was that memory could primarily be understood as a transition from nonstrategic to strategic behavior. Age of "spontaneous" strategy use seemed to vary (e.g., rehearsal strategies appeared developmentally earlier than sorting-clustering strategies). A positive sign was that children who did not use strategies on their own could profitably be instructed to execute them. That is, they could execute the strategies and their performance went up when they did so. More negatively, however, it was apparent even in these early studies that continued use of strategies was not an automatic byproduct of instruction.

Flavell's (1970) summary of his early work and a Society for Research in Child Development symposium organized by Flavell (1971; Belmont & Butterfield, 1971; Hagen, 1971) stimulated a great deal of memory development research during the next decade. The developmental psychology of memory that followed was dominated by studies assessing the use and significance of strategies, the role of the knowledge base in memory and strategy use, and the relationship of strategy use to knowledge of memory (i.e., metamemory).

Brown (1975) laid out five ways to classify memory development research, relying on dichotomous distinctions that seemed to characterize the work. These five dichotomies permit organization of the research and they highlight that workers in memory development have been very selective about the problems that they have studied: (1) Although there were experiments on both intentional and incidental learning, research on intentional learning predominated following Flavell's lead. (2) Although memory development was sometimes studied as a means to an end following Soviet suggestions (e.g., Smirnov & Zinchenko, 1969), more often it was studied as an end in itself. Again this was consistent with Flavell's early work. (3) Studies of exact recall were complemented by studies of not-so-exact recall (e.g., gist recall of text)—ones involving constructive errors that reflected the learner's knowledge base. Nonetheless, there were many more experiments that focused on exact learning compared to constructive memory. (4) The effects of strategies that produced "deep" compared to "shallow" comprehension were assessed, although this problem did not command the attention that it did in the adult literature. (5) Although the difference between memory for particular episodes versus semantic memory (memory of definitions, concepts, relationships, which is not tied to memory of particular exemplars of the concepts or relationships) was recognized following Tulving's (e.g., 1972) lead, most of the developmental work focused on episodic memory. Again, this was due in part to the fact that the earliest, seminal developmental studies were exclusively concerned with episodic memory.

Since Flavell's seminal work, there has been an enormous amount of research on children's use of memory strategies. It is certainly not possible to review all of this work, especially given the diversity of strategies that were studied (e.g., Pressley, Heisel, McCormick, & Nakamura, 1982). Instead, the tactic that we take in this chapter is to review two particular approaches to encoding (one other approach, elaboration, is considered in some detail in Chapter 6) and the development of retrieval skills, as well as issues surrounding the development of encoding and retrieval strategies.

Before turning to strategy development, however, the defining characteristics of memory strategies should be considered. For a long time, there was little controversy about the nature of strategies. It was assumed that strategies were task-relevant cognitive activities that were under conscious control. Strategies facilitated attainment of various goals (Naus & Ornstein, 1983; Ornstein, Baker-Ward, & Naus, in press; Paris, Newman, & Jacobs, 1985). Recently, however, there is more debate about the fundamental nature of strategies. For instance, in Pressley and Levin's two-volume set on cognitive strategies (Pressley & Levin, 1983a, 1983b), many different definitions of strategy were provided by the various contributors to the books.

There are two important factors contributing to the confusion about the definition of strategy. First, automatic information processing can produce the same effects as conscious use of strategies (e.g., Hasher & Zacks, 1979; Naus & Halasz, 1979; Walter Schneider, & Shiffrin, 1977; Shiffrin & Walter Schneider, 1977). Uncon-

scious activities sometimes produce performance that is even better than that
obtained by conscious efforts. Second, it is possible that some of the activities interpreted as conscious strategies actually reflect automatic processes. A typical situation is the one described by Lange (1973, 1978). He demonstrated that the category
clustering observed in young students performing sort-recall tasks was due to automatically activated associations rather than strategic activities. (More about this
example later in the chapter.)

Nonetheless, some researchers continue to argue that memory strategies must be
conscious (e.g., Paris, Lipson, & Wixson, 1983; Paris et al., 1985). The majority of
memory development researchers (e.g., Brown, 1978; Brown, Bransford, Ferrara,
& Campione, 1983; especially Campione & Armbruster, 1985; Flavell, 1985),
however, employ a much less restrictive criterion regarding intentionality. Pressley,
Forrest-Pressley, Elliott-Faust, and Miller (1985) provided one of the more detailed
of the new definitions of strategy:

A strategy is composed of cognitive operations over and above the processes that are natural
consequences of carrying out the task, ranging from one such operation to a sequence of
interdependent operations. Strategies achieve cognitive purposes (e.g., comprehending,
memorizing) and are potentially conscious and controllable activities (p. 4).

There is no doubt, of course, that this definition is fairly imprecise. That was
Pressley, Forrest-Pressley, Elliott-Faust, and Miller's (1985) intention, because they
conceptualized strategy as a "fuzzy set" of activities. The nature of that fuzzy set will
be more obvious after some particular examples are considered in detail.

Strategic Behaviors in Very Young Children

We know much more about strategy use by school age children than by preschoolers.
In part this is because the early American work (e.g., Keeney et al., 1967; Hagen &
Kingsley, 1968) and Soviet research (e.g., Yendovitskaya, 1971) provided little
evidence that intentional, strategic memorizing occurred before six years of age.
In fact, it is fairly easy to produce data consistent with this conclusion by using
the "modal memory" study model (Brown & DeLoache, 1978; DeLoache, 1980).
That approach involves presenting a sample of very young children with a memory
task that is composed of unfamiliar materials that are presented in an unfamiliar
context. In general, researchers have used the nonstrategic behavior produced by
preschoolers in such situations as a baseline against which the progress of older
subjects has been demonstrated. The basic problem with such an approach is that we
find out little about preschoolers (e.g., Gelman, 1978)—we only know what they
cannot or will not do.

There is another reason why there is so little understanding of early strategy use,
however. It is very hard to carry out studies with children two to five years of age
compared to older subjects. It is both difficult to get children to understand what you
want them to do and it is difficult to get them to do it (DeLoache, 1980). These
difficulties make obvious that standard techniques for analyzing the memory

behaviors of older children are not appropriate with preschoolers. Fortunately, there are other methods available, especially adaptations of ones used to study memory in infants. Use of these procedures seemed especially appropriate since there was the possibility of finding developmental connections between infancy and the preschool years (e.g., Sophian, 1984).

Thus, recall in preschoolers has been studied with retrieval-of-hidden objects, memory-for-events, and memory-for-objects paradigms, all approaches that were used in one form or another to study infant cognition (Daehler & Greco, 1985). The main issue addressed in these studies was whether, and at which age, conscious, intentional memory activities are observable in very young children. Memory activities were judged to be intentional in these experiments if they developed out of knowledge about a particular memory goal and were selectively employed (e.g., in the context of memory instructions; Wellman, 1977a).

Retrieval of Hidden Objects

Two different research strategies have been used to study memory for location in small children. There are "naturalistic" studies, which are based on daily observations that are recorded in diaries or observation protocols. This approach was first applied with infants and small children by Stern and Stern (1909; also Bühler, 1930) and with preschoolers by Hurlock and Schwartz (1932). The second method is the "delayed reaction," or "hide-and-seek" task (DeLoache, 1984). In its simplest form the child first observes an object being hidden. After a period of time that is filled with other activities, the child is requested to locate the hidden object.

The naturalistic studies provide anecdotal evidence of intact memory for location in one year olds. Bühler (1930) reported a case where a ball rolled under a cabinet during play. When asked to look for the ball about an hour later, the child was able to find it immediately although he had been occupied with other things since the disappearance of the ball. When Ashmead and Perlmutter (1980) analyzed entries in mothers' diaries, they found evidence of development between 7 and 11 months of age. The younger children were observed remembering the locations of objects that had relatively fixed positions (e.g., telephone, closet). Older subjects were better able to recall objects with changing positions. Nelson and Ross (1980) also used the diary method and determined that toddlers (who had just turned two) employed more intentional memory activities for recall of events than for the location of meaningful objects. The older children were able to recall both objects and events accurately after a relatively long period of time (i.e., up to three months). Although these diary studies provide valuable information about infants, there are methodological problems with them. Mothers' motivations and/or subjective interpretations cannot be evaluated reliably (Nelson & Ross, 1980). In contrast, reliability of measurement is no problem when memory for location is studied with hide-and-seek tasks, situations that permit examination of a naturalistic behavior in a controlled setting.

A simple version of the hide-and-seek task, the "perseveration" task (Sophian, 1984), has been used in a number of studies and is useful for illustrating conscious decision-making processes during search. The task consists of two trials. During the first, an object is hidden at place A; during the second, it is hidden at place B. Very young children (i.e., 6 to 9 months old) make the perseveration error or AB mistake (Daehler & Greco, 1985). Although they observe the object being hidden at place B on trial 2, they again search for the object at position A. This error is obtained even with a short retention interval following hiding at B. Sophian (1984) suggested that this phenomenon was due to the inability of very young children to differentiate between present and past behavior. By age 1½, children ignore the A position in favor of B, although this competency can be disrupted if complications are introduced, for example, by decreasing the explicitness of information about hiding and retrieval (Sophian & Wellman, 1980, 1983). In contrast, slightly older children (i.e., 3- and 4-year-olds) perform well in this situation even when things are complicated.

Intentional memory for location has been researched intensively in recent studies with many of these studies framed as research on the development of retrieval skills. The results of the early studies were ambiguous. Although Horn and Myers (1978), Loughlin and Daehler (1973), and Ratner and Myers (1980) found almost no evidence that children under three years of age profit from the presentation of retrieval cues, Perlmutter and her associates provided demonstrations that 2- to 3-year-olds make use of retrieval cues under certain conditions. For instance, Blair, Perlmutter, and Myers (1978) showed children colored pictures one at a time. Then the picture was hidden in one of nine drawers in a small filing cabinet. In the retrieval-cue conditions, another picture of another object was attached to the front of the relevant drawer. In the control condition, no picture was attached to the front of the drawer. The children then looked away from the filing cabinets for 25 seconds before attempting to retrieve the hidden picture. Provision of a retrieval cue aided the search of the 27- to 45-month-old participants in the study. Perlmutter et al. (1981) obtained comparable results in a similar paradigm and concluded that even 2-year-olds can use picture cues to encode location and search for objects.

A variety of other issues concerning search and retrieval have been investigated in studies of memory for location. For instance, Sophian and Wellman (1983) focused on children's emerging understanding that objects are not always found where they were hidden. If an object is hidden under a cup at place A, and the cup is then exchanged with the cup at place B, looking at place A will not produce the hidden object. Children who are 30 months old understand this fact better than do children who are 24 months old (Sophian, Larkin, & Kadane, 1985). It is now well established that visible retrieval cues that are strongly associated with the hidden object are readily used by preschoolers. For instance, Gordon and Flavell (1977) demonstrated that finding a picture of a fireman that was hidden in one of four folders was easy for 3-year-olds when a picture of a fire hat was placed on the outside of the folder containing the fireman.

One of the most impressive studies of preschoolers' use of retrieval cues was conducted by Ritter, Kaprove, Fitch, and Flavell (1973), who demonstrated that younger preschool children's (i.e., 3-year-olds) effective use of retrieval cues occurred *only* when the task was *very* simple. They observed substantial development of retrieval cue use during the preschool years. In Ritter et al. (1973) the test material consisted of six pictures of people (e.g., a soccer player) and six small toys (e.g., a soccer ball)—each person was functionally related to one of the toys. The 3- to 5-year-old subjects watched as each person entered one of six houses and put their toy in a box with the toy in the box visible at all times. In contrast, the people were placed out of sight in the house. The child's task was to show a "twin" of each person (6 pictures identical to the 6 people pictures that were hidden), the way to their partner. After this task, all materials were removed except for a single set of people pictures that were placed face down in front of the child. The children were then asked to recall the names of the toys. The children were free to use the picture retrieval cues if they chose to do so. The majority of children at each age level made use of the visible toys as retrieval cues during the first task, with no striking age differences. The second task yielded a clear developmental pattern, however. Approximately 20% of the 3-year-olds turned over the pictures of the people and used them as retrieval cues. In contrast, about 75% of the 5-year-olds used this device. See Geis and Lange (1976) and Schneider and Sodian (1988) for complementary results.

It is one thing to use retrieval cues that are provided. It is quite another for children to prepare for retrieval themselves. Ritter (1978) conducted a now classic study that is relevant to this point. The task was to prepare to find a piece of candy hidden in one cup on a turntable containing six cups. Paper clips and gold stars that could potentially be used to mark the relevant cup were placed near the turntable. The children were aware of the memory requirement and of the fact that they would have to close their eyes as the turntable was spun. The child would then be given an opportunity to retrieve the candy.

After placing the candy in the cup but before spinning the turntable, the experimenter asked the child, "Is there something you can do to help you find the candy right away?" Using the paper clips or gold stars to mark the appropriate cup was defined as spontaneous preparation for retrieval. If the child failed to mark the cup following this nondirective question, graded prompts were provided to induce preparation for later retrieval. The least explicit of these consisted of the experimenter pointing to the clips and stars and saying, "Can these help you to find the candy right away?" A slightly more explicit prompt consisted of the experimenter pointing to the clips and stars and commenting, "Can you use these over here to help you find the candy right away?" More explicit still was the experimenter putting a marker on the cup and asking, "Will this help you find the candy right away?" and "Do you want to leave the marker there or put it some other place?"

Although third-grade subjects placed the retrieval cues spontaneously without prompting to do so, all preschoolers required prompting with 3-year-olds needing more than 5-year-olds. Although all the third graders and 90% of the older preschoolers (4½ to 5½) used the retrieval cues at testing to find the candies, approximately one-third of the younger preschoolers (aged 3 to 4½) failed to prepare retrieval cues given even the most explicit prompting.

Others have produced data generally confirming the pattern of outcomes reported by Ritter (1978). For instance, Beal and Fleisig (1987) reported that preschoolers needed several prompts before they would use retrieval cues in search tasks structurally identical to the task studied by Ritter. This was despite the fact that Beal and

Fleisig made certain that their subjects were aware that retrieval would be difficult without cues. Whittaker, McShane, and Dunn (1985) also used a task that was structurally similar to the one employed by Ritter. They observed that 3-year-olds did not make use of strategies spontaneously to remember locations, with many failing to place a retrieval cue after several prompts. By 9 years of age, half the children prepared retrieval cues without a prompt to do so, and seven of the remaining eight children in the sample did so following some prompting. In short, there are observable improvements between the preschool and grade-school years in children's robust and flexible use of retrieval strategies.

In interpreting the memory-for-location and retrieval results, we point out that looking for coins under a cup (as well as most of the other laboratory tasks used in these investigations) is not a particularly common behavior for children, and it might be expected that greater strategic activity would be obtained with more naturalistically valid search tasks. A study by DeLoache, Cassidy, and Brown (1985) is particularly interesting in this regard, offering evidence that precursors of strategic behavior in location tasks are observable in children between 18 and 24 months of age. The most important data were collected between the hiding of a Big Bird doll by an experimenter (e.g., under a pillow in the living room where the study took place) and the time when the children were asked to retrieve the toy from the hiding place. Although the children were occupied with very attractive toys during this interval, they frequently interrupted their activities to look at the hiding place, to point at it, or to repeat the name of the hidden object. A follow-up study provided data making clear that these were actually memory-related activities. In that study, when Big Bird was placed in the environment, but not hidden (e.g., put on top of a pillow in sight of the child) so that no remembering was required to retrieve the doll, few orienting behaviors occurred.

The DeLoache et al. (1985) data support the hypothesis that children as young as 2 years of age can use rudimentary memory strategies. These strategic behaviors were only observed in tasks with very simple structures, however. With harder tasks, intentional preparation for retrieval is not observed until later. Consider a study by Wellman, Ritter, and Flavell (1975). The goal in that study was to remember where an object was hidden — under one of three identical cups — from the time an experimenter left the room until her return. Three-year-olds but not 2-year-olds exhibited what appeared to be consciously intentional memory behaviors including watching and touching the correct cup. In fact, 3-year-olds seem to be strategic across various types of hide-and-seek games and location tasks (e.g., Haake, Somerville, & Wellman, 1980; Wellman & Somerville, 1982; Wellman, Somerville, & Haake, 1979).

Memory for Events and Event Sequences

Diary entries have provided much evidence of very early memory for everyday events. Bühler (1930) pointed out that 2-year-olds sometimes remember even infrequent events for a long period of time. There are similar reports in more recent studies (e.g., Nelson & Ross, 1980; Todd & Perlmutter, 1980).

Whereas Todd and Perlmutter (1980) characterized the memories of 3- to 5-year-olds for everyday events as examples of "nondeliberate" memory, Somerville, Wellman, and Cultice (1983) studied children's prospective memory for everyday activities in an effort to find deliberate memory behavior by preschoolers. Parents cooperated in this study of 2- to 4-year-olds. The parents instructed their children to carry out a particular activity at a specified future time. The to-be-remembered event was either one that was highly interesting and appealing to the child (e.g., getting candy) or one that would be of little interest to the child. The child either had to remember the event for a short period of time or for a long time. There was better memory at all age levels in the study for the interesting event and when the time interval was short, with the interest variable having a greater impact on performance. That there were no significant effects in Somerville et al. that involved the age factor suggests that even 2-year-olds are capable of intentional memory, at least when given an interesting event to remember. See Renninger and Wozniak (1985) for complementary evidence documenting that interesting stimuli can prompt deliberate memory behaviors in children.

What are children's representations of everyday events like? Katherine Nelson (Nelson, 1978; Nelson, Fivush, Hudson, & Lucariello, 1983; Nelson & Gründel, 1981) and Jean Mandler (Fivush & Mandler, 1985; Mandler, 1983, 1984, 1986) have studied this problem. Both researchers believe that the script model developed by Schank and Abelson (1977) can provide an explanation of children's memory of everyday routines. Scripts are general representations of events, a type of generalized knowledge about temporal and causal relations between event and action components. For instance, there are "going to a restaurant" and "birthday party" scripts that specify how to reach certain goals in predictable fashions. These generalized scripts are believed to develop out of specific (episodic) experiences.

Nelson and Mandler and their associates have provided many empirical confirmations that even very young children organize their memories of daily events via scripts (Mandler, 1983, 1984; Nelson, Fivush, Hudson, & Lucariello, 1983; Nelson & Gründel, 1981). For instance, materials that can be related to a common script are remembered better by young children than materials that are taxonomically related (e.g., Lucariello & Nelson, 1985). Although the scripts possessed by 3- to 4-year-old children are very general, they become increasingly specific and complete with development (e.g., Adams & Worden, 1986).

Memory for Lists of Objects, Pictures, and Words

When preschoolers are presented lists of objects, pictures, or words to learn, they typically can recognize many more of these items later than they can recall, with recall often very poor (e.g., Myers & Perlmutter, 1978; Perlmutter, 1984; Perlmutter & Myers, 1979). That stimuli can be recognized suggests that the children have encoded the materials that were presented for learning; that they cannot recall them suggests that preschoolers are not very proficient at searching their memories and self-prompting themselves about events that they have experienced. Thus, an hypothesis advanced in a number of studies was that preschoolers' recall might be improved if they were provided prompts (e.g., category clues for recall of categorizable lists). Consistent with this hypothesis, semantic prompts (like category cues) improve recall by 3- to 5-year-olds (e.g., Ceci, Lea, & Howe, 1980; Davies & Brown, 1978; Emmerich & Ackerman, 1978; Morrison & Lord, 1982; Perlmutter & Myers, 1979; Perlmutter, Schork, & Lewis, 1982; Sophian & Hagen, 1978; Wingard, Buchanan, & Burnell, 1978).

Although cue manipulations at retrieval seem to produce dramatic and generally consistent effects, encoding manipulations (e.g., blocked versus nonblocked presentation of categorizable items for study) have been more variably successful. Thus, some investigators have reported facilitation due to blocking of categorizable items (e.g., Kobasigawa & Orr, 1973; Perlmutter & Myers, 1979; Morrison & Lord, 1982), whereas others have failed to observe benefits due to blocking (Emmerich & Ackerman, 1978; Garrison, 1980). Very salient prompts during encoding do seem to affect memory, however. Thus, requiring 4- to 5-year-olds to sort to-be-learned lists into semantic categories enhances memory of the material (e.g., Moely et al. 1969; Lange & Griffith, 1977). These sort-recall results make clear that even very young children can be led to employ organizational strategies profitably, although nonprompted, intentional use of such strategies has never been observed with 2- to 5-year-olds (Perlmutter & Myers, 1979).

Analyses of children's sorting have produced evidence that preschoolers' classification behaviors are more dominated by perceptual than taxonomic criteria, consistent with Piagetian theory (e.g., Piaget, 1970). Preschoolers tend to classify according to color rather than according to semantic or taxonomic characteristics (Melkman, Tversky, & Baratz, 1981; Perlmutter & Ricks, 1979). Perlmutter, Schork, and Lewis (1982) studied the effects of perceptual versus conceptual orienting questions during encoding. That the preschoolers in the study benefited from both color *and* category cues permits the conclusion that even very young children can use semantic category knowledge when encoding information.

A difficulty with the studies by Melkman et al., Perlmutter and Ricks (1979), and Perlmutter et al. (1982), however, was that children were not aware at encoding that they would be required to recall material later. What do sorting preferences look like when preschoolers and kindergarten children are aware of an upcoming test? Sodian, Schneider, and Perlmutter (1986) presented 4- and 6-year-olds with 16 toys that could be classified according to taxonomic and color criteria. The subjects in the "sort-and-remember" condition were told to code items into memory by putting them into groups that they felt belonged together. Subjects in a "play-and-remember" condition were given no instructions specific to sorting but rather were told that they were allowed to play with the items awhile before they would be given a memory test. All subjects categorized more according to taxonomic classification than according to color. Not surprisingly, the provision of category cues at recall had a more positive effect than provision of color cues. An especially important finding was that there was significantly more categorical clustering in the sorting condition than in the play condition during both encoding and recall. A significant memorizing versus playing effect in favor of the memorizing condition was obtained, but only with the 4-year-olds.

Although the average categorical clustering value differed significantly from zero during the sorting condition for both age groups, the design of the study by Sodian et al. (1986) did not permit conclusions about whether the organizational behaviors could be interpreted as intentional memory strategies. This was due to the fact that the play condition also included mention of later recall. Intentional memory strategies in young children can be most safely inferred when encoding behaviors occur following instructions that indicate a future memory requirement, and the same behaviors do not occur following instructions that do not indicate that a memory test will occur (i.e., following intentional but not incidental learning instructions; Wellman, 1977a).

One of the earliest studies with an intentional versus incidental instructional manipulation was reported by Appel et al. (1972). They observed no differences in the behaviors of preschoolers who were provided intentional versus incidental learning instructions (a result generally comparable to some of the Soviet data discussed in Chapter 1). Appel et al.'s (1972) initial study of the "differentiation hypothesis" stimulated a number of follow-up studies (e.g., Galbraith, Olsen, Duerden, & Harris, 1982; Yussen, Gagné, Gargiulo, & Kunen, 1974; Yussen, Kunen, & Buss, 1975). In contrast to Appel et al. (1972), there was clear differentiation between intentional and incidental learning situations throughout childhood in most of these followup investigations, most critically, even with preschoolers.

Baker-Ward, Ornstein, and Holden (1984) offered especially convincing evidence that preschoolers consciously memorize. Children in that experiment were presented either memory-neutral (play) or memory-relevant instructions. The subjects in the two play conditions were given no indication that they would have to recall information later. Children in the memory condition were informed that they could play with the toys awhile, but they should also do all that they could to remember a specified subsample of the toys (i.e., the to-be-remembered items). Subjects in the memory condition played significantly less than subjects in the play condition. Children in the memory condition were more likely than play subjects to name the to-be-remembered objects or look at them intensely. These differences in the frequency of memory-related behaviors as a function of experimental condition were found at all age levels and increased with age. These memory-related behaviors only affected the recall of the 6-year-olds in the study, however. Baker-Ward et al. (1984) speculated that this might be because the newly learned strategies were not routinized to the point that they could actually be useful to subjects.

Evidence of strategy development between the preschool years and kindergarten was also obtained in a study by Hudson and Fivush (1983). Kindergarten children in that study strategically used the structures of word lists that they were presented to learn whereas the preschool children did not.

The studies reviewed in this subsection make clear that rudimentary memory strategies can be observed when preschoolers prepare for recall. Preschoolers are more competent than was assumed just a few years ago (cf., Myers & Perlmutter, 1978; Perlmutter, 1980).

Summary

The empirical studies conducted in the last decade have concentrated on the identification of competencies in preschoolers more than deficits. The hypothesis that there is a "five-to-seven" shift from nonstrategic to strategic (coincidental with the onset of schooling) is no longer tenable (Brown, Bransford, Ferrara, & Campione, 1983). Many strategic behaviors have been identified in preschoolers, behaviors that indicate self-directed, goal-oriented actions. These behaviors are especially obvious when children are studied in familiar surroundings and with familiar tasks (characteristic of many of the studies considered in this section). For instance, strategic behavior can be observed with some variations of the hide-and-seek task when cognitive demands are low. With less familiar tasks, the results can be quite different:

The fact that the child thinks to prepare for retrieval in a toy hiding game does not necessarily mean that he will select a suitable cue to bait the correct container in a very similar retrieval-cue-selection task (Brown et al., 1983, p. 94).

For instance, see Whittaker et al. (1985) for direct evidence that laboratory hide-and-seek tasks are more complex than toy finding, and that the laboratory tasks can only be solved by school-age children. Even though preschoolers have some strategic skills, the ones they possess are extremely limited in scope of application.

Development of an Encoding Strategy: Rehearsal

It is not easy to determine that a strategy affects encoding only, and in fact, may be impossible to do so (Waters & Andreassen, 1983), since the advantages conferred by encoding strategies are often not realized until retrieval is required. Encoding strategies refer to procedures that are deployed during study of material in preparation for a subsequent test. Although there are many encoding strategies, a few have received much more attention from developmental psychologists than have others. We review two of the more prominently researched procedures in this section.

Rehearsal has been studied very intensely by developmental psychologists. This interest was partially motivated by the criticality of rehearsal in both multi-store memory models (Atkinson & Shiffrin, 1968, 1971) and "levels of processing" models (Craik & Lockhart, 1972) and by Flavell's early work establishing rehearsal as a strategy that developed between 5 and 10 years of age.

Flavell, Beach, and Chinsky (1966) studied list learning by 5-, 7-, and 10-year-olds. The children wore space helmets while they prepared for serial recall of picture lists. The helmets were constructed so that the experimenter could see the child's mouth and thus determine if the subject was verbally rehearsing the materials as they were presented. Only a very few 5-year-olds displayed multiple-item rehearsal strategies; in contrast, most of the oldest subjects cumulatively rehearsed the list items.

Direct measurement of rehearsal was complemented in Flavell et al. (1966) and in other studies by less direct indicators of cumulative rehearsal. The most important of these was analysis of recall by serial position in the list. When especially good recall occurred for items early in the list (primacy effect), rehearsal processes were assumed (Belmont & Butterfield, 1977; Hagen & Stanovich, 1977). Primacy effects were generally not found when preschoolers and younger school children were left to their own devices to learn material. It is, however, relatively easy to evoke primacy in these nonproducers by training them to use rehearsal strategies (Gruenenfelder & Borkowski, 1975; Hagen & Kingsley, 1968; Hagen, Hargrave, & Ross, 1973; Keeney et al., 1967; Kingsley & Hagen, 1969). Clear primacy during uninstructed learning can be observed from about 8 to 10 years of age.

In addition to correlations between primacy effects, use of rehearsal, and age, researchers who were interested in rehearsal were able to confirm a causal link between rehearsal and primacy through experimental manipulations. For instance, primacy effects are reduced among older but not among younger children when rehearsal opportunities are limited by time constraints (Allik & Siegel, 1976; Hagen & Kail, 1973).

Other measures of input activity also supported the conclusion that rehearsal develops. One of the most important of these involved analyses of subjects' pauses while they studied (Ashcraft & Kellas, 1974; Belmont & Butterfield, 1969, 1971). Although 13-year-olds in Belmont and Butterfield's study displayed progressively longer pause times with the presentation of each new item on a serial list, pause times were more uniform as a function of list condition with younger children (i.e., 9-year-olds). It was inferred from these results that the older subjects used an active, cumulative rehearsal strategy but that the younger subjects probably did little more than verbally label individual items as they were presented.

Data obtained using the overt rehearsal technique developed by Rundus (1971) permitted even more detailed developmental conclusions (Cuvo, 1975; Kellas, Ashcraft, & Johnson, 1973; Ornstein, Naus, & Liberty, 1975). The advantages of the overt rehearsal method, which requires that subjects memorize all items out loud, are that the quantity and quality of rehearsal activities can be directly measured and evaluated. The work of Peter Ornstein, Mary Naus, and their associates (Naus & Ornstein, 1983; Ornstein & Naus, 1978, 1985; Ornstein, Baker-Ward, & Naus, in press) using this method have been especially revealing, and thus will be considered in detail in the remainder of this subsection. Ornstein and his associates studied whether changes in rehearsal were more qualitative or quantitative in nature; the importance of encoding and retrieval processes for the efficiency of memorization; and contextual conditions that are necessary and sufficient to induce active memorization strategies in younger children.

Ornstein et al. (1975) made a detailed study of qualitative differences in the rehearsal of third, sixth, and eighth graders. The subjects were instructed to rehearse serial list items out loud, with five seconds provided between the presentation of each item. The typical age effects for serial recall were obtained. Older subjects both recalled more items and exhibited a primacy effect. In contrast, there were no age differences in the total amount of rehearsal nor was the correlation between amount of rehearsal and recall very large. Qualitative analyses of the rehearsal sets, however, were much more informative, with a rehearsal set defined as the number of items rehearsed together. Third graders tended to rehearse single items (rote repetition). The older subjects, however, put more items together in each rehearsal set. Ornstein et al. (1975) argued that older subjects' active rehearsal accounted for both their greater recall and the primacy effect that was obtained in their data.

Naus, Ornstein, and Aivano (1977) provided clear evidence that the difference in rehearsal between third graders and older children reflected a production deficiency by the younger children. When they trained third graders to use three-item rehearsal sets, third graders displayed the primacy effect typical of older children. In addition, their recall was approximately at the level of grade-6 children (also Ornstein, Naus, & Stone, 1977). A more thorough analysis of the third-grade rehearsal revealed more rigidity in the younger subjects than in older children, however, with younger children tending to form a single three-item set following each item and repeating it until the next item was presented. Older children tended to vary their three-item sets more.

When all of the relevant data are considered, it seems that the essential difference between the memorization processes of younger compared to older children are qualitative rather than quantitative. Passive one-word memorization strategies are replaced by cumulative rehearsal strategies, with the number of different items in a rehearsal set eventually reaching three or four (Ornstein & Naus, 1978). These cross-sectional results were recently complemented by longitudinal analyses. In Kunzinger (1985) an overt rehearsal task was presented to 7-year-olds who were retested two years later. There was an increase in the rehearsal set size with development (from 1.7 to 2.6 items). Rehearsal frequency never correlated with recall. The size of the rehearsal set correlated only at the second measurement point. An especially interesting finding was the high stability in performance. Children who had larger rehearsal sets at the initial measurement also had larger sets at test point 2. Guttentag, Ornstein, and Siemens (1987) observed comparable longitudinal stability between 8½ and 9½ years of age.

All of the relevant data suggest that developmental increases in active, cumulative rehearsal play a crucial role in the explanation of age differences in free and serial recall tasks. The question remains, however, about the degree that cumulative rehearsal facilitates encoding of information versus retrieval of it. Perhaps only active rehearsal transfers information from short-term memory into long-term memory. Alternatively, perhaps both forms of rehearsal permit transfer of information to long-term memory, but that active rehearsal makes it easier to retrieve the information later. An experiment that would test these two possibilities would compare the effects of various types of rehearsal under testing conditions that differ with respect to retrieval demands.

Comparison of recognition versus recall testing provides such an opportunity. Recognition tests reduce retrieval demands considerably, but provide information about what is available in long-term memory. If developmental differences occur on recall tests, but there are none on recognition tests, it can be assumed that the material was encoded into long-term memory at all age levels, but that younger children experience retrieval difficulties that are somehow linked to their failure to use cumulative rehearsal. If, however, there are also developmental differences in recognition, this could be taken as evidence that different repetition strategies produce different encodings – that is, the amount and quality of information in long-term memory depends on the strategy used to code the material.

Naus, Ornstein, and Kreshtool (1977) conducted an experiment along these lines. Third and sixth graders learned a word list and then took either a recognition or a recall test. Consistent with other developmental data, there were significant developmental differences in recall, especially due to developmental differences in recall of items at the beginning of the word lists. No age differences were found in the recognition data, however. Both active and passive rehearsal seemed to produce transfer of information from short- to long-term memory.

There probably are different types of representations in long-term memory following passive versus active rehearsal, however. Naus et al. (1977) discussed the possibility that the overt cumulative rehearsal strategies build inter-item associations that make it easier to retrieve them during recall. Compatible with this assumption, the effects produced by active rehearsal strategies are considerably reduced when to-be-learned material is presented in a blocked fashion (e.g., by category). Presumably, salient list structure produces inter-item associations automatically (Ornstein et al., 1975; Ornstein, 1977). An additional mechanism that may account for the retrieval benefits produced by cumulative rehearsal is the self-testing that is part of cumulative rehearsal. Thus, cumulative rehearsers have practice with recall more than passive rehearsers before the actual recall test takes place (Naus & Ornstein, 1983; Ornstein & Naus, 1978).

Possible Explanations of Young Children's Failures to Use Rehearsal Strategies

Studies of the content of older children's rehearsal sets reveals that better retention occurs when items are produced in groups that include both recently encountered items and items from earlier list positions (Cuvo, 1974, 1975) – that is, when rehearsal is cumulative. An interesting observation by Cuvo (1974) was that older school children and college students were more likely to include items that they liked in cumulative rehearsal sets. They focused on these items and that seemed to result in them being rehearsed more. Thus, one possible explanation of cumulative rehearsal is that *motivation* plays a role.

Kunzinger and Witryol (1984) believed that motivational stimulation of items would also affect younger children who normally prefer passive rehearsal strategies. They believed that the younger children might be motivated to pay more attention to the items that they were interested in. Motivation was manipulated by assigning a monetary value to items on the list, with some worth 1¢ and others worth 10¢. The second graders in the study were told that they would receive the amount of money associated with the items that were recalled later. In the control group, 5¢ was associated with each item. There were important differences in recall between the experimental and control conditions. The size of the rehearsal sets was doubled in the experimental condition to an average of more than two highly valued items.

There was also a clear primacy effect in the experimental condition. The differential motivation condition thus produced effects that are compatible with those of direct training procedures (Ornstein, Naus, & Stone, 1977).

A second hypothesis is that *specific prior knowledge* can activate memory strategies (Bjorklund, 1985, 1987; Chi, 1978, 1985b; Naus & Ornstein, 1983; Ornstein & Naus, 1985). Older children's cumulative rehearsal may be tied to the development of semantic memory, with older children having more concepts and interconceptual associations to trigger use of strategies. Tarkin, Myers, and Ornstein (reported in Ornstein & Naus, 1985) tested this hypothesis directly, examining the influence of the knowledge base on the rehearsal activities of young children. Eight-year-olds were presented word lists that varied in their meaningfulness and familiarity to children (even the least meaningful words, however, were known by all children). The children displayed age-typical rehearsal (i.e., less than two items per rehearsal set) for nonmeaningful items. In contrast, the learning sets for meaningful items contained more than three items. Memorization behavior with meaningful materials was comparable to the behavior of 11- to 12-year-olds with normal word lists (Ornstein & Naus, 1985). Highly meaningful stimulus materials make rehearsal processes and retrieval easier in that the learner profits from associations between the individual items that are activated automatically. Ornstein and Naus (1985) also demonstrated in a second example (the comparison of adult football experts and novices) that especially meaningful material increases the size of rehearsal sets. The familiarity of material seems to be an important determinant of use of more efficient and effective rehearsal procedures.

Guttentag (1984, 1985) proposed that young children do not employ cumulative rehearsal strategies spontaneously because the *mental effort* required to do so strains their functional capacity. Guttentag studied this hypothesis with a dual-task procedure. In addition to rehearsing to-be-recalled items overtly, subjects simultaneously performed key tapping. The subjects were informed that rehearsing was the more important task, although they should try to do both at once. Mental effort was operationalized as the interference on key tapping produced by cumulative rehearsal. Interference was measured as the difference between normal tapping during a baseline period when simultaneous rehearsal was not required and tapping during rehearsal.

In Guttentag's first experiment, second, third, and sixth graders were instructed to employ the overt cumulative rehearsal strategy and to perform the motor task simultaneously. Even the youngest subjects were able to do this with no age differences in performance. There were, however, significant differences in the degree of interference experienced. Motoric performance was clearly disrupted more when younger children rehearsed compared to when older children did so. There were no age differences in interference when children were instructed to rehearse passively, however (experiment 2). Based on these data, Guttentag (1984, 1985) argued that age differences in spontaneous use of cumulative rehearsal strategies may in part be due to the enormous effort required of young children in order to employ complex strategies. See Bjorklund and Harnishfeger (1987) for a similar finding concerning the role of mental effort in the use of categorization strategies.

A study conducted by Ornstein, Medlin, Stone, and Naus (1985) is interesting because it not only confirms the interference detected by Guttentag, but also provides a more exact analysis of the components of cumulative rehearsal that pose special difficulties for younger grade-school children (i.e., those that cause the mental effort). Ornstein et al. (1985) demonstrated that the efficiency of cumulative rehearsal improved considerably when second graders were provided additional visual cues as they rehearsed, that is, when previously presented items continued to be visible (thus, reducing the pressure on working memory to hold previously presented material in consciousness). It was clear in this study that cumulative rehearsal was easier for second graders given the visual cues; with the visual cues, they cumulatively rehearsed almost five items per set in response to the cumulative rehearsal instruction compared to about three items per set given the cumulative rehearsal instruction without pictorial support. Guttentag et al. (1987) used a similar manipulation and produced complementary data with children in grades 3, 4, and 6.

In summary, rehearsal is an "ill-defined group of memory strategies" (Brown, Bransford, Ferrara, & Campione, 1983; Flavell, 1985, p. 218). Thus, 5- and 6-year-olds often respond with single verbal labels in response to each item on a serial list. Slightly older children repeat the labels several times while an item is in view. The majority of 10-year-olds use cumulative rehearsal to learn serial lists. Although not considered in this section, more complex rehearsal tactics are evidenced by even older subjects. For instance, many university-age subjects use cumulative rehearsal for early list items followed by a fast-finish approach to final list items (e.g., Barclay, 1979).

Our understanding of rehearsal strategies was made possible by use of observational methods, especially when overt rehearsal was required of subjects. These analyses revealed that quantitative increases in rehearsal played little role in explaining recall data. In contrast, use of cumulative rehearsal has strikingly positive effects on recall.

Instructional experiments made clear than even children in grade 1 can carry out cumulative rehearsal strategies when taught to do so, even though very few first-grade children use cumulative rehearsal spontaneously. Procedures and materials can sometimes be modified, however, so that children who are normally production deficient with respect to cumulative rehearsal will employ more active rehearsal strategies. This occurs when there is high motivation for learning and when particularly meaningful or familiar material is employed. An important difficulty for younger children seems to be the mental effort required to carry out cumulative rehearsal. This is probably due to inefficient use of strategy components, such as maintaining previously presented items in short-term memory so that they can be included in rehearsal sets.

Development of Another Encoding Strategy: Organization

Bousfield's (1953) work on subjective organization during learning was pioneering work on subject-controlled memorizing activities (Murphy, 1979; Murphy & Puff,

1982; Pellegrino & Hubert, 1982). Bousfield's methods permitted many inferences about processes that mediate learning and recall. In general, subjects were presented a list of words or pictures in a random order in preparation for free recall. Organization of the materials at output were presumed to reflect processes that occurred during study. For example, if a word could be categorized according to semantic categories and recall was organized following these categories, it would be inferred that the learner engaged in intervening organizational processes. In many cases, however, subjects were presented lists that did not contain items that went together in any concensually meaningful way. Nonetheless, when subjects attempt to recall such lists several times, it is often the case that there is trial-to-trial regularities in recall (i.e., subjective organization).

Development of organizational strategies was studied with picture and word lists, usually ones containing items that could be categorized. The items were often selected using age-appropriate norms (e.g., Posnansky, 1978b; Bjorklund, Thompson, & Ornstein, 1983) with common items from familiar categories (e.g., animals, furniture, professions). Depending on the age of the subjects, three to 12 categories were used, each containing three to five items (Murphy & Puff, 1982). Subjective organization was most often measured in developmental studies using the adjusted ratio clustering (ARC) measure (Roenker, Thompson, & Brown, 1971) and the ratio of repetition measure (Bousfield & Bousfield, 1966). For both of these measures, values close to 1 represent almost perfect organization and 0 indicate random responding.

Bousfield, Esterson, and Whitmarsh's (1958) study on conceptual and perceptual clustering stimulated a flood of developmental work assessing factors that affect organization. Many of the early developmental studies on semantic grouping during free recall reported greater output clustering with increasing age. The inference was that older children organized input more in preparation for recall (e.g., Cole, Frankel, & Sharp, 1971; Moely et al., 1969; Neimark, Slotnick, & Ulrich, 1971). A frequently cited result is Moely et al.'s (1969) finding that only the 10- to 11-year-old children in that study organized at a level that was significantly greater than chance (index of organization = .6). This finding suggested that organizational strategies develop somewhat later than the passive rehearsal strategies reviewed in the last section, and probably even a little later than cumulative rehearsal. This makes sense since the discovery or creation of semantic relations between items seems like a more complex and demanding process than rehearsal.

On the other hand, even young children's recall contains a lot of organization when lists containing highly associated items are learned (Myers & Perlmutter, 1978; Rossi & Wittrock, 1971; Sodian et al., 1986). For example, Haynes and Kulhavy (1976, experiment 1) varied whether subjects studied a list composed of highly associated items or items that were not associated. There were clear age trends in recall and clustering with the low association lists. In contrast, there was a great deal of clustering at all age levels for lists composed of highly associated items. There are now many demonstrations that the degree of output organization systematically covaries with association and typicalness values of the item lists (Bjorklund, 1985; Corsale, 1981; Frankel & Rollins, 1985; Hasselhorn, 1986;

Schneider, 1986). Lange (1973, 1978) argued, based on this type of result, that the output cluster values are less an indicator of conscious strategic operations than the inter-item associations in the to-be-learned materials. A high degree of output organization for highly associated items probably occurs because recall of any particular item more or less automatically triggers recall of closely associated words. No consciously controlled strategic processes are necessary for this mechanism to work. Associative effects can occur at both encoding and retrieval:

The subject is "struck" by the organization he perceives, and he encodes and stores organizational units as a direct and automatic function of their perceived structure. Assuming the validity of this analysis, it is reasonable to point further than the recall organization we sometimes see in preschool and elementary school children. . . [organization] occurs through a series of involuntary actions that can operate at both the perceptual-encoding and retrieval phases of processes (Lange, 1978, p. 107).

A recent study by Schneider (1986) summarizes well the development of children's use of organizational strategies. Second- and fourth-grade children were given a recall task, with categorizable pictures serving as the stimulus materials. The pictures were movable (and thus, could be sorted into piles). Subjects were permitted to do anything that they wanted to learn these items. Four different types of lists were used in the study. One list contained items that were highly related to the category (Battig & Montague, 1969), with high interassociations (Marshall & Cofer, 1970; Palermo, Flamer, & Jenkins, 1964) between some of the items on the list (hereafter the High Related-High Associated list). Thus, the animals on this list included dog, cat, mouse, horse, cow, and pig. The second list was composed of items highly related to the category, but with low inter-item associations (High Related-Low Associated). The animals on this list included tiger, elephant, cow, pig, bear, and dog. The third list was composed of items that were weakly related to the category, although there were some high inter-item associations (Low Related-High Associated). Animals on that list were goat, deer, buffalo, hippopotamus, monkey, and lamb. The Low Related-Low Associated list included the animals beaver, rat, alligator, camel, squirrel, and giraffe.

In general, the fourth graders in the study employed much more categorical sorting during study than did the second graders. Not surprisingly, the fourth graders also clustered more at recall and recalled more than the second graders. In addition, there was a main effect on clustering for inter-item associativity at recall, with highly associated lists producing more clustering. Most importantly, there was a striking age by list associativity interaction in the clustering data, such that low associativity especially penalized younger compared to older subjects. In fact, the clustering of high and low associated lists was approximately equal for the older subjects in the study. Although the main effect for associativity and the age by associativity interaction were not significant in the recall data, there were strong trends in the recall data mirroring the clustering data. In general, there were significant correlations between clustering at study, clustering at recall, and recall.

What emerges from Schneider's study is a portrait of second graders who use organizational strategies much less than fourth graders. On the other hand, younger children's use of the clustering strategy can be evoked when the categories contain highly associated items.

Effects of Input Organization

A typical procedure in early studies of organization was to present children with lists composed of items from a few categories with the items in random order. In general, there was little evidence in these experiments that 6- to 8-year-olds used available categories to reorganize to-be-learned lists (e.g., Moely et al., 1969; Neimark et al., 1971).

These failures were followed by studies in which children were prompted to make use of potential organizational features through directions to sort to-be-learned materials into meaningful groups. In general, when children were asked to sort a list several times, the items were sorted into stable groups after a few trials—that is, sorting became consistent from trial to trial, with these sorts generally (although not perfectly) consistent with the categorical structures of the lists (Lange & Griffith, 1977; Lange & Jackson, 1974; Worden, 1975). A main hypothesis in these studies was that these subject-determined sorts would positively affect recall of material. Prompted sorting during study did in fact produce high clustering at output and improved recall (e.g., Lange & Griffith, 1977). In short, instructions to young grade-school children to sort during study seemed to overcome a production deficiency with respect to use of organizational information in lists (see also Black & Rollins, 1982; Frankel, Hagan, & Rollins, 1984; Moely et al., 1969; Schneider, 1985b; Schneider, Borkowski, Kurtz, & Kerwin, 1986).

Lange (1978) proposed two possible explanations for young children's failures to organize their free recall when left to their own devices to learn potentially categorizable lists. One possibility was input failure, or the failure to group stimulus materials clearly and stably during encoding. The other involved failures during the retrieval phase to make use of groupings that were constructed at encoding. Lange's own work (Lange & Griffith, 1977) favored the former interpretation, since he obtained strong covariation between children's input organization and their recall.

The two alternative explanations proposed by Lange could be evaluated most unambiguously by considering actual sorting behaviors generated during study and the relationships between organization of sorts during study and organization of recall. Neimark, Ulrich, and Slotnick (1971) observed very early that young grade-school children often failed to sort classifiable materials according to semantic categories and that there was often poor concordance between the spontaneous organization of young grade-school children's sorting during study and the organization of their subsequent recall. Unfortunately, the analyses in this early work do not permit detailed description of the relationship between sorting and recall organizations.

Later research was more analytical. Consider Kee and Bell's (1981) study that included subjects from grades 2 and 6 as well as university students. They measured the ARC cluster values for both encoding and recall. The oldest subjects in the study had high ARC cluster scores at both input and output. In contrast, the grade-2 and grade-6 subjects had low ARC scores during input, but higher ones at output (a finding generally consistent with the results reported by Neimark et al., 1971). Kee and Bell's (1981) study also included an instructional component. When the child subjects were instructed to sort into experimenter-specified categories during encoding, their ARC scores at encoding and output were high. Instructions to use categories at testing had a much less pronounced effect on organization than did the study instruction. The study instruction generally improved the children's recall performance, especially at the grade-2 level. Kee and Bell (1981) concluded that variations in organizational behaviors during encoding and not during testing produced differences in memory performance in the sort-recall task. Kee and Bell's (1981) conclusion has been supported in more recent studies that used multiple regression procedures to estimate effects of organization at input and organization at output on memory performances in children of various ages (Black & Rollins, 1982; Weinert, Knopf, and Körkel, 1983; Schneider, 1985b, 1986; Schneider et al., 1986).

Thus far, the discussion has focused on lists that were organizable along taxonomic lines. There are other potential dimensions to organize input, however. In addition, there have been proposals over the years that although use of taxonomic criteria might be a classification criterion that would be used by older children and adults, younger subjects might prefer to group items using other standards. The next subsection takes up this hypothesis in some detail.

Developmental Changes in Classification Styles

The assumption that memory processes in young children are determined by the available knowledge base goes back to Piaget (1970; Piaget & Inhelder, 1973). In its most stringent form, Piaget argued that preschool children could not profit from the provision of taxonomical organization since categorical knowledge is not available during the preoperational stage. A more lenient version of this hypothesis is that younger children have organizational preferences, such that perceptual or functional stimulus dimensions are more likely to be noticed by preschoolers, and thus, can be used more meaningfully than taxonomic attributes (Markman & Callanan, 1984; Worden, 1976). A more specific hypothesis that follows from this general position is that preschoolers and kindergarten children should tend to categorize objects or pictures by color or functional attributes (e.g., hammer with nails) rather than regarding taxonomic relationships.

There is experimental evidence relevant to both the strict and more lenient versions of the "developmental shift" hypothesis. It was apparent from Melkman et al., (1981) and Perlmutter and Ricks (1979) that 3- and 4-year-olds considered perceptual as well as conceptual stimulus dimensions during sorting (see also Kobasigawa & Middleton, 1972; Moely, 1977). Categories seem to figure more prominently in children's sorting, however, when they know that they are sorting in preparation for a memory task (Sodian et al., 1986). In addition, categorical prompting at recall is more efficient than color prompting even for very young children (Melkman et al., 1981; Sodian et al., 1986). Data generated in sorting tasks certainly do not seem consistent with the stringent version of the knowledge hypothesis.

Investigations of the "syntagmatic-paradigmatic shift" (i.e., children prefer to group objects on the basis of functional relatedness before they organize using taxonomic criteria) are relevant to the lenient version of the hypothesis. Consistent with this hypothesis, Denney and Ziobrowski (1972) reported that first graders preferred to organize sorts using functional attributes (e.g., grouping knife and cake together because a knife can cut a cake) in contrast to categorical dimensions (sorting knife with other instruments and cake with other foods) used by adults. Worden (1976) compared sorting and recall by second and fifth graders. She included a condition in which children were permitted to sort any way that they wished, as well as conditions in which sorting was taxonomically constrained and functionally constrained. Worden believed that there would be a qualitative shift between second and fifth grade from preference for functional to taxonomical organization. Her results, however, were not consistent with this position. At both age levels, subjects who sorted following their own preferences recalled more material than subjects who sorted into experimenter-determined categories. At both age levels, spontaneous sorts reflected preference for functional (thematic) grouping compared to taxonomic organization. Siaw (1984) provided data consistent with Worden (1976), in that his subjects did not benefit from instructions to sort into categories. Nonetheless, Siaw did not observe much use of thematic sorting at either the 7- or 10-year-old levels in his study, with use of taxonomic organization in free sorts increasing with age. Other results are also antagonistic to the syntagmatic-paradigmatic shift hypothesis (Bjorklund, 1976; Cox & Paris, 1976; Lange & Jackson, 1974). For example, Bjorklund (1976) was able to show in a series of experiments that kindergarten, third-grade, and sixth-grade children could identify more taxonomic than thematic categories prior to recall. In short, although there are some differences between studies in the conclusion that is reached about children's preference (i.e., thematic versus taxonomic, with most of the data favoring taxonomic), there is little evidence within these experiments for a developmental shift from thematic to taxonomic.

An alternative hypothesis to explain apparent developmental differences in organization is that young children do organize, but do so using categories that are consistent with their knowledge of the world rather than the taxonomic knowledge of adults. Rosch (1973, 1975; Mervis & Rosch, 1981) provided data supporting the hypothesis that semantic categories in younger children are at first represented by prototypical examples. Given that the typical list in sort-recall experiments is composed of both prototypic and nonprototypic exemplars, there is the possibility that young children's failure to use categorization may be tied to their lack of knowledge of noncentral category members.

This type of thinking stimulated research on recall in which children's knowledge of category members was examined as a possible determinant of categorization strategy use. Chechile and Richman (1982) and Richman, Nida, and Pitman (1976) found, for example, that the usual age differences in recall of categorizable lists could be reduced by constructing lists that were equally meaningful to the various ages of children, with meaningfulness of items determined through use of age-specific norms rather than adult meaningfulness norms. In fact, when lists are composed of material that is more meaningful to children than adults, it is possible to reverse the usual age-recall relationship. For instance, Lindberg (1980) reported that the third graders in his sample remembered significantly more items than college students and had higher cluster values when the items were extremely salient and meaningful for the younger subjects compared to the older ones. This result is similar to Chi's (1978) observation that child chess experts remember meaningful chess positions better than do adult chess novices. In addition to Haynes and Kulhavy's (1976) study that was taken up earlier, Bjorklund and Thompson (1983) demonstrated that the ease with which categorical relations could be identified directly influenced recall organization and level in first, third, and sixth graders. Nonetheless, because retrieval cues were provided by both Haynes and Kulhavy (1976) and Bjorklund and Thompson (1983), it was difficult to conclude based on their data that meaningfulness necessarily affected children's encoding (i.e., most of the effect could have been due to the influence of retrieval cue). Rabinowitz (1984) tackled this problem through the addition of a "cue neutral" experimental condition. Groups of second and fifth graders were better able to organize and recall more prototypic than category-nontypic items when no retrieval cues were present. The influence of meaningfulness of organization on recall seemed to be clear in this study.

The role of associative and categorical processes on children's memory performance have been analyzed especially carefully by David Bjorklund and his associates (Bjorklund, 1985, 1987; Bjorklund & de Marchena, 1984; Bjorklund & Jacobs, 1985; Bjorklund & Thompson, 1983; Bjorklund et al., 1983). Their basic hypothesis was that there was a developmental shift in list learning during the grade-school years that was mediated by changes in the knowledge base. This shift is from use of salient associative relationships during encoding to the use of taxonomic categories, a shift mediated by changes in the organization of children's semantic memory rather than increased use of conscious organizational strategies. A variety of evidence supports this hypothesis. In a study of the sort-recall task, Bjorklund and de Marchena (1984) reported that younger children (first graders) relied primarily on associative grouping principles to organize their sorting and continued to use this strategy even when the list structure permitted several ways to exploit category cues. In contrast, fourth and sixth graders used taxonomic information alone. Bjorklund and de Marchena concluded that the greater-than-chance clustering values in the younger children's recall were not due to the processing of taxonomic-conceptual relationships, but rather were caused by the inter-item associativity of the material. Consistent with Lange's (1973, 1978) hypothesis, it seemed that associative-organizational processes occur relatively automatically.

Other studies provide additional support for Lange's position. Frankel and Rollins (1982) discovered, for example, that in recalling material that could be semantically categorized, young children produced categorizable material in pairs, with older subjects remembering longer "strings" per category. Frankel and Rollins argued that this pattern of performance indicated that younger children's internal organization of categorizable information is more associative than categorical. A more direct test of the associativity theory is possible when children learn lists that vary systematically in their item prototypicality (high vs. low) and their inter-item associativities (high vs. low). Using such lists, Frankel and Rollins (1985) were able to show clearly that high cluster values occurred with kindergarten children only when both inter-item associativity and prototypicality was high. High clustering was found with older children regardless of list structure. Similar effects of inter-item associativity on organization of item sets were found by Schneider (1986) in German second graders.

Bjorklund and Jacobs (1985) constructed lists of categorizable items, some of which were highly associated with the category items and others of which were low category associations. Words that were recalled contiguously could be classified according to whether they (1) belonged to different categories (e.g., dog-apple) and (2) were highly associated (dog-cat) or poorly associated (dog-tiger) category members. Subjects at all grade levels in the study (third, fifth, seventh, and ninth graders) had lower latency for contiguous recall of highly associated items in a category than for contiguous recall of low associated category members. There were significant age differences in contiguous recall latencies of low associates. Only the two oldest groups of children were able to process these more quickly than words from different categories. These results are quite compatible with those obtained by Frankel and Rollins (1985) and Schneider (1986) and can be interpreted to mean that younger children benefit little from categorical information when inter-item associations between items are low.

Most of the data reviewed in this subsection support the position that children's systematic application of categorical information in the recall of word lists clearly covaries with the familiarity of the stimulus material (especially Bjorklund & Thompson, 1983; Corsale, 1981; Hasselhorn, 1986; Rabinowitz, 1984; Schneider, 1986). Hasselhorn (1986), who made use of latent variables path analysis (Lohmöller, 1984), provided additional support for this conclusion. He examined relationships between the quality of prior knowledge, organizational behavior at recall, and memory performance. The quality of grade-4 children's prior knowledge directly influenced both the organization and level of recall.

Are developmental improvements in recall of categorizable lists due only to changes in the child's knowledge base (see Chapter 4 for discussion of knowledge base effects), or do developmental increases in use of intentional organizational strategies account for at least some of the memory improvement? Bjorklund (1985) took a clear stand, favoring the position that most of the improvement in memory during the grade-school years at least is tied to changes in the child's knowledge base:

I dispute this position [strategy development hypothesis], arguing instead that most of the age changes in the organization of children's recall are not strategic, but rather can be attributed to developmental changes in the structure and content of children's conceptual representation. Organization in memory does become strategic, I believe, sometime during adolescence, resulting in a qualitatively different type of memory functioning. However, I argue that the regular improvements observed in memory organization over the course of the preschool and elementary school years can most parsimoniously be attributed to developmental differences in the structure of semantic memory and the ease with which certain types of semantic relationships can be activated (p. 103).

One of Bjorklund's (1985) main assumptions was that with increasing age, the inter-item relationships in semantic memory become more elaborate and could be activated relatively automatically. He presumed, based on Case et al., (1982), that with development the functional mental space becomes larger, in part because of increasingly automatic access of relevant knowledge. With increases in efficiency of knowledge access, and hence increases in functional capacity, older children can deal with to-be-learned material at a more abstract level (i.e., taxonomically). Eventually, access to higher order categorical information also become very automatic. At that point (sometime in adolescence), there is excess capacity that could be used in the service of strategies.

Every aspect of Bjorklund's (1985) position was extreme (cf., Rabinowitz, 1984). Developmental increases during childhood in use of categorical relations were interpreted solely as a function of the knowledge base. Semantic relationships that could mediate the learning of children were activated unconsciously. No hint of intentionality was apparent until adolescence. Bjorklund contended that conscious strategies, when they eventually did occur, were in fact stimulated by the knowledge base. He argued that at some point subjects will notice the cluster structure of their output and in turn recognize the gains associated with clustering. This would stimulate the 13- to 15-year-old children to use clustering in the future.

Many of Bjorklund's (1985) claims were speculative, although there are data that support his portrait of memory development in part. For example, at least for free recall and sort-recall tasks, there is evidence that automatic, associative use of semantic relationships occurs (Lange, 1973, 1978). Nonetheless, this does not imply that intentional strategic behavior does not occur, a point raised by many critics (Hasselhorn, 1986; Ornstein & Naus, 1985; Ornstein et al., in press; Schneider, 1986; Zembar & Naus, 1985a). In fact, there was plenty of reason to doubt the conclusion that conscious use of organizational strategies does not occur until adolescence.

Studies that examined organization at input rather than at output (Bjorklund's focus) produced data suggesting more use of strategies than Bjorklund's (1985) framework permitted (Ornstein et al., in press; Schneider, 1986). Investigators studying input assumed that intentional memorization processes during encoding could be presumed when spontaneous sortings by categories or other efficient learning processes were observed at study. Thus, Schneider (1986) recorded sorting and other memorization activities used by second and fourth graders. One of the most interesting aspects of the data was that the children who used sorting behaviors were also the ones who engaged in other strategic activities like rehearsal and self-testing. One possible conclusion suggested by this outcome was that the children who sorted realized that sorting would positively affect memory. This hypothesis was evaluated by Schneider (1986) by examining children's metacognition about strategies. If sorting behaviors at study are only a side effect of an increasingly elaborate knowledge base, then knowledge of taxonomic sorting as a strategy should show no substantial relationship to sorting during study. On the other hand, correlation between strategy metamemory and sorting would be expected if children were engaging in intentional sorting in the service of a memory goal. Although there does not seem to be a correlation between strategy metamemory and sorting with 7- to 8-year-old children (Schneider, 1985b, 1986; Weinert et al., 1984), there are consistently significant correlations (averaging between .3 and .4) among third and fourth graders (Andreassen & Waters, 1984; Hasselhorn, 1986; Schneider, 1985b, 1986). This pattern of correlations is consistent with the hypothesis that intentional use of organizational strategies as mediators of sort-recall tasks develops during the grade-school years.

An additional important point that became obvious in Schneider's investigations was that it is very difficult to conclude a lack of strategy knowledge by a subject simply because the child fails to evidence sorting during study. Consider the study behaviors and comments of a second grader (Schneider, 1986), a subject who made no obvious attempt to sort a list of low prototypic and low associated items:

They're all animals, clothes, furniture, and things to drive. Probably it helps if I put the animals and other things together that belong together. But these here? I don't know. Maybe it's just as good if I try to remember where each picture was located?

This child clearly knew more about strategic use of categorization than indicated by input or output organization. What this case suggests is that effective use of categorization as a strategy depends on a well-developed knowledge base that includes remote associations and nonprototypic category members.

It seems not to be very sensible to conclude that memory development boils down either to development of semantic knowledge or development of intentionally deployed strategies. The literature reviewed here suggests that realistic models of memory development during preschool and the grade-school years should consider both the nonstrategic knowledge base and use of memory strategies (Ornstein & Naus, 1985; Ornstein et al., in press; Rabinowitz & Chi, 1987; Zembar & Naus, 1985a, 1985b). In particular, there is a lot of evidence consistent with the developmental portrait of memory development suggested by Ornstein and Naus (1985). They argued that younger children's attempts at sort-recall tasks are stimulus driven in that strong associative inter-item relations automatically induce some semantic encoding. Ornstein et al. (in press) assume further that during grade school, children experience enough memory tasks to discover strategic information, like the utility of exploiting categorical and associative relations between items. These observations fuel attempts to organize to-be-learned materials even when inter-item associations are not salient (Best & Ornstein, 1986). Efficient use of organization depends on the elaborateness of the available knowledge base. Thus, Ornstein and his associates emphasize the relevance of intentional and automatic factors on memory performance.

We note in closing this subsection that even Bjorklund is now accepting that both intentional and automatic factors are important in memory development (Bjorklund & Muir, 1988). It is notable that this most recent paper by Bjorklund cites prominently many of the studies of strategy development that are included here, including those that suggest that strategy use occurs even in very young children. Bjorklund and Muir develop in detail potential theoretical relationships between strategies and the knowledge base. Although first attempts have been made at elucidating such knowledge by strategy interactions (e.g., Zembar & Naus, 1985a, 1985b), much more research is needed on this problem. For instance, there have been few comparisons of normal and learning-disabled children. The work that has been done (Ceci, 1983, 1984; Ceci & Howe, 1982) has lead to better understanding of the nature of deficits in learning-disabled children in terms of their use of automatic and intentional processes. We suspect that Bjorklund and Muir's chapter will be an important source of hypotheses for future work relating automatic to intentional processes.

Summary

In general, the development of organizational strategies resembles the development of rehearsal strategies, although rehearsal is an earlier acquisition — production deficiencies are obtained during sort-recall tasks with low prototypical and low associated materials well after cumulative rehearsal skills are used consistently and profitably.

One methodological conclusion is especially striking. The use of output organization as a sole indicator of strategic behavior is generally misleading. Output organization reflects more characteristics of the to-be-learned materials than intentional strategic processes. The merit of the work done by David Bjorklund and Frankel and Rollins (1985) is that they demonstrated that material parameters like category prototypicality or inter-item associativity can play a role in determining recall. These variables greatly influence both input and output organization. Sometimes the organization of input is so striking that even very young children use strategies like sorting at input. This is not intentional study behavior.

Determining whether input behaviors are intentional requires additional assessments that can be related to the memorizing behaviors. In addition to observing whether sorting occurs, use of other strategies should also be assessed and the subjects should be questioned about their knowledge of sorting as a strategy and its effects on memory. If sorting is one of several strategies that a child is attempting to use, and if the child reports that sorting does increase recall, and if the child states that sorting is being used to prepare for the test, it seems fair to conclude that sorting is being used intentionally (along with other strategies) in the service of memory.

We believe that the evidence considered as a whole suggests that both the increased knowledge base and the gradual development of flexible and intentionally used organizational strategies contribute to developmental improvements in learning of categorizable lists. Categorization strategies are extremely interesting because they depend on a well-developed knowledge base for their efficient execution (i.e., one cannot categorize if one does not have knowledge of the relevant categories). Interactions between strategy use and the knowledge base will be considered further in Chapters 4 and 6.

Development of Retrieval Strategies

Although rehearsal and organization have been described as encoding strategies, their effects become apparent during retrieval (Flavell, 1985; Kail, 1984). Sometimes children fail to recall all that they have encoded, however. On those occasions, it is sometimes possible to increase the probability of recall through strategic efforts at the time of testing, through the use of retrieval procedures.

Some anecdotal evidence from Schneider (1986) makes clear the importance of retrieval strategies for recall. Two fourth graders attracted some attention during the sort-recall task described earlier because both of them very purposely sorted the 24 to-be-learned pictures into the four categories represented on the list. These two subjects were not similar at all, however, in how they went about trying to recall the items on the test. One seemed to generate test answers in a random order, an observation supported by very low clustering in the recall data. This child's memory performance was slightly below average for grade-4 subjects. In contrast, the commentary made by the other child implicated a more sophisticated retrieval strategy. He first recalled the four category names and thought about how six items had to be remembered for each one. He began recall with one category and shifted categories only after all six items were recalled. His memory test performance was perfect. Since the subjects did not differ in intelligence or memory span or in any other obvious way, it seems likely that the difference in their memory performances was due to their use of different approaches to retrieval.

In this section we consider in detail whether there are age differences in the use of retrieval strategies, and if so, whether development of retrieval skills improves memory performance. Kobasigawa (1977) analyzed in detail potential deficiencies in children's retrieval: (1) Children can fail to perceive that internal or external memory cues are potential memory aids; (2) they may lack strategies for locating target information in memory; (3) they may not have enough experience with the problem to evaluate when the search process should be considered finished.

There are many studies of the first potential deficiency cited by Kobasigawa, especially with respect to recognition and use of external memory aids. For instance, Kobasigawa (1974) presented lists of categorizable items to 6- to 11-year-olds to learn for subsequent free recall. He also provided picture cards to the children during learning and recall. Each picture represented one of the categories on the test (i.e., a picture of a zoo for zoo animals). Six-year-olds generally did not use these retrieval cues at testing, but 8- to 11-year-olds used the cues more systematically. Developmental improvements in recall were interpreted by Kobasigawa (1974, 1977) to mean that there was a developmental difference in efficient use of retrieval cues.

Retrieval deficits in grade-school children are also evident with respect to use of internal cues in the form of category names. An early example was provided by Scribner and Cole (1972). Second, fourth, and sixth graders were presented categorizable words in a random order. As in Kobasigawa (1974), the subjects were aware of the category names during learning and recall. The subjects in the control condition were simply instructed to recall the items given the category cues. In contrast, subjects in the experimental condition had to recall all the items from one category before they were allowed to proceed to the next category (constrained recall). The constrained recall condition evoked exactly the sophisticated behavior used by the retrieval-talented fourth grader in the Schneider (1986) study (discussed earlier), and produced memory performance that was significantly better than occurred in the cued recall condition. Moreover, this held at all age levels. None of the children transferred the constrained strategy, however, when given a transfer list consisting of to-be-learned-and-recalled items from new categories. Generally comparable results were reported by Lange (1973) whose procedure was similar except that he used pictures rather than verbal materials and used the same categories for the transfer task.

How should these results be interpreted? Methodological problems in these studies preclude a definitive conclusion. First, including a free recall condition without retrieval cues would have improved both studies. Such a condition would have made it possible to estimate better the age-specific effect of cue presentation, particularly during the transfer phase. In addition, nothing was known about how subjects behaved during the encoding phase. Age-correlated differences could be due to the older subjects already having created better conditions for retrieval, that is, by organizing the learning material into categories during the encoding phase. Finally, the to-be-remembered lists were presented several times in succession in these studies, with items presented in a random order on each trial. Such a design increases the probability of encoding variability (Waters & McAlaster, 1983; Waters & Waters, 1976, 1979), since subjects encounter each item in the encoding context and then again in a subject-determined retrieval context (i.e., the item is retrieved with other items with the order of retrieved items often quite different than the order at encoding). Great encoding variability affects younger children more negatively than older children, so that these experiments may have provided poorer conditions for effective learning by younger compared to older children. In short, it is difficult to differentiate between the quality of encoding and retrieval processes in the experiments performed by Kobasigawa (1974), Lange (1973), and Scribner and Cole (1972), although all of the studies suggest retrieval deficiencies in young children.

One solution to this problem is to minimize age-correlated differences in encoding strategies, for example, by having the items sorted exactly according to their taxonomic groups during the learning phase. A number of studies (Ceci & Howe, 1978a; Ceci et al., 1980; Williams & Goulet, 1975; Worden, 1974) have used such a procedure. The study by Ceci and Howe (1978a) is especially relevant. They employed to-be-learned lists that could be organized thematically and taxonomically and determined that their 4-, 7-, and 10-year-old subjects could organize the stimuli perfectly in both modalities. A cued-recall test given immediately following sorting employed taxonomic cues for half of the subjects at each age level and thematic cues for the remaining subjects. Free recall was measured one day later. Table 3.1 summarizes the main results.

First of all, note that cued recall varied little as a function of developmental level, suggesting that about the same number of items was available in memory for each of the age groups. The free recall results were quite different. Older children spontaneously generated many of the taxonomic and thematic cues and used them to mediate free recall, but younger children did not do so. A "modal switching index" was calculated (also shown in Table 3.1) to index the degree to which subjects switched between taxonomic and thematic modalities during free recall. Although

TABLE 3.1. Mean numbers of pictures cue recalled and free recalled along with the proportion of mode switching as a function of age.*

Age (yr)	Cued recall	Free recall	Proportional amount of modal switching
4	20.15	12.25	.14
7	21.20	16.75	.29
10	21.79	18.50	.66

*Data from Ceci & Howe, 1978a.

the 10-year-olds made such a shift for 66% of all possible cases, younger children did less switching. Within each age level there was a significant positive relationship between this index and the total number of items recalled. Additional analyses led Ceci and Howe (1978a) to conclude that the age differences in free recall were due primarily to use of more flexible retrieval strategies by the older children (see also Hasher & Clifton, 1974) rather than to several alternative interpretations (ones too complicated to be considered here).

Age differences in the flexibility of retrieval strategies were also demonstrated by Salatas and Flavell (1976a). They attempted to control the developmental differences in encoding strategies by having the subjects (6- and 9-year-olds, college students) learn all items to a high level of performance – to the point that they could perfectly recall all list items (all of which could be categorized) during constrained recall (i.e., with category cues provided and exhaustive recall of category members required). At the end of this phase, the subjects were asked indirect retrieval questions that required searching through the items using dimensions other than the categories specified during study. For instance, one question was, "Which items are small enough to be put in this carton (box)?" An optimal retrieval plan for this situation consists of the following: (1) Recall the category names used during encoding; (2) search in each of these categories exhaustively; (3) evaluate each item in each category to see if it meets the requirements mentioned in the question; (4) tell the selected items to the experimenter.

Given the complicated nature of the optimal retrieval strategy, it is not surprising that only a few of the school children used it. Most of the college students, however, did retrieve using the optimal approach. For another example of the development of a complex retrieval heuristic, see Keniston and Flavell (1979).

Although precautions were taken in studies like Ceci and Howe (1978a) and Salatas and Flavell (1976a) to minimize the older children's encoding advantages, some encoding differences may have remained that favored the older compared to the younger children (Sophian & Hagen, 1978). Hall, Murphy, Humphreys, and Wilson (1979) attempted to eliminate further the influence of developmental differences of during-the-experiment learning processes. They used items from different semantic categories that had comparable associativity values for second and fifth graders. In order to preclude the older children's encoding advantages, the analyses focused on recall of the items in the middle of the list rather than at the beginning or the end (i.e., so that primacy and recency effects that might occur as a function of encoding strategies could be eliminated). These middle-list items were free recalled to the same degree by both the younger and older children in the sample. The most important results were on a cued recall test that followed free recall. Highly associated cues produced better memory at both age levels. Fifth graders as a whole remembered more cued items than second graders. A comparison of the cued recall probabilities to the cue-word associative strength values revealed an especially interesting age difference. The cued recall probabilities were significantly higher than associative probabilities at the grade 5 level, but not at the grade 2 level. Hall et al. (1979) concluded that intentional, strategic retrieval operations could only be inferred for the older children. Younger children's cued recall reflected associative processes more than efficient retrieval.

We conclude that there are developmental differences in the efficient use of retrieval strategies. The attempts to isolate retrieval that were summarized in this section consistently revealed clear trends in the development of efficient retrieval processes from 4 to 12 years of age. The spontaneous application of simple retrieval strategies such as the use of external associative cues can be observed in kindergarten or early grade-school years. Really complex retrieval strategies, such as reorganization of the stored information combined with exhaustive search and thorough evaluation (e.g., Salatas & Flavell, 1976a) does not enter the strategic repertoire until the late grade-school or adolescent years. In general, older children are much better than younger children at employing flexible and exhaustive search procedures. That encoding and retrieval processes cannot be studied independently makes it difficult to determine the proportion of memory due to use of encoding compared to retrieval heuristics, although this problem is being tackled using some ingenious methodologies, ones reviewed briefly in the next section.

Encoding Versus Retrieval Strategies as Determinants of Memory Development

The Descriptions Model

How should an experiment be designed in order to determine the interaction between encoding and retrieval processes and their effects on recall? A balanced factorial design would be preferred by many, where subjects of various age groups are assigned to conditions that vary systematically with respect to the use of encoding and retrieval strategies. Emmerich and Ackerman (1978) used this approach with first and fifth graders as well as college students. At encoding, the to-be-learned items were either presented randomly, blocked into categories, or subjects sorted them into categories. Testing involved either free recall, categorically cued recall, or categorically constrained cued recall (i.e., all items from a category had to be recalled before moving to another category).

The encoding and retrieval factors influenced recall performance independently and in interaction. Both factors seemed to contribute to age-related performance improvement. That the independent effect of encoding on children's performance was quite modest compared to the effect of retrieval, led Emmerich and Ackerman to conclude that encoding processes are only efficient inasmuch as they support the generation of effective retrieval strategies.

Brian Ackerman has recently taken a different approach to the study of encoding-retrieval interactions, generating data relevant to a "descriptions" model (Ackerman, 1987; Norman & Bobrow, 1979). Ackerman assumes that encoding of stimulus information depends on the context in which the information is encountered, and that the representation of an event (description) that is constructed reflects only a subset of the information in the original stimulus, a subset determined by biasing cues that are present during encoding. The adequacy of a representational description is a function of whether it contains functionally important properties of the stimulus that permit adequate retrieval.

Consider the pair *knife/axe*. Suppose that when these items are presented at study, subjects are asked a categorical question, "Are these weapons?" Presumably that biases information that is stored about these objects, such that the encoding of knife and axe includes information about their weapon status. At testing, subjects would be presented *knife* and be required to recall *axe*. Recall of *axe* should be increased if the retrieval context biases the subjects toward cues that were encoded at study. Thus, posing the question about weapons at retrieval might be expected to facilitate recall of axe. Posing a question that focussed on some other attribute (e.g., "Is this a kitchen utensil?) would be expected, if anything, to reduce the likelihood of recalling axe since the subject would be oriented away from cues that were salient at original encoding.

Ackerman and his colleagues (1982, 1983, 1984; 1985a, 1985b, 1985c, 1985d, 1985e; 1986a, 1986b; Ackerman & Hess, 1982; Ackerman & Rathburn, 1984; Ackerman & Rust-Kahl, 1982) have studied in detail the dependency of children and adults on identical study and retrieval environments. One tactic has been to vary the types of questions asked at encoding and retrieval (e.g., either identical ones at study and testing or different ones). Are there developmental differences in the need for compatible encoding and retrieval environments? In general, stimulus recall is lower following different questions than following same questions. Ackerman calculated the difference in recall performance for both types of orientation questions in order to determine the degree of performance decrease (encoding penalty shift) resulting from the presentation of incompatible cues. The encoding penalty decreased with increasing age, suggesting that the recall performance of younger children is more strongly dependent on compatible study and testing cues.

Ackerman has obtained other developmental interactions that are interesting as well. For instance, when children were given categorical orientation questions at encoding and retrieval (i.e., there was compatibility), there was a developmental increase in recall. This suggested that second graders may have difficulty with categorical orientation questions. If so, perhaps younger children would do better with more specific questions that did not require evaluation of category membership, but instead tapped relationships that are salient to young children (e.g., functional relationships). For instance, would asking a question like, "Could a prince use this object to fight his enemies?" (a specific, function question) be more helpful than asking, "Is this a kitchen utensil?" (a categorical question)? Ackerman (1985b) determined that even though there are age-correlated differences in recall given compatible categorical questions, there are none with more specific compatible questions. Young children could competently employ compatible specific retrieval cues.

Ackerman and his colleagues (1983; Ackerman & Hess, 1982; especially Ackerman & Rathburn, 1984) evaluated one possible explanation of why same-categorical questions produce lower recall with younger compared to older children. Perhaps categorization questions do not permit discrimination of category members that are stored in memory? If so, Ackerman and Rathburn reasoned that compatible questions about smaller categories should have a larger effect with young grade-school children than compatible questions about large categories. After all larger category questions specify many more possibilities that must be considered and discriminated from the correct answer than do smaller category questions. Ackerman and Rathburn presented pairs to second graders, fourth graders, and college students (e.g., knife/axe). The manipulations relevant to the present discussion were that pairs (a) were accompanied either by large category questions (Are these weapons?) or small category questions (Are these small hand weapons?) at acquisition and (b) were accompanied by either large category, small category, or specific questions (Might a prince use these to slash his enemies?) at retrieval. The results supported the conclusion that part of the problem with large category questions is related to discriminability in that same small category questions produced better recall than large same-category questions. Nonetheless, there was no support for the hypothesis that this could account for developmental differences in the effectiveness of large category questions in that there was a main effect for same small versus same large category questions that was not qualified by an age by category size interaction.

A strength of Ackerman's approach is that there is a serious search for encoding by retrieval interactions. That there are generally consistent advantages for same compared to different questions is consistent with the conclusion that orienting activities at encoding produces a trace that is best retrieved by comparable orienting cues at recall. That younger children are more dependent on compatible encoding and retrieval cues is supportive of the general conclusion in the last section that there are developmental improvements in children's retrieval skills. In closing this discussion of Ackerman's work, we emphasize that we only scratched the surface of his theory and data (see Ackerman, 1987, for more complete details), which we view as extremely impressive evidence that the relationships between encoding and retrieval can be tapped and studied developmentally.

Mathematical Modeling Approaches

Those who subscribe to mathematical modeling approaches for the analysis of encoding and retrieval make minimum theoretical assumptions about the nature of these processes. Their emphasis is on the analyses of probability parameters that describe learning and retention (e.g., the probability of an item being stored on a first trial, the probability of an item being stored on any trial after the first trial, probability of consistently recalling an item given that it was recalled on the first trial). In particular, study and comparison of these parameters should permit more complete description of learning and the pinpointing of effects produced by various manipulations.

Three different groups have proposed mathematical models for separating encoding and retrieval processes. The approaches all build on Markovian probability models and use memory tasks where the to-be-learned material is presented over a number of trials. These three models can be differentiated in that they seem to emphasize different aspects of memory. Following Brainerd's (1985a) classification, we refer to them as short-term memory, long-term memory, and retention models.

Chechile and Meyer's (1976) model was designed to answer questions about short-term memory. The main question was whether forgetting in short-term memory was due to the loss of traces that had been encoded or failures to retrieve traces that remained available (perhaps retrieval failures mediated by retroactive or proactive inhibition). Chechile and Meyer generally assumed that traces were either encoded or they were not, with a parameter θ_s that specified whether items were stored. In a similar manner, retrieval was conceived of as either adequate or inadequate and the parameter θ_r specified the probability across several trials that memory traces that were stored could be recalled. The probability of forgetting (θ_f) can be determined in a straightforward fashion given these two parameters as $1 - \theta_s \theta_r$.

Chechile and Meyers (1976) used an experimental paradigm consisting of a mixture of recall and recognition tasks. It was a modified version of the Brown-Peterson distractor task. Each trial consisted of a subspan recall test and two recognition tests. During the recognition test subjects judged confidence in their recognition decision on a 3-point scale. The data yielded a total of 11 independent empirical probabilities (for details, Brainerd, 1985a, 1985b; Chechile & Meyers, 1976).

Chechile, Richman, Topinka, and Ehrensbeck (1981) completed the first developmental study using this approach. First and sixth graders and college students learned 18 different sets of five items over the course of five trials. It was a serial probe task where five hidden pictures were turned over one after the other, each for approximately half a second, and then returned to their original position. A short distractor task followed the presentations, with recall and recognition subsequently assessed. Recall consisted of responding to the question, "What was here?" as the experimenter pointed to each location. Recognition required responding to the question, "Was this picture here?"

At all age levels, storage proved easier as reflected by mean values of the storage and retrieval parameters (i.e., $\theta_s > \theta_r$). Particularly important from a developmental point of view, the value of the forgetting parameter increased between the first and sixth-grade levels, but with no additional improvement between sixth grade and the undergraduate level. The retrieval parameter, however, increased consistently across the three age groups. Chechile et al. (1981) concluded that storage and retrieval processes develop at different rates. The storage processes are at a relatively high level early and seem to stabilize in late childhood. In contrast, young children evidence low levels of retrieval with improvement into adulthood.

A follow-up study by Chechile and Richman (1982) with kindergarten and second-grade children was conducted to determine the influence of the meaningfulness of materials on encoding and retrieval. The children were presented nine-item (supraspan) lists, again with both recall and recognition assessed. Two groups of second graders served in the study, one that learned exactly the same materials as the kindergarten subjects and another who received a different set of items. This different list was constructed by selecting items that were as meaningful to second graders as were the items on the kindergarten list to kindergarten children. The most important result was that when meaning was controlled, there were no recall differences as a function of developmental level. Chechile and Richman interpreted this result in terms of their "hardware invariance" hypothesis. They believed that these data supported the position that many age differences in short-term memory performance are mediated by developmental changes in the knowledge base.

In contrast to the focus on short-term recall in Chechile and Richman's work, Brainerd and his colleagues (Brainerd, 1982; Brainerd & Howe, 1982; Brainerd, Howe, & Desrochers, 1982; Brainerd, Howe, & Kingma, 1982; Brainerd, Howe, Kingma, & Brainerd, 1984) have studied long-term memory. Much of their developmental work has been based on a Markovian model first used by Greeno (1968, 1970; Greeno, James, Da Polito, & Polson, 1978) to measure encoding and retrieval processes. The model has the advantage that it can be used for a variety of list-learning tasks where recall is measured (e.g., free recall, cued recall, paired-associate learning, serial recall). It assumes two discrete phases in the learning process that can be characterized by the transition between three states. There is an initial "unlearned" state (U), where only errors occur. The intermediate partially learned state (P) is where errors (substate E) and successes (substate C) can occur. Only success occurs in the final, learned (L) state. It is assumed that transitions between these states occur in discrete (all-or-none) jumps. Brainerd's model has 11 independent parameters described in Table 3.2. In general, these parameters are distinguished by stage of learning that they refer to, with some indexing transitions from one stage to the next. Thus, the transition from U to P is due to the encoding of a trace in long-term memory. Here, the three parameters a', a, and f are relevant. Following initial storage, the trace may not be readily retrievable. Thus, there is a mixture of recall successes and failures. The transition from stage P to L is characterized psychologically as retrieval learning, where the parameters b', b, c, and d index the probability of reliable retrieval. During this phase, when recall is still characterized by mistakes, one speaks of heuristic retrieval. Reliable retrieval (referred to as algorithmic retrieval) during state P is described by the parameters e, g, h, and r.

Brainerd and his colleagues have carried out many necessity and sufficiency tests (Greeno, 1968) of this two-stage model (e.g., Brainerd, Howe, & Kingma, 1982). Necessity tests determine whether the assumptions of a two-stage process model produce better explanations of a set of data than would a one-stage model. Sufficiency tests are used to decide whether more than two stages are required to account for the data. In general, good fits to the two-stage model have been obtained for both children's and adults' recall data.

Particularly relevant here, Brainerd and his colleagues have offered a great deal of evidence that encoding and retrieval parameters measure independent processes. The majority of the developmental studies were conducted using second- and sixth-

TABLE 3.2. Theoretical interpretations of the 11 parameters of the two-stage model.*

Parameter	Interpretation
Storage	
a′	Probability of storing a trace on Trial 1
a	Probability of storing a trace on any trial after Trial 1
f	Probability of losing a previously stored trace
Retrieval learning	
b′	For traces stored on Trial 1, the probability that no further retrieval learning is needed
b	For traces stored after Trial 1, the probability that no further retrieval learning is needed
c	The probability of learning a retrieval algorithm after a success in State P
d	The probability of learning a retrieval algorithm after an error in State P
Retrieval performance	
1-r	For items entering State P on Trial 1, the probability of a success
1-e	For items entering State P after Trial 1, the probability of a success
g	For two consecutive trials in State P, the probability that a success follows an error
h	For two consecutive trials in State P, the probability that a success follows a success

*Adapted from Brainerd, 1985a.

grade subjects (e.g., Brainerd, Howe, & Kingma, 1982; Brainerd et al., 1984; Howe et al., 1985a, 1985b), although several have included other age groups (adults in Brainerd, Howe, & Desrochers, 1982; kindergarten children in Brainerd, 1982, and Brainerd & Howe, 1982). Much (but certainly not all) of the work has been concerned with free recall. For instance, subjects were often asked to learn n-item word lists over the course of several learning-testing cycles. Learning ended only after all items could be reproduced without error on two successive trials. We review here only the most important developmental trends.

Similar to Chechile and Meyers, developmental trends were found for both encoding and retrieval parameters. The most important result, which was again consistent with Chechile and Meyer's outcomes, was that encoding developed faster than retrieval. A number of developmental invariances were detected. For instance, the values for the parameter a were always higher than those for a', indicating that all subjects found it easier to store a memory trace on later trials compared to storing it on the first trial. It was always more difficult to store a trace on the first trial (parameter a') than it was to retain a trace (parameter $1-f$).

A few of the results produced by Howe, Brainerd, and Kingma (1985a, 1985b) provide interesting information about the development of encoding and retrieval parameters in learning of taxonomically structured lists. Howe et al.'s (1985a) most important experimental manipulations were list structure (unrelated words vs. taxonomically-related items), the number of categories in taxonomically organizable lists (two vs. four), and whether recall was free or cued. Consistent with other findings, developmental differences in the retrieval-learning parameters were greater than the developmental differences for the encoding parameters. Although the presentation of a cue during the test phase affected both the encoding and retrieval parameters, the size of these effects varied with age. With younger children, cuing had the greatest effect on the encoding parameters. In contrast, the retrieval-learning parameters were most affected in the older sample. Increasing the number of taxonomic categories has a positive effect on retrieval learning (following success) in the cued-recall condition for second graders. For sixth graders it had a positive effect during free recall for both the encoding and retrieval parameters. In general, it was clear that developmental improvements in recall were due both to encoding and retrieval-learning components, but not to forgetting or retrieval-performance parameters following successful storage.

The third research program on mathematical modeling that we consider was conducted by Alex Wilkinson and his associates. Wilkinson, De Marinis, and Riley (1983) and Wilkinson and Koestler (1983, 1984) studied the "repeated recall" paradigm, in which a single short learning trial is followed by three test trials with no further opportunity for study of the target lists. Because there is only one opportunity for encoding at the beginning of the session, the focus of this model is on retention, although it is possible to analyze performance in terms of encoding, retrieval, and forgetting processes. Encoding was considered the establishment of a memory trace. Retrieval in this study was roughly comparable to what Brainerd and his colleagues referred to as retrieval learning. Retrieval and forgetting processes were viewed as complementary aspects of learning lists.

The clearest developmental results produced by Wilkinson occurred in Wilkinson et al. (1983). The values for the storage parameters increased significantly between fourth and ninth grade in that study. The retrieval and forgetting parameters did not vary significantly with age. The same pattern of outcomes was also found by Wilkinson and Koestler (1983). Thus, the ability of a subject to store a durable trace following a single trial is age dependent, although there seems to be no development in the tendencies to retain a trace.

Summary

The three models converge in supporting the conclusion that there are developmental differences between childhood and adulthood in encoding. On the other hand, although Chechile and Richman and Brainerd and his associates report data suggesting that developmental retrieval functions are more striking than developmental encoding functions, Wilkinson detected little development of retrieval in the paradigm that he studied. In addition, the relative contributions of encoding and retrieval components as explanations of memory development seem quite different in Chechile and Richman's model compared to Brainerd's work, and thus, there is no clear, simple answer that emerges from this work as to whether encoding or retrieval processes drive memory development. Brainerd (1985a) examined these data and concluded that the relative contribution of encoding and retrieval development may be task specific.

We believe that mathematical models of the type described here will prove additionally useful in analyses of the development of encoding and retrieval processes. Brainerd's group especially seems to be developing procedures that can be used with a variety of paradigms that have traditionally interested workers in memory development (i.e., free and serial recall, paired-associate learning). Brainerd's group has also showed how investigation of mathematical modeling parameters can be illuminating about traditional experimental manipulations, for example, picture versus word effects on learning (Brainerd, Desrochers, & Howe, 1981). Given the enthusiasm and commitment of researchers working in this area, we expect a great deal of developmental work from them in the future.

In applauding this research approach, we do not believe that it can in any way replace the alternative methods of analyses reviewed in this chapter. We are struck that the mathematical modelers focus on analyses of memory output, completely ignoring measurable encoding and retrieval activities of the learners that they are studying. In this regard, they seem to be making the same mistake that Bjorklund and his associates made, and in doing so, risk missing many important developments. More positively for the math modelers, there seems to be no reason that their exceptionally analytical skills cannot be put to work analyzing the differences in output for more versus less behaviorally active encoders and retrievers. The mathematical modelers are providing tremendously powerful methods of decomposing the typical dependent variable in memory experiments—memory output. If combined with clever ways of determining individual differences between learners that can be measured independently of the memory outcome variable, our understanding of within-age and between-age differences in children may increase dramatically. See Howe, Brainerd, and Kingma (1985b) for an interesting first example of this type of work, with the differences between learning disabled and normal learning children analyzed into a number of components in that study.

Cross-Cultural Studies of Strategy Development

How typical or universal is the development of strategic competence? Because school is an institution where memory performances are expected and rewarded, there is the possibility that schooling affects the development of memory and memory strategies. Because amount of schooling and chronological age are completely confounded in western culture, it is impossible to decide on the basis of western data alone whether strategy development is a function of maturation, schooling, or age-correlated environmental experience other than schooling. There is an important role for cross-cultural experiments here.

The research strategy most frequently used in cross-cultural studies of memory consists of measuring memory performance in American and non-western samples. Much of this work has been conducted with the Kpelle and Vai in Liberia, with Mayas and Mestizos in Mexico, and Guatemala, and with the Aboriginals in Australia. We discuss briefly some of the most important of these studies.

For instance, Cole, Gay, Glick, and Sharp (1971) studied the development of free recall of lists of categorically related words, providing some of the most complete cross-cultural information on memory development. The well-known advantages of free recall consist of being able to assess both recall and the amount of clustering during recall (which can be taken as one indicator of the use of organizational strategies). To-be-learned materials were carefully selected to ensure that the subjects (Kpelle from Liberia) would be quite familiar with them. Both lists of words and objects were used in these studies. For one series of experiments, three age groups were involved, 6- to 8-year-olds, 10- to 14-year-olds, and 18- to 50-year-olds. The two younger groups included approximately equal numbers of schooled and nonschooled subjects. None of the adults had attended school. A group of California children (in school, of course) served as the comparison group. The memory differences between the American and African samples were enormous. The usual adult versus child differences in memory were obtained in the American sample. In the Kpelle sample, however, the adults and children did not differ significantly. It was particularly noticable in the African subjects that they did not improve much over trials. Finally, it was also apparent that the American 11-year-olds and adults used categorical information to mediate recall. In contrast, low clustering was found for all ages within the Kpelle sample, suggesting that these subjects did not organize the to-be-learned material semantically. Taken as a whole, these results indicate that semantic organization strategies are not spontaneously employed by the Kpelle.

Wagner (1974) examined the degree to which intentional memory strategies were spontaneously employed in nonwestern cultures. Wagner used a serial-memory task. It was assumed that the analysis of serial position curves would enable conclusions about intentional rehearsal processes (Atkinson & Shiffrin, 1968). The subjects were presented seven cards, each of which depicted two objects (an animal and a household object). The picture cards were only presented briefly and then turned over one by one. Following this, a test stimulus was presented containing one of the two items on one of the cards, with the child's task to identify which of the seven turned-over cards included this item.

Inferences about rehearsal strategies and structural memory characteristics were made by analyzing primacy and recency effects respectively. Beginning at about 14 years of age, there were memory differences between the educated and noneducated samples that were primarily due to differences in the first few items in the list. That is, there was a primacy effect. Following Atkinson and Shiffrin's (1968) logic, Wagner (1974) assumed that the differential primacy effects reflected greater use of rehearsal in the educated compared to the noneducated sample. Wagner concluded from these results that memory strategies for serial recall are only employed spontaneously by subjects with schooling. The invariance of the recency effects across age groups and educational levels can, on the other hand, be interpreted to mean that structurally-mediated parameters (i.e., short-term memory) should probably be considered universal.

Wagner (1978) pointed out an important problem with Wagner (1974). The effects of education and urbanization were confounded in the earlier study. Whereas the subjects with school experience came from the capital of the Yucatan province in Mexico, the non-schooled subjects were recruited from the country. Thus, the between-group differences could have been due to educational or urban-rural differences. These two factors have been separated carefully in more recent studies including Wagner (1978).

Wagner's (1978) study included the serial task described previously. There were four age groups in the study (6- to 9-year-olds, 10- to 12-year-olds, 13- to 16-year-olds, and 17- to 22-year-olds). There were equal numbers of males in each age group with subsamples of schooled and nonschooled subjects and subsamples of urban and rural subjects. Thus, it was possible to analyze age, educational, and urbanization effects separately. For the serial recall task, Wagner's (1974) results were replicated in the Wagner (1978) study. In addition, however, both education and urbanization proved to be contributors to serial recall performance. The city versus country effect was especially apparent in the younger children. Younger city children remembered more regardless of schooling status. The educational effect was apparent among the older subjects, starting at about 13 years of age, with the effect of rural versus urban environment decreasing in importance with increasing age. The superiority of the schooled groups was reflected mainly in a primacy effect that was not apparent in the recall of the non-schooled subjects. This was interpreted by Wagner as additional evidence that rehearsal strategies are a byproduct of schooling.

All of the research reviewed up to this point in this subsection has involved laboratory tasks. Perhaps memory for everyday materials is mediated by strategies and processes that are universal in their development. Some of the best and most interesting of this research involves memory for text. Most of the text research does not support the position that cultural background determines memory performance. On the contrary, they tend to show that universal schemata are operative during the encoding and recall of stories so that almost no differences are observed as a function of culture or level of formal education.

For instance, in Mandler, Scribner, Cole, and DeForest (1980), children and adults from the Vai tribe of Liberia, with and without schooling were presented with a total of five stories, four of which were western in origin and one of which was from the Vai tribe. Significant differences were found between children and adults with regard to total recall of the stories. More importantly, however, there were no differences found in recall of familiar and unfamiliar types of stories (i.e., no tendency for cultural-specific results). Finally, a comparison of these results and those of earlier studies with American grade-school children and college students (Mandler & Johnson, 1977) also provided clear evidence that the recall patterns of the stories (in terms of the structural elements of the stories that were recalled) remained relatively invariant in both cultures. Mandler et al. (1980) concluded from these results that the general schematic structure of stories was an important determinant of recall performance. The results supported the assumption that story schematic elements are important mediators of text learning and recall. (See Chapter 4 for more on structural-schematic qualities of text as a determinant of memory.)

Further support for this conclusion was provided by Dube (1982) in a study of African and American junior high school students and African adolescents without school experience. All groups were presented two stories of African and two of European origin. The African groups demonstrated better memory performance as a whole. Consistent with Mandler et al. (1980), Dube found no difference in memory of the European and African stories. The superior memory performance of the African subjects was interpreted by Dube as possibly being due to the African's greater experience with oral storytelling and retelling. Ross and Millson (1970) obtained a comparable result in a comparison of adults from Ghana and New York. The Africans outperformed the Americans in story recall.

In drawing general conclusions about the cross-cultural text recall data, we would be remiss if we did not point out that there are some results that differ from the ones reviewed thus far. For instance, Kintsch and Greene (1978) found that American students were much worse recalling an Indian story than Grimms' fairy tales. Rogoff (1981) found that memory performance of young children varies with whether they have had formal education or not. Multiple regression analyses established that memory performance for two mythological stories was better predicted by number of years in school than by age or social background variables. When taken as a whole, however, the cross-cultural text studies provide clear evidence that recall of meaningful stories depends less on education than recall of unrelated materials. With respect to children, it seems likely that this effect may reflect the fact that children rarely use the types of sophisticated strategies that really efficient learning and memory of text requires (e.g., Bereiter & Bird, 1985). Because many stories in many cultures have structural-schematic properties, children throughout the world have opportunities to experience and learn these structures that can mediate learning and recall of text (e.g., Mandler, 1984).

A comparable analysis can be applied to other ecologically meaningful tasks, ones for which there are few or small cross-cultural effects. Consider a study conducted by Rogoff and Waddell (1982). School children from Guatemala and North America (8 to 10 years of age) demonstrated comparable memory performance in reconstruction of a miniature scene. The children's task was to place 20 familiar objects in a three-dimensional panorama representing a location familiar to children. The slight (although not statistically significant) superiority of the Mayan children seemed to be particularly interesting because the Mayans were recruited from the same area that provided Kagan, Klein, Finley, Rogoff, & Nolan's (1979) sample. In that study, the Mayans performed more poorly than Americans in a traditional memory span task. Given that both Mayan and North American children have many opportunities to experience scenes during development, there seems to be equivalent opportunity to learn the memory and retrieval skills necessary to mediate such tasks.

That memory performance depends greatly on prior familiarity with to-be-learned stimulus materials has been established especially clearly in studies on visual-spatial memory (e.g., Drinkwater, 1976; Kearins, 1981; Kleinfield, 1971). A main premise in all of these investigations was that the survival chances for the populations in question (eskimos in Kleinfeld's work, Australian aboriginals in the studies by Drinkwater & Kearins) depended greatly on their visual-spatial skills (i.e., their ability to orient themselves spatially in relatively monotonous terrain). When similar abilities are required in memory tests, children from Eskimo and aboriginal groups clearly outperform Caucasians from civilized regions. Kearins (1981, 1983) work is a particularly good example of this type of research.

Kearins (1981) required subjects to look at an array of objects for about 30 seconds. Then, subjects were required to place the objects back into their array positions. Regardless of the types of objects in the arrays (i.e., civilized items like bottles and knives or natural items like stones and leaves), the aboriginal children were consistently better at remembering array locations. Kearins (1983) provided additional data supporting the criticality of stimulus familiarity, reporting differences favoring aboriginal children over civilized children in verbal recall of wild animals. Kearins hypothesized that aboriginal children's interest in and knowledge about wild animals promoted their memory in this task. Kearins reported a variety of data suggesting that Anglo-Australian children were more likely to attempt verbal rehearsal strategies, whereas aboriginal children seemed to rely more on spatial-imaginal strategies. In summary, Kearins data clearly support the hypothesis that prior knowledge and culturally-supported visual-spatial skills can more than compensate for verbal strategies.

In summary, cross-cultural differences in children's memory seem to be very specific. It seems that use of rehearsal and organizational strategies during list learning is more common in western cultures than in nonschooled societies. The development of the strategic skills that mediate strong performance on list-like tasks seem to be tied to schooling. Materials that possess similar meaningful structures that children experience universally (e.g., stories, scenes) are more likely to be remembered equally in schooled and nonschooled cultures than are materials that are not experienced universally.

The results presented here can be reconciled with Oerter's (1985) thesis that school and instruction not only influence human development in the form of knowledge expansion and the development of specific capabilities, but also basically change that development. Thus, the development of some memorization strategies represents school-dependent developmental change. It is impressive that the effects of formal education on the performance of various memory tasks can be shown more clearly than the effects of chronological age, social environment, social class, and urbanization.

We must caution, however, that the methodological problems involved in this cross-cultural research are enormous. For instance, the schooled and nonschooled children in a particular region may differ on many characteristics besides schooling—that is, there are obviously selection factors in determining who will go to school in these regions and who will not. Sometimes culturally specific personality characteristics undermine attempts to conduct comparisons. For instance, Rogoff and Mistry (1985) found that young Mayan children demonstrated poorer memory of stories than young American children. As it turned out, the Mayan children were extremely uncomfortable in the experimental situation because they are usually not permitted to speak freely with adults. An anecdote like this suggests that other cross-cultural data may be tainted by social interaction effects not understood by westerners. The general conclusion that formal education probably has specific effects on memory rather than a general one seems fair enough given the data that are on hand, and it is is a very important finding.

Closing Comment

Reseachers interested in memory development have spent a lot of time studying the development of encoding and retrieval strategies, with some of the more important developments and issues taken up in this chapter. The development of strategic competence was probably attractive to memory development researchers at the end of the 1960s and beginning of the 1970s, in part because it seemed at that time that there were qualitative differences in strategy use as a function of age. At the end of the 1980s, strategy development appears more continuous. For instance, there is gradual development of rehearsal skills. Even preschoolers rehearse the location of a hidden object by looking at the hiding place during a retention interval. Single-item repetition of to-be-learned words on lists is gradually replaced by increasingly complex cumulative rehearsal.

Early work on strategies was characterised by a narrow focus on strategies only, and then only in western cultures. There is now a realization that use of encoding and retrieval strategies must be considered in interaction, and that use of these strategies depends on nonstrategic knowledge. Some of the strategies that have commanded the greatest attention by workers in memory development seem to be ones that are most sensitive to schooling effects. That is, they do not develop universally, but rather are observed more in schooled societies than in nonschooled societies.

New methodologies are opening exciting possibilities for increasing understanding of strategic development. For instance, mathematical modeling and the descriptions approach permit analyses of encoding versus retrieval. Math modeling in particular permits more complete analysis of the dependent measures that has been the case in much of the previous research. Researchers have also become very clever at coding overt memorizing and retrieving behaviors and relating these to memory performance. The identification of observable behaviors that are telling about strategy use is a major advance.

In subsequent chapters, strategy use will be considered additionally with respect to knowledge and metacognitive factors, especially the dependency of strategy use on these factors. The immediate concerns in the next chapter, however, are occasions when the knowledge base predominantly determines memory. This discussion will make clear that those (e.g., Bjorklund) who believe that the knowledge base can produce important main effects on memory are correct, even if some of the specific hypotheses about knowledge main effects discussed in this chapter proved not to be correct.

4. The Knowledge Base

The nature of the contents of the knowledge base is more than a little bit fuzzy. It certainly contains information about how to do things (i.e., procedural knowledge) and nonprocedural facts about the world (declarative knowledge) (e.g., Siegler, 1983). Although there is not an exact equivalence between procedural knowledge and strategies, the most important procedural knowledge considered in this book is memory strategies, which were considered in detail in the last chapter. Thus, the concern in this chapter is more on the declarative knowledge base and how it affects memory directly (i.e., through mechanisms other than facilitating the use of strategies as discussed in Chapters 3, 6, and 7).

Even restricting discussion to the declarative knowledge base does little to reduce the uncertainties concerning the nature of the memory base. For instance, there are great debates about the modes of representation in the base (e.g., imagery, Paivio, 1986; propositions, Pylyshyn, 1984) and the organization of information (e.g., categorical versus schematic, Mandler, 1983, 1984). Not surprisingly, there are also a variety of models about how the long-term knowledge base changes with development. Although it is not our purpose to review these conceptions in any detail, a brief review of the available alternatives makes clear that developmentalists have been considering potential changes in knowledge from a variety of perspectives.

Both Bjorklund and Chi posit modified network models of semantic memory (cf., Anderson, 1976; Collins & Loftus, 1975; Norman & Rumelhart, 1975). They assume that every item (concept) in semantic memory is represented by nodes that are connected to each other by means of links. The connections between the nodes are determined by various relations, with inter-item associativity considered a fundamental one. Bjorklund (1987) in particular assumes that characteristic features are stored for every item, features that mediate inter-item associative processes (e.g., a child can associate a cat and a dog by recognition of the common features "four legs," "domestic pets," or "friendly"). Knowledge structures are viewed as hierarchic (i.e., some aspects of knowledge are subordinate to others – "cats," "dogs," and "frogs" are categories that are subordinate to the category "animals," which is subordinate to the category "living things." The probability that a specific item will be activated and transferred to the short-term memory is viewed as a function of context, inter-item associativity, the number of characteristic item features, and the frequency with which this specific item was activated in the past. Developmental changes in this network affect the number of available items and their accessibility. Bjorklund (1987) assumes that developmental changes in concept representations follow from additional encounters with items. New features are added with experience, with the additional features permitting more elaborate codings when items are presented as to-be-learned information. The enriched encodings that follow permit better accessibility of the items during retrieval. In addition to the number of characteristic item features, the strength of the relation between the individual nodes can vary. Bjorklund assumes that the strength of relations between nodes increase (a) with additional encounters of the items and (b) because the encoding preferences for objects change from more imaginal to more linguistic and semantic (e.g., Bruner, Olver, & Greenfield, 1966).

The basic assumptions made by Chi and Rees (1983) are quite similar to ones made by Bjorklund. Chi and Rees are more strongly oriented to computer models, however. In addition to networks, they focus on production rules (if-then relationships). In contrast to the factual knowledge represented by semantic networks, these production rules portray procedural knowledge. Such production rules are elements of a production system that generates and activates the system activities as well as generating new rules. Furthermore, Chi and Rees include schema in their model of children's knowledge. If a new situation resembles previous situations that are represented in the generalized schema, the schema may be activated, permitting organization and interpretation of all of the incoming information according to the schema. Thus, consider a child who is led by a parent from a parking lot into a building that has a counter with people who order food and receive it. This information should be more than enough to activate the fast-food restaurant schema, at least by children residing in western, industrialized economies who are permitted frequent opportunities to dine at McDonalds, Burger King, and Wendy's. In turn, the child has no problem responding, "Burger, fries, and a Coke," when the parent asks what the child would like – even if the child is not old enough to read the menu! In addition, the child may not wait for a waitress to clear the table, but instead beg to be the one who carries the tray to the trash can. Chi and Rees (1983) emphasize that with development, there are changes in both procedural and declarative knowledge. Consistent with Bjorklund (1987), they also assume a shift in the preferred mode of representation from predominantly imaginal to linguistic and semantic.

Mandler (1983) designed a rudimentary model of the development of knowledge organization that took into consideration both categorical and schematic representations. Both categorical and schematic knowledge are assumed to be established in the daily episodes of early childhood. The child registers the similarity of episodes that are repeated regularly and learns to categorize various objects that are encountered in the world. Classifications are attempted as part of everyday functioning, thus, explaining the dominant functional character of young children's classification systems (Chapter 3). On the other hand, classifications become more independent of context with opportunities to judge objects free of context, solely on the basis of similarity (as occurs in formal educational settings).

In short, there are a variety of positions about changes in the knowledge base with development, with changes in knowledge about facts, procedures, and scripts considered explicitly. The life episodes that young children experience provide a rich data base for establishing representations, especially ones that emphasize functional properties of objects and how to function in particular settings (i.e., everyday scripts). Young children's representations also seemed to be dominated by perceptual information. In contrast, older children's representations are more complete, and with development, they resemble increasingly the knowledge base of adults. Thus, older children can classify materials taxonomically rather on the basis of their function alone. Scripts become increasingly general, and thus, more flexible. Whereas the 3-year-old's restaurant script might be adequate to mediate understanding of McDonald's and Burger King, but nothing else, the older child's fast-food restaurant script is elaborate enough to assimilate new instances from White Castle to a sit-down-but-decidedly-fast-food steak house. These changes in knowledge are important to understand, given that it is clear that knowledge plays a major role in determining memory of at least some newly encountered content, a main theme developed in this chapter.

It has been recognized for some time that memory performance is highly dependent on the developing knowledge base. Flavell (1985) eloquently describes the situation:

Thus, what the head knows has an enormous effect on what the head learns and remembers. But, of course, what the head knows changes enormously in the course of development, and these changes consequently make for changes in memory behavior (p. 213).

Systematic studies on the influence of task-relevant prior knowledge on memory behavior and performance have only been carried out in the last decade. The results have been so striking that the knowledge factor has been portrayed in recent descriptions of memory development as an extremely important explanatory component of memory performance (e.g., Bjorklund, 1985; Howe, 1985; Kail, 1984; Körkel, 1987; Oerter & Schuster-Oeltzschner, 1987; Ornstein & Naus, 1985).

Some coverage of knowledge effects on memory was appropriate in the previous chapters (i.e., knowledge effects on the development of functional capacity and the use of particular strategies), and the points covered there will not be re-reviewed here. Rather, in this chapter we consider evidence that task-specific prior knowledge can affect memory performance directly—that is, when developmental improvements in memory performance may be due to development and application of the knowledge base predominantly rather than due to development of strategic competence. There have been empirical studies of diverse types of prior knowledge.

Whenever researchers have looked, it has proven possible to identify prior knowledge influences on memory.

That prior knowledge can affect children's memory was confirmed in studies of "inferential" memory, with Scott Paris and his colleagues providing especially telling data (Paris, 1975, 1978; Paris & Lindauer, 1977, 1982; see also Trabasso & Nicholas, 1980). Children in the Paris' experiments (e.g., Paris & Carter, 1973; Paris & Lindauer, 1976; Paris & Upton, 1976; Schmidt, Paris, & Stober, 1979) were presented mini-stories that were followed by memory tests. Constructive, inferential processes in remembering texts (processes driven by prior knowledge of relationships in the world) were assumed whenever there was incorrect memory of sentences that were not actually included in the original stories but were consistent with the meaning of the material in the text (i.e., when true inferences were made). In general, there were clear developmental increases in inference skills. For instance, Paris and Upton (1976) reported a developmental increase in inferring instruments used to perform actions (e.g., inferring a shovel was used by a boy who was reported to be digging a hole). In general, others have been able to replicate this development (e.g., Omanson, Warren, & Trabasso, 1978). The conclusion that follows from all of this work is that older children are more likely than younger children to use their general knowledge and go beyond the facts presented in text to fill in the gaps in information that is to be remembered.

A study of prior knowledge that was conducted by Brown, Smiley, Day, Townsend, and Lawton (1977, experiment 2) is especially interesting in that specific prior knowledge was experimentally induced in subjects. The second-, fourth-, and sixth-grade participants received information about a topic a week before they were presented a text passage that could be interpreted in light of this prior knowledge. The memory of even the youngest subjects in the study was affected by the prior knowledge manipulation. Particularly relevant here, the children made many constructive errors in recalling the text passage, making inferences that were consistent with the prior knowledge they had acquired the week before. The presence of relevant prior knowledge clearly affected the children's learning of related but "new" material.

Perhaps the most robust finding in the literature on knowledge effects is that experts in an area learn more when studying "new" information in their domain of expertise than do nonexperts. For instance, the second graders in Pearson, Hansen, and Gordon (1979) could be categorized as snake experts or novices. Questions on a short text about snakes dealt with information explicitly presented in text, as well as facts that were only implied in text, but could be deduced based on prior knowledge. As expected, the experts answered the questions much better than the novices. The relatively greater superiority of experts on text-implicit questions was considered due to the operation of snake-content schema possessed by the experts but not the novices.

Schneider, Körkel, and Weinert (1987a) presented grade-3, grade-5, and grade-7 children a story about a soccer game, with the participants classifiable as soccer experts or novices. The children could further be classified with respect to general ability, either as poor learners or good learners. The results were generally consistent across a variety of measures that tapped both exact memory of the text and memory for appropriate inferences. There were clear main effects for expertise such that soccer experts outperformed novices. Even more striking, the expertise classification was much more predictive of performance than was the general ability classification. Low general ability experts descriptively outperformed high general ability novices on every memory and comprehension measure included in the study.

A third dramatic demonstration of the effects of the knowledge base on children's learning was provided by Chi and Koeske (1983). A 5-year-old dinosaur expert was asked to retain two lists of dinosaur names of equal length, one list consisting of familiar names. The same pattern of results was found in a post-test about a year later, which can be interpreted to mean that a direct relationship does indeed exist between the degree of prior knowledge and the ability to memorize.

Other studies contrasting experts and novices have provided additional impressive demonstrations of factual knowledge effects on memory performance. Superior memory performance by experts are almost always limited to areas of expertise, however (Chase & Simon, 1973; Chi, Feltovich, & Glaser, 1981; Chiesi, Spilich, & Voss, 1979). In particular, Chi (1978, 1981, 1985b) has produced striking developmental data consistent with this conclusion.

Chi (1978) recruited experienced and inexperienced chess players and gave them the task of recalling various chess positions presented to them briefly. The most interesting aspect of this research was that subjects' knowledge correlated negatively with age — the children (average age = 10 yrs) were the experts and the adults were the novices. Although the children performed significantly worse on traditional memory-span tests than the adults, they averaged much better on the chess-related memory tasks. They were able to remember more chess positions correctly, needed fewer trials to reach the learning criteria, and predicted their performance more accurately.

Chi (1978) has stimulated follow-up studies. For instance, the reversal of the usual age effect was also demonstrated by Weinert et al. (1984) for text learning. The subjects in that study were fourth, sixth, and eighth graders, half of whom could be classified as soccer experts and half of whom were soccer novices. The expected differences between experts and novices were especially evident in the comprehension of a soccer-related passage, particularly in the importance ratings given to individual parts of the text. The youngest experts (fourth graders) were clearly superior to the oldest novices (eighth graders) in recognizing the important compared to the less important aspects of text.

In general, all of the effects referred to in the last few paragraphs have been attributed to possession of a well-developed knowledge base. One possibility is that many of these effects are actually a combination of greater knowledge and greater interest in the content in question, however. After all, it seems a safe bet that the experts in these studies were probably both knowledgable and interested in the content of expertise, and there is a literature substantiating that children learn more content when reading text that is interesting to them (Asher, Hymel, & Wigfield, 1978; Belloni & Jongsma, 1978; Bernstein, 1955; Ceci, 1984; Estes & Vaughan, 1973; Stevens, 1980) The separation of knowledge and interest effects is important, because children often acquire knowledge about material that really does not fascinate them (i.e., elementary schools often require specific contents to be learned regardless of student interest). The small amount of research that does exist in fact suggests that children's interest and knowledge probably both contribute to comprehension and learning of text (Baldwin, Peleg-Bruckner, & McClintock, 1985), and thus, our suspicion is that work on interest will prove complementary rather than antagonistic to the theoretical position that the knowledge base is an important determinant of memory.

In contrast to the studies of children with expertise not possessed by most children, Bjorklund and his colleagues (Bjorklund & Zeman, 1982, 1983; Bjorklund & Bjorklund, 1985) concentrated on knowledge that is more universally acquired. For instance, Bjorklund and Zeman presented 7-, 9-, and 11-year-old children with two structurally similar memory tasks. The subjects were supposed to (a) remember the names of their classmates (class recall task) and (b) memorize and recall a list of taxonomically classifiable items. Although the usual age differences in recall and clustering were found in the traditional list learning task, subjects of all ages could remember the names of their classmates equally well. It has also become apparent that the cluster values computed for seating arrangements, reading groups, and sex were comparable at each of the age levels. Since a post-recall metamemory interview did not provide much evidence that the children's behavior in the class recall task reflected conscious memory strategies, Bjorklund and Zeman (1982, 1983; also Bjorklund, 1985, 1987) concluded that children's performance on the class recall task was mostly due to the automatic activation of associative relations. In a follow-up study, Bjorklund and Bjorklund (1985) induced subjects to use a specific retrieval strategy (i.e., use seating arrangement to mediate recall). Organizational measures (clustering) were affected by use of this strategy (in fact, organization was maximized). Consistent with other observations that young children can learn some retrieval strategies to a high level of competence with little effort (e.g., an alphabetical retrieval strategy in Chi, 1985b), even young children could follow the new retrieval instructions and produced clustering values comparable to those of the older subjects. Nonetheless, there was no improvement in level of recall as a function of use of the strategy. Bjorklund and Bjorklund (1985) argued that this result was consistent with their position (reviewed in Chapter 3) that the employment of intentional memory strategies only has a minimal effect on performance in this type of task.

Even more abstract and general forms of long-term knowledge can have an effect on children's learning and memory. Traditional stories have become a favorite research stimulus in psychology of memory, mainly because they have a typical or "canonical" form independent of content. There is an initiating event (usually a problem) to which the protagonist of the story reacts emotionally (internal response). Attempts to solve the problem produce consequences to which the protagonist must react. Formal story grammars have been developed that describe story structures (e.g., Johnson & Mandler, 1980; Mandler & Johnson, 1977; Stein & Glenn, 1979), accompanied by specific tests of the effects of children's story grammar knowledge on memory performance.

When stories conform almost perfectly to ideal story grammar forms, developmental differences in recall are less striking than when stories deviate from the ideal structure. For instance, even preschool children are capable of recalling temporal sequences in ideally structured stories (Wimmer, 1980). When stories differ from stereotypic story grammatical format, children as well as adults have a tendency to recall the stories in their canonical form, that is, the order of story elements is transformed as part of the encoding and retrieval processes (Mandler, 1978; Mandler & DeForest, 1979; Stein & Glenn, 1975, 1979). The structural similarity of story recall in normal children, learning-disabled children, and adults from different cultures (Bower, Black, & Turner, 1979; Nelson, 1978; Mandler et al., 1980; Weaver & Dickinson, 1984) suggests that certain general structural schema have universal meaning.

Age differences in *quantity* of recall are striking, nonetheless, when story elements are presented in other than canonical order (McClure, Mason, & Barnitz, 1979; Stein & Nezworski, 1978). The ability to recall such stories increases with age, with children having greater difficulty remembering stories that deviate from the canonical form than they do remembering stories that are consistent with conventional story grammar structures (e.g., Mandler, 1978; Nelson & Gründel, 1981). Adults who process such stories seem to be able to reorder and shuffle the information that they are presented to make the story consistent with story grammar conventions, at least when prompted to do so (e.g., Stein & Nezworski, 1978). Children on the other hand seem not to be able to reorder story elements (Buss, Yussen, Mathews, Miller, & Rembold, 1983). Consistent with the theme that various types of knowledge can affect memory performance, there is an important exception to this generalization. Children have less difficulty processing and remembering noncanonical presentations when they are presented content that can be related to scripts that are already very familiar to them (Nelson, 1978; Nelson et al., 1983; Nelson & Gründel, 1981; Nelson & Hudson, in press).

On the other hand, possessing familiar scripts can cause memory problems. Fivush, Hudson, and Nelson (1984) compared children's general "museum script" with kindergarten children's report of their own visit to a museum. Memory tests after six weeks or a year showed that the general script had changed very little. The memory of the personal museum visit was also astonishingly accurate after six weeks or even after a year. All subjects were capable of differentiating the visit from the general museum script. On the other hand, less special events (e.g., memory of a specific dinner) share more features with generalized script memory. Nelson and Hudson (in press) report on an unpublished study in which they obtained no structural differences between 3- to 5-year-olds' general scripts about birthday parties and their reports about specific birthday parties. Nelson and Hudson argued that this represented a fusion process in memory, a blending of the specific episode with the general script. That this process is not limited to young children is suggested by recent data reported by Gehringer and Strube (1985). Their study included 10- to 11-year-old students, as well as samples of 18- to 20-year-old adults and 35- to 40-year-old adults. They found that all groups in their study distorted both biographic and autobiographic information to conform to stereotypic scripts, with few and not very striking developmental differences in the structure of recall.

Taken as a whole, the results in this chapter provide impressive evidence that a child's knowledge base can have a great effect on memory. There are many challenges that remain in elucidating knowledge-base effects, however. For instance, as the knowledge base develops, there is more complete coding of concepts and stronger interconnections between them, and thus, long-term memory should be more accessible with increasing age. With increased accessibility, both automatic and strategic processes should be facilitated. Nonetheless, at all age levels, there are important differences between people in the degree of accessibility that they have to what is stored in long-term memory (Brown et al., 1983, p. 99). What determines these differences? That there are differences in accessibility makes clear that knowledge alone can never be a sufficient explanation of memory performance. Since conscious and systematic search of long-term memory for possible knowledge that could mediate memory is an important learning strategy (e.g., schema activation; e.g., Levin & Pressley, 1981), we close by noting that the inclusion of a separate chapter on knowledge does not mean to imply that we view knowledge as a component that operates autonomously most of the time (a point that was discussed in detail in Chapter 3). It is often used in conjunction with strategies. On the other hand, most of the effects reviewed in this chapter probably were mediated rather directly by the knowledge base, with conscious use of strategies playing a minor role.

One strategy that is often recommended in the literature (e.g., Tierney & Cunningham, 1984), however, boils down to activating the background knowledge that one has (e.g., as an aid to comprehension and memory of text). When people possess background knowledge that is consistent with the content of the text, there is plenty of reason to expect that prior knowledge activation should increase learning, for at a minimum the reader is thinking "deeply" about the topic of the upcoming text (cf., Rickards, 1976; Rickards & Divesta, 1974; Watts & Anderson, 1971). Not suprisingly, people do remember more that they read if they possess and have activated relevant knowledge (e.g., Anderson & Pearson, 1984; Arnold & Brooks, 1976; Bransford & Johnson, 1972; Brown et al., 1977; Levin & Pressley, 1981; Pearson et al., 1979; Tierney & Cunningham, 1984). But what if the person does not possess relevant prior knowledge, and in fact, has misconceptions about the topic covered in the text? Positive effects following activation of incorrect prior knowledge is predicted by the theoretical view that information conflicting with prior knowledge and expectations is especially noticable and noted, and thus, should be especially memorable (e.g., Graesser & Nakamura, 1982; Mandler, 1984; O'Brien & Myers, 1985; Peeck, van den Bosch, & Kreupeling, 1982; Schank, 1982). On the other hand, there is also the possibility of negative effects when a flawed knowledge base is activated. Interference, inferences, and intrusions from errant prior knowledge can follow (e.g., Anderson & Pearson, 1984; Brown et al., 1977; Lipson, 1982; Pichert & Anderson, 1977; Smith, Readence, & Alvermann, 1984).

A study by Alvermann, Smith, and Readence (1985) illustrates the potential negative impact of activation of errant prior knowledge on children's comprehension and learning from text. Grade-6 children either activated or did not activate prior knowledge about a passage before reading it. Thus, prior-knowledge-activation subjects who subsequently read a passage about light and heat from the sun (a passage containing information that clashed with prior knowledge typically possessed by grade-6 students) were first asked to write down all that they knew about the topic. After writing the essay, the subjects read the text. Following completion of reading, subjects were first asked to write down everything that they could remember from the passage and then were given 10 multiple-choice questions, some of which were explicitly designed to contain foils consistent with misconceptions about light and heat from the sun possessed by grade-6 students (determined by pilot testing). Procedures in the nonactivation condition were identical to those in the activation condition, except that there was no essay writing before reading.

The outcomes were rather striking in Alvermann et al. (1985). Free recall of the text was better when children did not activate the prior knowledge. Specifically, there was significantly less recall of text ideas that were incompatible with grade-6 children's prior knowledge, and a trend toward less recall of the remainder of the passage (our reanalyses). In addition, multiple-choice questions that included misconception foils were less likely to be answered correctly in the prior-knowledge-activation condition. When contrasted to the positive effects produced by congruent prior knowledge in other studies, Alvermann et al.'s (1985) data make clear that prior knowledge activation is a double-edged sword. Activation of misconceptions can significantly interfere with learning of objectively more correct perspectives. Complicating the situation even more, Pressley, McDaniel, Tanenbaum, and Wood (1988) recently produced facilitation when correct prior knowledge was activated in adults, but observed no interference from activation of incorrect prior knowledge (in fact, there was some evidence of slight facilitation). We suspect that quite a bit of research will be conducted in the near future on acquisition of new information when the learner possesses inconsistent prior knowledge, for it is apparent that both children and adults often know less than they think with respect to important contents such as basic scientific information (e.g., Anderson, 1987). A hypothesis suggested by comparison of Alvermann et al.'s (1985) results with Pressley et al.'s (1988) data is that adults are better than children at subsequently managing an errant knowledge base that is activated. A lot of work relevant to both theoretical and educational issues could be generated in response to this issue alone.

5. Metamemory

Metamemory is knowledge about memory. It resembles constructs advanced by earlier theoretical traditions (Cavanaugh & Perlmutter, 1982), such as systematic introspection as defined by the "Würzburg School" (Ach, 1905). Otto Selz (1913) made assumptions about self-regulating processes. He specified evaluation and selection mechanisms that resemble processes that are central to contemporary theory. Despite reservations about introspective data throughout the 20th century (e.g., Lyons, 1986), the potential importance of modern research on metacognition was anticipated enthusiastically by some experimental psychologists, including Tulving and Madigan (1970):

> Why not start looking for ways of experimentally studying and incorporating into theories and models of memory one of the truly unique characteristics of human memory: its knowledge of its own knowledge . . . We cannot help but feel that if there is ever going to be a genuine breakthrough in the psychological study of memory . . . it will, among other things, relate the knowledge stored in the individual's memory to his knowledge of that knowledge (p. 477).

At about the same time, John Flavell (1971) introduced the term metamemory for knowledge about memory processes and contents and gave it special status in his taxonomy of memory phenomena (Flavell & Wellman, 1977). There was great expansion of metamemory theory in the ensuing decade.

Introduction to Metamemory Theory

Metamemory was viewed by Flavell as one of four broad, somewhat overlapping memory categories—structurally-determined capacity, strategies, the nonstrategic knowledge base, and metamemory (i.e., the topics covered in Chapters 2 through

5 respectively of this volume). Flavell's (1971) conception of metamemory was global, encompassing knowledge of all possible aspects of information storage and retrieval. Metamemory included (but was not limited to) knowledge about memory functioning, limitations, difficulties, and strategies. Flavell and Wellman's taxonomy parsed metamemory into two main categories, "sensitivity" and "variables." The *sensitivity* category included knowledge of when memory activity is necessary (e.g., awareness that a particular task in a particular setting requires the use of memory strategies). The *variables* category was divided into three subcategories: (a) characteristics of a person relevant to memory, (b) characteristics of a task relevant to memory, and (c) potentially applicable memory strategies. An example of a person variable is the child's mnemonic self-concept, including clear ideas about his or her own memory strengths and weaknesses. Task variables include factors that make a memory task easier (e.g., familiar materials, high interitem associations) or harder (e.g., longer lists, when study time is short). The strategies variable includes all changes in knowledge about encoding and retrieval strategies, including the many strategies considered in Chapter 4.

Flavell and Wellman (1977) assumed that metamemorially sophisticated people did not view the metamemory categories and subcategories as independent of one another, but rather as overlapping and in interaction. People with well-developed metamemory know, for instance, that different individuals do not always solve a problem equally well (i.e., there are person by task interactions) and that the strategy chosen to solve a particular problem depends largely on person and task characteristics (i.e., there are person by strategy by task interactions). Flavell (1979, 1981, 1984) also argued that metamemory was not isolated from knowledge about other aspects of mind, and he generalized the metamemory taxonomy developed in Flavell and Wellman (1977) to metacognition in general. As in the metamemory classification, general metacognitive knowledge about persons, tasks, and strategies was differentiated. Flavell also introduced the term *metacognitive experiences* to refer to occasions during cognitive processing when new insights about cognition arose. Thus, a university student might try a method of outlining in order to learn textbook content. If, after using the method, the student realized that a lot of effort had been expended and little was learned, that would qualify as a metacognitive experience. The student would have gained insight into the utility of the outlining strategy. Flavell's theory was that metacognitive knowledge, metacognitive experiences, and cognitive behaviors constantly interact, as illustrated in Fig. 5.1.

An impression that could be gleaned from some of Flavell's early research was that a lot of metacognitive development was complete by age 8 or 9 (e.g., Kreutzer, Leonard, & Flavell, 1975). One motivation for Ann Brown's (1978; Brown & DeLoache, 1978) reconceptualization of metamemory was to counteract this impression, which followed largely from analyses of isolated pieces of metacognitive knowledge (i.e., children's knowledge of particular person, task, and strategy variables). In contrast to Flavell, Brown focused on the component that Flavell and Wellman (1977) labeled "here and now memory monitoring." Her frame of reference was the competent information processor, one possessing an efficient "executive" that regulated cognitive behaviors. This executive is aware of the system's capacity

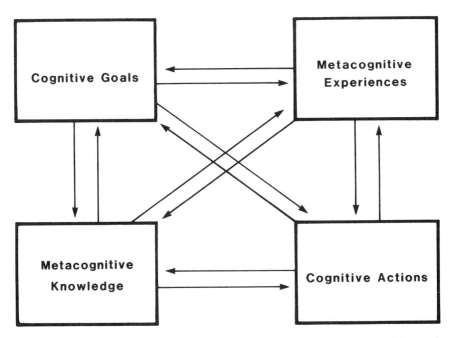

FIGURE 5.1. Flavell's model of metacognition and cognitive control. From Cognitive monitoring, by J.H. Flavell. In W.P. Dickson (Ed.), *Children's oral communication skills*, New York: Academic Press, 1981, p. 40.

limits and strategies. The executive can analyze new problems and select appropriate strategies and attempt solutions. Very importantly, the executive monitors the success or failure of ongoing performance, deciding which strategies to continue and which to replace with potentially more effective and appropriate procedures. In addition, the efficient executive knows when one knows and when one does not know, an important requirement for competent learning (e.g., Holt, 1964, pp. 28–29). Brown took the perspective that memory monitoring played a large role in these executive actions, and that metacognitive effects on cognitive regulation were more important than other metacognitive functions. In contrast to metacognitively mature adults (and many adults do not qualify; see Chapter 7) who possess proficient executive capabilities, children do not monitor well and often fail to make appropriate executive decisions. For instance, children often do not monitor comprehension problems when reading text (e.g., Baker & Brown, 1984; Garner, 1987; Körkel, 1987), and they fail to recognize when they do not have enough information to complete a task (e.g., Beal & Flavell, 1982; Flavell, Speer, Green, & August, 1981). (More discussion of children's monitoring deficiencies is presented in Chapter 7.)

Brown's contributions to the development of metacognitive theory are enormous. Like Flavell, Brown recognized that memory and other cognitive activities (e.g., learning, attention, & problem solving) were inextricably intertwined and that a theory of metacognition should capture a variety of cognitive phenomena in relation to one another. For instance, personality traits like self-concept and achievement motivation are part of metamemory in that they include knowledge about the self as a learner. Brown also mapped out some of the educational implications of metacognition (e.g., analyses of metacognitive processing during comprehension of text). She has developed the case explicitly that metacognitive abilities develop quite slowly during the school years. In addition, she has compared the metacognitive competencies of retarded and learning-disabled children to those of normal children.

Other theorists have also contributed substantially to the development of metacognitive theory, and metamemory theory in particular. For instance, there has been additional study of preschoolers' metacognition, with Wellman's (1983, 1985a, 1985b, in press) "theory of mind" particularly emphasizing the development of metacognition in early childhood. Wellman differentiates five partially overlapping classes of knowledge that develop during the preschool years. *Knowledge about existence* is the most basic category. Children know by about 2 to 3 years of age that there is an inner mental world. They have a rudimentary understanding of mental verbs like "thinking" or "remembering" and can separate mental processes from external behaviors associated with them (although not with absolute certainty or accuracy). Children gradually learn to recognize that the mental world can be differentiated into processes such as remembering, knowing, and guessing (i.e., they acquire *knowledge of distinct mental processes*). Although 3- to 4-year-olds are not generally capable of differentiating these processes, older preschool children make differentiations that are quite similar to those of adults. Although there are numerous differentiation possibilities between individual mental processes, these processes also have a number of things in common. The category *knowledge about integration* attempts to represent the growing understanding of the similarity between certain mental activities, such as thinking and remembering. There are clear developmental improvements in integration during the preschool years. Categories 4 and 5 are *knowledge about variables* (e.g., task, strategy) and *cognitive monitoring* (i.e., awareness of their mental condition relative to task demands) and are based on the categories of the same name in the Flavell and Wellman (1977) model.

A great deal of attention has been given to more advanced metacognition in older children. Kluwe (1980, 1981, 1982; Kluwe & Friedrichsen, 1984; Kluwe & Schiebler, 1984) developed a more complete and more differentiated description of metacognition than provided by either Brown or Flavell. Kluwe's model includes knowledge about minds in general (i.e., how all minds operate) and knowledge about individual differences in cognition. Kluwe's conception borrowed heavily from general theories of information processing. For instance, the concepts *declarative* and *procedural* knowledge were introduced to represent the ideas that *knowledge of data* (i.e., knowing "that") and *knowledge of processes* (i.e., knowing "how") are both necessary in human thinking. Kluwe considered analysis of knowledge about processes to be particularly important. These procedural components are active agents in Kluwe's framework. He incorporates ideas about executive and control processes that are similar to Brown's, although more elaborate. Kluwe identifies control processes that evaluate ongoing cognition (i.e., monitor current perfor-

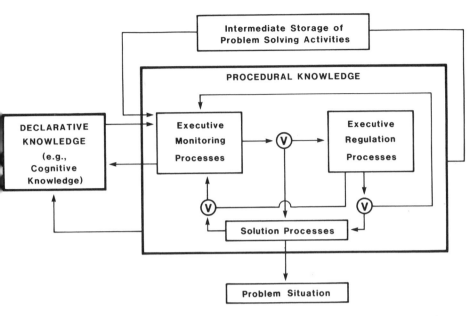

FigURE 5.2. Hypothetical model of executive activity in problem solving. From Cognitive knowledge and executive control: Metacognition, by R.H. Kluwe. In D. Griffin (Ed.) *Animal mind—human mind*. New York: Springer, 1982.

mance). Other control processes are more directed at regulation, allocating attention and selecting other processes to be applied in given situations, as well as determining the intensity with which strategic processes are to be applied. Figure 5.2 illustrates Kluwe's thinking about the complex interactions that exist between declarative and procedural processes.

Scott Paris and his associates (e.g., Paris & Lindauer, 1982; Paris et al., 1983; Paris & Jacobs, 1984; Paris & Oka, 1986) also proposed a taxonomy of metacognitive variables. There are two particularly important categories of metacognition in the Paris model. *Awareness of cognition* includes knowledge about task and strategy characteristics in the sense of Flavell and Wellman (1977). It also includes knowledge about when, where, and why to use particular strategies (i.e., the conditional knowledge that a person requires in order to use a strategy). The second major category is *self-monitoring*, which includes evaluation of ongoing cognitive processes, planning to use cognitive processes, and regulation of those processes.

Pressley, Borkowski, and their colleagues (e.g., Borkowski, Johnston, & Reid, 1987; Pressley, Borkowski, & O'Sullivan, 1984, 1985; Pressley, Borkowski, & Schneider, 1987; Pressley, Goodchild, Fleet, Zajchowski, & Evans, in press; Pressley, Snyder, & Cariglia-Bull, 1987) have proposed an elaborate model of metacognition, the Good Strategy User Model, with only a small part of it reviewed here. *Strategies* are the fundamental elements in this framework. Good strategy users also have *general strategy knowledge*, that is, they understand general principles about strategy functioning (e.g., mental effort is necessary to deploy most strategies). In contrast, *metacognitive knowledge about specific strategies* (often abbreviated to *specific strategy knowledge*) refers to knowledge about particular strategies (e.g., when and where to use a strategy). Good strategy users also possess skills that permit them to acquire additional metacognition. In particular, *metacognitive acquisition procedures* take other strategies as input and evaluate them. For instance, self-testing procedures can be metacognitive acquisition procedures, such as when self-testing is undertaken to judge the efficiency of a new strategy or when performance comparisons are made to determine which of several memory strategies is most powerful as a mediator of a particular type of memory problem (e.g., Neuringer, 1981). All of the components of good strategy use interact. For instance, specific strategy knowledge influences the adequate application of memory strategies. As the strategies are carried out, they can be evaluated, which leads to expansion and refinement of specific strategy knowledge (i.e., perhaps that the strategy in use is particularly helpful in this situation). The Good Strategy User Model is taken up in greater detail in Chapters 6 and 7.

In summary, metamemory theory continues to evolve, with this evolution both motivating additional research and being motivated by research outcomes. Given the complexity of metamemory processes, it is not surprising that a variety of research approaches have been required to provide information about the many facets of metamemory. Explicit discussion of how metamemory is assessed sets the stage for discussion of the major findings to date.

Assessment of Metamemory

There are a variety of measures that have been used to capture what children know about memory. In reviewing the various measures, we rely on a distinction introduced by Cavanaugh and Perlmutter (1982). Some measures of metamemory are taken without concurrent memory assessment (independent measures), and others are collected simultaneously with the measurement of memory activity (concurrent measures). Independent measures usually tap pieces of information about memory that children possess, the facts that are known about memory capacities, tasks, strategies, and their interactions. In contrast, concurrent measures tap awareness of ongoing processing—They are measures of monitoring.

Independent Measures: Assessing Knowledge of Facts About Memory

Although paper-and-pencil metamemory questionnaires are often used with adolescents, adults, and elderly persons (see Dixon, 1985; Dixon & Hultsch, 1983a, 1983b; Herrmann, 1982, 1984; Perlmutter, 1978; Zelinski, Gilewski, & Thompson, 1980), they are almost never employed with children. Instead, verbal interviews are conducted with child subjects. Undoubtedly, the best known of these studies was Kreutzer et al. (1975). They interviewed children in kindergarten, grade 1, grade 3, and grade 5 about memory, using 14 items containing one or more questions about memory storage and retrieval. These items assessed knowledge of person variables, task demands, and strategies. Many of the questions involved a decision between two options (e.g., whether to dial a telephone number immediately after hearing it or to get a drink of water before dialing). Other questions demanded more of the children. For instance, children's knowledge of retrieval strategies was tested by asking them to think of all the things they could do to try and find a jacket they had lost while at kindergarten.

Cavanaugh and Borkowski (1980) conducted the only complete replication of Kreutzer et al.'s (1975) study, presumably because of the large number of items in the original research. Other studies (e.g., Borkowski, Peck, Reid, & Kurtz, 1983; Brown, 1978; Kurtz & Borkowski, 1984; Schneider, 1986; Schneider et al., 1986; Weinert et al., 1984) have incorporated some of the items, however, with most of the data consistent with Kreutzer et al.'s (1975) original findings. It has been established that the items used in the study are generally reliable (Kurtz, Reid, Borkowski, & Cavanaugh, 1982). More recent interview studies are even better from a psychometric perspective, however. Hasselhorn (1986) illustrates the improvement in assessment. He began with an extensive item pool and then conducted extensive pilot testing, dropping items that were not sufficiently reliable or did not seem to be otherwise valid.

Nonetheless, it must be admitted that there is a long history of skepticism about the validity of self-reports and interview data (see Brown et al., 1983; Ericsson & Simon, 1980, 1984). Many of the concerns are about the veridicality of verbal reports to actual cognitive processing. These problems are especially acute with children (Cavanaugh & Perlmutter, 1982). Young children's verbal skills are often inadequate for them to articulate their knowledge about memory (Cavanaugh & Perlmutter, 1982; Wellman, 1985a). For instance, do performance differences in metamemory interviews between preschoolers and grade-1 children indicate "true" differences in children's conceptions of memory or differences in the language skills of 5- compared to 6-year-old children? Young children are often less likely to answer at all, or they are less able to elaborate what they say. They are also less schooled in the verbal conventions (e.g., specialized vocabulary) that permit communication about complicated topics (like knowledge of memory). An anecdotal example makes clear that the problem of incomplete verbal reports is not limited to preschoolers, however. Brown (1978) reports that when a 7-year-old was asked what he would do to remember a list of taxonomically categorizable pictures, the child answered that he would look at them. Given the pictures, the child carefully placed them into taxonomic categories and then proceeded to scan them carefully. Asked what he had done to remember, the 7-year-old replied that he had looked at the pictures just like he said that he would. These remarks make evident the importance of converging measures rather than reliance on children's verbal reports alone (e.g., Brown, 1978; Brown et al., 1983; Cavanaugh & Perlmutter, 1982; Meichenbaum, Burland, Gruson, & Cameron, 1985; Schneider, 1985c). There are a number of other independent measures of metamemory that can be employed.

Wellman (1977b) developed a nonverbal technique to explore metacognition in preschoolers. Subjects were asked to make decisions about pairs of pictures, each of which portrayed characters in different memory-related situations. For instance, one picture depicted a girl trying to learn the names of five people and another showed a girl trying to learn the names of 15 people. The task was to answer a question about memory by picking one of the two pictures, with questions concerning memory-relevant variables like age and study time as well as memory irrelevant variables such as the color of the person's hair. Yussen and Bird (1979) developed a similar procedure to test the knowledge of younger subjects about how variables like noise or study time affect memory performance. Wellman (1978) used rank ordering of pictured situations instead of paired comparisons to assess children's knowledge about the interaction of memory variables (e.g., number of items and study time). In all of these studies, age differences in the number of correct solutions have been interpreted as representing developmental improvements in knowledge about memory.

Justice (1985, 1986) developed a procedure that involves presenting various memory strategies (looking, naming, rehearsal, and grouping) on a videotape. After watching the videotape and naming the four strategies (but without an opportunity to see the models attempting recall), the children make paired comparisons of the four strategies. For each pair, the children are asked to state which strategy is better for free recall of the items on a picture list. Investigators (Justice, 1985, 1986; Schneider, 1986; Schneider, Körkel, & Vogel, 1987) using this approach have produced consistent data. Kindergarten and young elementary-school children recognize differential effectiveness only when strategies produce dramatic differences in performance. Older elementary-school children, however, can detect more subtle differences in strategy effectiveness. The conclusion that older children have a better knowledge about the advantages or disadvantages of a particular strategy was validated in Schneider (1986) and in Schneider et al. (1987), with additional analyses in those studies involving the rank ordering of strategies.

Best and Ornstein (1986) have developed a method of assessment based on peer tutoring. The method requires that older children (e.g., third or sixth graders) be asked to tutor a young child (e.g., a first grader) about how to do a task (e.g., sort-recall; see p. 53, this volume) in order to maximize learning. The tutors' assignment is to describe to the younger children what they themselves would do when given a similar task. Tutors' instructions are taped and subjected to content analyses. The measure of metamemory is the extent to which the instructions include appropriate strategy instructions (e.g., appropriate use of organizational strategies for a sort-recall task).

Concurrent Measures: Assessing Memory Monitoring

Concurrent measures are characterized by the presence of simultaneous memory activity (see Cavanaugh & Perlmutter, 1982; Meichenbaum et al., 1985). The number of such measures have increased substantially in recent years, largely due to research efforts in the area of reading (see Baker & Brown, 1984; Brown, 1980; Forrest-Pressley & Waller, 1984; Garner, 1987; Körkel, 1987). We cover here only the concurrent measures used most frequently in metamemory research and that are most theoretically revealing.

Performance predictions, as the name implies, are made prior to study of to-be-remembered material and involve estimation of how much will be learned. A form of performance prediction that has been used often in developmental research is prediction of one's own memory span (e.g., Flavell et al., 1970). Subjects are presented incrementally longer lists of to-be-learned materials (pictures, words, or figures), with the task to indicate whether she or he could still recall a list that long. The child's memory span is then tapped using the same lists. Comparison of the prediction value with actual memory span yields the metamemory indicator, which is usually interpreted as a byproduct of memory monitoring (i.e., children who have monitored their memory proficiently in the past should be more aware of their memory span than children who have not monitored at all or not monitored well in the past). Performance prediction accuracy can be measured for a variety of memory tasks, with recent applications in text learning (e.g., Körkel, 1987; Uhl, 1986).

In contrast to performance predictions, which are made before studying occurs, recall readiness assessments are made after material has been studied at least one time. One variation involves asking subjects to continue studying until their memory of to-be-learned material is perfect. For instance, Flavell et al. (1970) found that 5- to 6-year-old children are often too optimistic about their readiness for a test, with low levels of recall occurring after they claim that they are prepared for a test. Much more realistic assessments can be obtained from older children.

A number of developmental studies have explored children's feeling of knowing (Brown & Lawton, 1977; Cultice, Somerville, & Wellman, 1983; Posnansky, 1978a, 1978b; Wellman, 1977a, 1979). Children are shown series of items and are asked to name them. When a child cannot recall the name of an object given its picture, she or he can be asked to indicate whether the name would be recognized if the experimenter provided it. These feeling-of-knowing ratings are then related to subsequent performance on a recognition test that includes nonrecalled items. Like performance predictions and recall readiness estimates, feeling-of-knowing judgments are taken before the test of interest.

In contrast, other concurrent measures tap memory behaviors as they occur. Thus, verbal protocol techniques (e.g., Ericsson & Simon, 1980, 1984) require subjects either to verbalize all thoughts that come to them while performing a task (i.e., think aloud) or to verbalize between trials.

Finally, children can be asked to judge their memory performance immediately after attempting a task (i.e., make postdictions) (e.g., Berch & Evans, 1973; Bisanz, Vesonder, & Voss, 1978; Kelly, Scholnick, Travers, & Johnson, 1976; Masur, McIntyre, & Flavell, 1973). This can involve estimating overall performance or estimating performance on an item-by-item basis.

Measurement Problems

All methods for assessing metamemory have problems. Some of these are very serious. The existence of such difficulties makes it especially imperative that converging measures be used as often as possible. We touch on some of the more serious difficulties associated with particular approaches.

As discussed already, differences in verbal skills can cloud interpretations of developmental differences obtained using interview measures. There are serious problems in asking children to comment on hypothetical situations (Ericsson & Simon, 1980, 1984), situations that they may have never experienced or may have little memory of experiencing. In addition, interviews usually involve subjects verbalizing about general rather than task-related cognitive processes, which limits the chances of verbal protocols being true reflections of the subjects' experiences (see Brown et al., 1983).

Verbal protocols are subject to many of the criticisms of other interview data (although they are better in that they pertain to a specific task that was just performed). Thinking aloud may also interfere with carrying out the task. The result can be either incomplete reports or changes in task performance from what would occur otherwise, although this is less of a problem if the verbal reports are solicited between trials.

Rank orderings have been criticized because these methods are procedurally complex. For instance, Wellman (1978) required children to compare depictions of three tasks. As it turns out, three-option problems are more difficult for young preschoolers than for older children, regardless of the content of the questions (Steuck, 1984). Individual paired comparisons are conceptually simpler, but often studies involve formidable numbers of comparisons (i.e., all possible paired comparisons are made, and each may be repeated several times in order to obtain reliable data). Fatigue can be a real issue.

Although peer tutoring seems to be a highly motivating situation, there is no guarantee that tutors express all that they know. One likely hypothesis is that they might bias their explanations of strategies downward to match their perceptions of the cognitive levels of tutees (e.g., Shatz & Gelman, 1973).

A number of concerns have been raised about the span estimation task (e.g., Brown, 1978; Cavanaugh & Perlmutter, 1982; Hasselhorn, 1986). For one, the competence of young children can be overestimated if the researcher stops taking estimates once the child indicates that a list is too long—Young children often respond inconsistently, and even if they indicated that they could not recall a list composed of five or six items, they might claim that seven- or eight-item lists would be no problem (Brown, 1978). Whether span estimates are accurate seems to vary with material and task familiarity (e.g., Körkel, 1987; Markman, 1973; Schneider, Körkel, & Weinert, 1987b) or whether children receive training on the task (Markman, 1973; Weaver & Cunningham, 1985). Mode of assessment seems to affect span estimations. For instance, Weaver and Cunningham (1985) found that preschoolers span predictions were more realistic when they listened to items on a tape and used a stop-key to indicate when the list was too long rather than when they responded to verbal probes.

Recall readiness measures can also be criticized. Might young children indicate that they are ready for a test because they understand the task to be one of learning quickly? It is known that younger and older children use different response criteria in evaluating their readiness, with younger children applying more liberal criteria than older children (Worden & Sladewski-Awig, 1982). A similar problem plagues feeling-of-knowing data. Nelson and Narens (1980) have shown that the feeling-of-knowing paradigm confounds the subject's threshold for "know" versus "do not know" responses with their knowledge about unrecalled items. This is a problem in developmental data since knowledge about unrecalled material varies with development.

In summary, there is not a perfect index of any aspect of metamemory. The candor of metamemory researchers about the limitations of their measures is commendable. If anything, they seem to be a little too self-critical, for many of the measurement problems that metamemory researchers confront are similar to measurement problems in other areas of psychology. The forthright approach to these methodological problems has led to considerable methodological progress. For instance, some problems associated with plotting the development of test monitoring have been solved. Pressley and Ghatala (in press; Pressley, Levin, Ghatala, & Ahmad, 1987) devised tests that tap prior knowledge (and thus, monitoring during study is eliminated) and that are equivalently difficult at each age level (and thus, confoundings between developmental level and the objective difficulty of the test are avoided). It is impossible to read the metamemory research produced in the last few years without being impressed at the methodological savvy of investigators overcoming what could have been viewed as insurmountable problems. Even more striking, diverse methodologies often produce converging data. For especially impressive evidence on this point, see Wagoner's (1983) or Garner's (1987) review of monitoring during text learning.

Development of Metamemory

A lot of metamemory data has been produced in the last decade, much of which was orderly and highly informative about children's knowledge about memory. We understand better both (a) children's long-term, factual knowledge about memory and (b) their abilities to monitor memory. Brief coverage of these two acquisitions is provided in this section, with findings organized on the basis of some of the major research directions pursued by metamemory researchers.

Children's Factual Knowledge About Memory

WHEN DO CHILDREN KNOW THE RELEVANT MENTAL VERBS?

A basic type of metamemory is understanding mental verbs, such as *thinking, forgetting,* or *knowing.* Although Kreutzer et al. (1975) provided evidence that the youngest participants in their study (kindergarten children) could properly apply mental verbs, it has proven more difficult to determine preschoolers' knowledge of mental verbs. Misciones, Marvin, O'Brien, and Greenburg (1978), who studied the verbs *knowing* and *guessing,* and Wellman and Johnson (1979), who conducted research on *remembering* and *forgetting,* asked preschoolers to judge the "mental status" of an agent who either watched an object be hidden or who was blindfolded as an object was hidden. The agent then searched for the object, sometimes finding it and sometimes not. Thus, the agent should have been labeled as *forgetting*, if he possessed the necessary prior knowledge but did not find the object; if the prior knowledge was available and the performance correct, then the agent should have been credited with *remembering* or *knowing*; and *guessing* was the appropriate label when there was no prior knowledge available, regardless of whether the object was located. In both studies, however, preschool children judged mental status more on the basis of whether the object was found than on the basis of the prior knowledge possessed by the agent. Whenever the agent in Misciones et al. (1978) performed correctly, the preschoolers used the label *knowing*; incorrect actions were labeled *guessing*. Correct actions (locating the object) were described as *remembering* by Wellman and Johnson's (1979) subjects; incorrect actions are consistently defined as *forgetting*.

In a follow-up study, Johnson and Wellman (1980) hypothesized that the ability of preschoolers to distinguish between internal and external worlds might be demonstrable using an additional "trick condition." The children observed as an object was hidden in one of three boxes. The children were then requested to tell where the object was and were immediately proven wrong. Instead of saying that this was due to *lack of knowledge*, the subjects stubbornly insisted that they *knew* and *remembered* where the object was, even though it was not found there. Mental verbs were correctly applied to mental states at all age levels (4-, 5-, 7-, and 9-year-olds) in this trick condition. Comparisons of the outcomes in Johnson and Wellman (1980) with Wellman and Johnson (1979) and Misciones et al. (1978) makes clear that different conclusions can follow from collection of data using different methods—although 4-year-olds in Johnson and Wellman (1980) used mental verbs correctly, the results in Wellman and Johnson (1979) and Misciones et al. (1978) establish that children's competent use of these verbs is highly constrained.

Knowledge of Person Variables

Knowledge about person variables includes knowledge about all variables or permanent personality attributes or states that can influence memory of information (Flavell & Wellman, 1977). Kreutzer et al. (1975) included only one item that tapped knowledge of person variables. They found that 9- and 11-year-olds could better conceptualize memory abilities in that they realized that memorization skills vary from person to person and from situation to situation. The 9- and 11-year-olds also knew that they did not have an equally good memory in all situations and it was quite possible that their friends had a better memory than they did. In contrast, most of the kindergarten and first-grade subjects were convinced that they always remembered well and that they were better at remembering than their friends. In fact, 30% of the kindergarten children were convinced that they never forgot anything. This finding is consistent with other demonstrations that the memory-related self-concept of young children is unrealistic (e.g., Schneider, 1985b; Schneider et al., 1986; Weinert et al., 1984). Five- and 6-year-olds generally tend to overestimate their performance.

Wellman (1977b) included a total of four items that provided information about person-related metamemory possessed by preschool children. Three of these items were related to irrelevant personal characteristics such as hair color, clothing, or weight, whereas the fourth item was directed at a memory-relevant personal characteristic (age). A little more than 75% of the 3- and 4-year-olds and all of the 5-year-olds rated two of the three irrelevant factors as not important as determinants of memory (e.g., judged that whether a person was fat or thin would not influence memory performance). Even more impressive, most of the children were also able to provide appropriate reasoning for their decisions. In contrast, however, only about 50% of the children in the sample recognized that memory improves with increasing age.

Preliminary results from the Munich Longitudinal Study on the Development of Individual Competencies (Weinert & Schneider, 1987a, 1987b) also indicate that 4-year-old children do not know that chronological age is a correlate of memory performance. Only about 33% of the children in the study were able to judge correctly that there was an association between age and memory. In contrast to Wellman (1977b), however, almost half (49%) of the 4-year-old subjects in the Munich study assumed that hair color was correlated with memory performance.

In closing this subsection, it should be pointed out, however, that the modest knowledge about the effects of age on memory that is possessed by preschoolers is only evident when age is a salient variable in the metamemory assessment items. Much less awareness of the age-memory association is obtained with problems in which age is a less obvious factor (Wellman, 1977b; Yussen & Bird, 1979). Preschool children clearly have difficulty in determining the importance of relatively stable personal characteristics that determine memory performance.

KNOWLEDGE OF TASK VARIABLES

Although there is not much research on knowledge about person characteristics that determine memory, there are a number of studies evaluating children's knowledge of task factors that affect memory. Wellman (1977b) provided the first hints that knowledge of task characteristics is available at the preschool level. The study included items related to a variety of factors that can affect memory, such as properties of materials (e.g., how much material there is to learn), circumstances of the learning situation (e.g., noise & length of study time), and external supports (e.g., help from friends or retrieval cues). The clearest results supporting competency in preschool children were obtained for the "number of items" and "noise" variables. Eighty-two percent of the children were convinced that 18 items are more difficult to remember than 3 items; 66% of the subjects said that noise negatively influences memory performance. In contrast, only 37% of the subjects assumed that friends could be of help in retention, and only about 26% felt that the amount of total learning time would have an effect on memory performance.

Later studies (Weinert et al., 1984; Yussen & Bird, 1979) produced data suggesting that, if anything, Wellman (1977b) overestimated preschoolers' knowledge of task variables. For instance, in both the Munich longitudinal study and in Yussen and Bird's (1979) research, only about 40% of the 4-year-old subjects could judge correctly the effect of the number of items on the difficulty of memory problems. The 4-year-old subjects in the Yussen and Bird study also made fewer correct responses for the noise and time variables compared to the preschoolers in Wellman's (1977b) research (11% vs. 55%). Interpretation of Wellman's (1977b) data is especially clouded because he eliminated subjects who could not answer simple control questions correctly (i.e., 35% of the 3-year-olds, 25% of the 4-year-olds, and 10% of the 5-year-olds). If one assumes that these subjects probably would have made incorrect responses to the materials questions, Wellman's data are more compatible with those in the Munich study and in Yussen and Bird (1979).

Yussen and Bird reported that 6-year-olds' understanding of the significance of task characteristics is much more complete than the understanding of preschool children. About 78% of the grade-1, 6-year-olds in their study knew that the number of items affected memory performance. Eighty-nine percent of the grade-1 subjects indicated that noise negatively influences learning performance. Even the most difficult item (i.e., the relevancy of learning time for performance) was answered correctly by about half of the 6-year-olds.

Although these results seem to indicate that by grade 1, children know a great deal about the importance of some task characteristics on memory performance, it must be emphasized that other variables are poorly understood by young children. For instance, 7-, 9-, and 10-year-old students in Moynahan's (1978) study were asked to judge which of two lists would be easier to learn, one composed of taxonomically organized items or one composed of conceptually unrelated words. Although both older groups recognized the advantages conferred by taxonomic structure, this did not hold true for the 7-year-olds. This result has been confirmed in followup studies (Schneider, 1986; Schneider et al., 1987; Weinert et al., 1984). Grade-1 children also lack knowledge of retrieval factors and their effects on memory: (a) The majority of grade-1 children in Speer and Flavell (1979) did not recognize that recognition memory tasks are easier than recall tasks (i.e., recall requires more retrieval). (b) Fifty-five percent and 65% of Kreutzer et al.'s kindergarten and grade-1 subjects respectively knew that gist recall was easier than verbatim recall, compared to 100% of grade-5 children who understood that verbatim recall was a more difficult retrieval task. Other studies (Borkowski et al., 1983; Kurtz & Borkowski, 1987; Kurtz, Schneider, Turner, & Carr, 1986; Myers & Paris, 1978) suggest that, if anything, Kreutzer et al. (1975) overestimated kindergarten and grade-1 children's understanding of the relative ease of gist and verbatim recall. (c) Although the majority of preschool and kindergarten children know that memory tasks are easier when retrieval cues are available, sophisticated understanding of retrieval cues and how they work develops during the grade-school years (Beal, 1985; Schneider & Sodian, 1988).

KNOWLEDGE ABOUT AN ESPECIALLY IMPORTANT TASK: TEXT AND ITS STRUCTURE

One of the most common types of to-be-processed and to-be-learned materials in the real world is text. Thus, it may not be surprising that a good deal of effort has been expended determining children's knowledge of text structure. Brown and her colleagues (e.g., Brown & Smiley, 1977) have conducted very visible research on this problem. Students were asked to rate the pieces of information in text as most important (top one-fourth), slightly less important (second one-fourth), less important still (third one-fourth), and least important. Although grade-7 students provided importance ratings that were roughly equivalent to the ratings provided by college-student adults, grade-3 and grade-5 children's ratings differed greatly from those of adults. One possible explanation of the apparently late development of text knowledge in this study is that the texts were fairly long and complicated as was the rating procedure.

Investigators who have used shorter and less complicated texts as well as less complicated rating systems have produced data suggesting greater knowledge of text structure by elementary-school children. Unlike Brown's research, most of the follow-up studies used texts constructed on the basis of formal story grammars (Kintsch & van Dijk, 1978; Stein & Glenn, 1979). (See Chapter 4 for a brief discussion of story grammar.) High metacognitive knowledge was assumed in these studies when children identified the most important elements in text to be the ones that are more central according to story grammar models.

For instance, Yussen, Mathews, Buss, and Kane (1980) showed that fifth graders could differentiate central information from less important information in text, but that grade-2 children could not do so. Hoppe-Graff and Schöler (1980) obtained comparable results, as did Denhiere and Le Ny (1980). Recent studies have suggested, not surprisingly, that children are more proficient at differentiating important from less important information when reading text based on contents in which they possess expertise (Denhiere, Cession, & Deschene, 1986; Körkel, 1987).

Perhaps the most impressive demonstration of early knowledge of the relative importance of text elements was provided by Young and Schumacher (1983). Even 4- and 6-year-old children were sensitive to relative importance levels within simple picture stories. The importance ratings of preschool children correlated significantly with those of adults; the ratings of 6-year-olds were very similar to those of adults. Young and Schumacher's (1983) study is a clear example of the great effect that materials modifications can have on task difficulty. A finding such as this one prompts skepticism when researchers try to set an absolute age limit for certain abilities.

KNOWLEDGE ABOUT STRATEGIES THAT ARE USEFUL FOR "NATURAL" MEMORY TASKS

Since simple strategies are used in natural settings as early as the second year of life (see Chapter 3), it might be surmised that preschool and kindergarten children would possess elementary knowledge of memory strategies, particularly ones that could be used in real-world memory tasks.

Kreutzer et al. (1975) included one item to assess knowledge of strategies that could be used in preparation for future retrieval. Participants were asked to tell everything that they could do in order to be sure that they would remember to take their ice skates to school the next day. The answers could be placed into four main categories. The three *external* categories involved manipulation of the skates (e.g., putting them near the door), use of external memory cues (e.g., notes), and relying on cues provided by other people (e.g., asking a parent to provide a reminder). The fourth category of answers involved *internal* processes that the child could carry out (e.g., rehearsal of the fact that the skates needed to be taken to school). There was a significant developmental increase in the number of strategies reported, although even kindergarten children were able to come up with at least one strategy each. All age groups reported more external than internal strategies. The strategies reported by grade-3 and grade-5 children seemed more clearcut and efficient than those provided by kindergarten and grade-1 participants. In their replication work, Borkowski and his associates (Borkowski et al., 1983; Cavanaugh & Borkowski, 1980; Kurtz & Borkowski, 1987) have obtained generally comparable data in response to the "skates" question.

A similar strategy question was included in the Munich Longitudinal Study (Weinert & Schneider, 1986, 1987a, 1987b). Four-year-olds were asked what they could do in order to remember to take their snack to preschool the next day. Children in this age group reported only external strategies, with 14% of the children suggesting a manipulation of the snack (e.g., put it near the door); 3% suggested construction of a note; and 3% said that they would ask someone else to help.

Kreutzer et al. (1975) also included an item to assess knowledge of retrieval strategies. the question was, "What would one do to find a jacket that had been lost in school?" The answers were classified by Kreutzer et al. (1975) in two main categories, "search" referring to search procedures carried out by the child and "other" strategies referring to solutions that involved other people. Subjects at all age levels suggested looking places where the jacket would be likely to be found (e.g., the cloakroom) and asking people who would be likely to be helpful (e.g., the teacher). Every kindergarten child offered at least one solution, with grade-1 children averaging two solutions. Suggestions to search systematically and elaborately were offered more often by older (grade-5 children) compared to the younger participants. Follow-up research has provided data that complements the Kreutzer et al. (1975) findings. Only about 25% of the 4-year-olds in the Munich Longitudinal Study generated retrieval strategies. Yussen and Levy (1977) reported that the number of reported strategies for retrieval of a lost object increased up until about 10-years of age; the number of strategies for finding an internal piece of information (how can one remember a birthday present that one thought to be a good idea but has forgotten in the meantime) increases well into adolescence according to the Yussen and Levy (1977) data.

Kreutzer et al.'s (1975) study also included problems that required subjects to make preparations to remember an upcoming event (i.e., the birthday party of a friend) and to retrieve information about an event that had already happened (i.e., to remember that Christmas when a particular present was received). The birthday party problem produced data that was similar to the data generated for the ice skates problem. Even the youngest children could come up with a strategy or two, with more and increasingly sophisticated strategies reported by the older children. In contrast, the memory-of-Christmas problem was extremely difficult. Kreutzer et al. (1975) reported that kindergarten children could hardly understand the task. First graders said that they would seek assistance from other people, as did third graders. Although fifth-grade subjects produced more strategies and more varied strategies, there was still room for improvement. Others (Cavanaugh & Borkowski, 1980; Kurtz & Borkowski, 1987) have confirmed that very few adequate responses are generated for the memory-of-Christmas item until the end of the grade-school years.

What emerges from the Kreutzer et al. (1975) data and the follow-up research is a portrait of developing knowledge of strategies from 4 years of age through the grade-school years and into adolescence. The development of knowledge about strategies during the grade-school years has been confirmed in other research aimed at elucidating children's understanding of strategies suitable for performing laboratory tasks.

KNOWLEDGE ABOUT STRATEGIES THAT ARE USEFUL FOR FREE RECALL TASKS

Children's knowledge about organizational strategies was tapped by a single item in Kreutzer et al. (1975). The subjects were shown nine picture cards (three from each of three categories), and they were told to imagine that these items had to be learned in a few minutes. They were also told that they could do anything they wished to acquire the items. There was a clear age trend. Only one kindergarten child used a categorization strategy, although many grade-5 subjects did so. When partial category use was scored, 35% of the kindergarten children, 40% of the grade-1 subjects, 70% of the grade-3 participants, and 80% of the grade-5 subjects evidenced rudimentary knowledge of organizational strategies.

Data on knowledge of categorization strategies has also been generated by comparing videotaped presentations of strategies pairwise. Sodian et al. (1986) presented lists containing items that could be categorized taxonomically or by color. The 4- and 6-year-olds made pairwise comparisons between taxonomic sorting, color sorting, random sorting, and looking strategies. The judgments of the 4- and 6-year-olds differed little, with only one significant difference between the two age groups. The taxonomic sorting strategy was judged much more positively by the older children. More negatively, the 6-year-olds did not realize that the taxonomic-sorting strategy was more potent than the color-sorting approach.

The shift in knowledge about free recall strategies between kindergarten and grade 6 was obvious in three studies using the paired-comparison method (Justice, 1985, 1986; Schneider, 1986). In general, preschoolers considered "looking at" as the best strategy, with taxonomic sorting, rehearsal, and naming trailing in popularity. Kindergarten children were more likely to view all four strategies as equally effective. Second and fourth graders preferred grouping and rehearsal, but did not differentiate between these two. By grade 6 there is clear understanding that semantic-grouping strategies are superior to rehearsal, naming, and looking.

KNOWLEDGE ABOUT THE INTERACTION OF MEMORY VARIABLES

Until now, we have considered children's knowledge of task, person, and strategy variables separately. Wellman in particular has assessed children's knowledge of how these variables interact, however. Wellman (1978) presented memory problems to 5- and 10-year-olds. Each problem consisted of ranking three picture cards, each of which contained a memorizing scenario (the three scenarios differing with respect to the likelihood of successful memory performance). For instance, one set consisted of pictures of three boys, each of whom was supposed to remember some items, either three, nine, or 18 items. Thus, this was a simple problem tapping a single task variable (i.e., number of items). A complicated interaction problem (item by strategy interaction) was depicted with the following three cards: (a) boy A who was to remember 18 items merely by looking at them; (b) boy B who just looked at three items; (c) boy C who wrote down the names of three items. This metamemory question was considered to be answered correctly if a subject indicated that boy A was less likely to do well than boy B who was less likely to do well compared to boy C.

Neither the 5- or 10-year-olds had any trouble solving the simple memory problems; there were, however, substantial developmental differences for the complex memory problems. Although the 10-year-olds performed almost perfectly, the 5-year-olds only answered 32% of the complex memory problems correctly. The younger children tended to estimate task difficulty by taking only one of the two relevant features into account.

Does Wellman's (1978) result mean that preschool children are not capable of considering and comparing two different features of memory problems at the same time? Probably not. Wellman, Collins, and Glieberman (1981) focused on knowledge about the combined effects of a task variable (i.e., the number of items to be remembered) and a person variable (i.e., the amount of effort expended). Three values of each of these variables were combined factorally to create nine different picture cards. The subjects' task (5-, 8-, 10-, and 19-year-olds) consisted of predicting how many items the boy on the card would remember. Prediction of memory performance served as the dependent variable. The most important result was that all of the children were aware of the combined influence of number of items and effort on probability of success, although there were differences between the age groups due to different weighting of the two factors as determinants of memory performance. Compared to the older children, younger children did not consider the amount to be learned to be a particularly important variable, weighting effort much more heavily. This result is consistent with young children's general tendency to attribute success to effort (Kun, 1977; Nicholls, 1978). Although the older children gave greater consideration to the amount that was to be learned, only the 19-year-olds made performance predictions that reflected appropriately balanced consideration of both variables in combination.

How can the apparent inconsistencies in Wellman (1978) and Wellman et al. (1981) be explained? Wellman (1978) required ranking of three scenes that varied with respect to two variables. Wellman et al. hypothesized that preschoolers in that situation concentrated on one variable and ignored the other one entirely. Thus, Wellman et al. presented only one value of each of the two variables at a time, which should have been easier than simultaneous consideration of three pairs of values, especially for younger subjects. Although Wellman et al. succeeded in showing that 5-year-olds possess at least elementary knowledge of the combined influence of two variables, Wellman's data (1978; Wellman et al., 1981) also make clear that interactive memory knowledge develops very slowly. This development continues well into adolescence.

Using sensitive methods that minimize demands on the child, it is possible to demonstrate some rudimentary knowledge of the metamemorial facts in pre-schoolers (e.g., some understanding of mental verbs, knowledge of important versus less important elements in picture stories). Knowledge of facts about memory is more impressive in the primary-grade years, and much more complete by 11 or 12 years of age. Nonetheless, knowledge of memory is not complete by the end of child-hood. For instance, understanding the relative importance of text elements con-tinues to develop, as does understanding of task and person-variable interactions that determine memory.

One of the most important findings produced by metamemory researchers is that there is increasing knowledge of strategies with increasing age. Nonetheless, although late grade-school children know most of the strategies covered by the metamemory measures reviewed in this section, there is increasing evidence that many adolescents (including college students) have little or no knowledge of some powerful and important memory strategies. There is also increasing knowledge about the characteristics of the strategies that children do know, including their rela-tive potencies—This is absolutely critical metamemory for efficient thinking to take place. The role of this type of metamemory will be discussed throughout the remainder of this book.

Memory Monitoring

PERFORMANCE PREDICTION ACCURACY

If people have monitored their previous performances adequately, they should be able to predict future memory performances, and be better able to do so than people who have not monitored in the past. That is the logic of accepting performance prediction accuracy as a measure of monitoring.

While preschool children overpredict their memory performance consistently, elementary-school children are much more accurate (e.g., Flavell et al., 1970; Kelly, Scholnick, Travers, & Johnston, 1976; Levin, Yussen, De Rose & Pressley, 1977; Markman, 1973; Monroe & Lange, 1977; Worden & Sladewski-Awig, 1982). Whether elementary-school children over- or underestimate performance seems to vary with the memory task. For instance, serial memory span is usually over-estimated (e.g., Flavell et al., 1970), whereas recall of categorizable lists is under-estimated (e.g., Worden & Sladewski-Awig, 1982). (The latter result is probably not surprising given elementary-school children's lack of awareness of the effects of categorizing on memory as discussed earlier in this chapter.)

Several studies have tried to pinpoint preschoolers' difficulties in making perfor-mance predictions. One likely possibility is that many memory tasks are completely unfamiliar to preschoolers. Thus, preschool children make more realistic predictions when asked how far they can jump (Markman, 1973). Predictions are also more accurate when the memory task is conducted in a familiar context, such as a game (Justice & Bray, 1979) or in a simulated shopping situation (Wippich, 1980).

A particularly interesting question is whether predictions of overall performance improve in accuracy as experience with the memory task increases. There seems to be developmental improvement here. Subjects in Schneider (1986), Schneider et al. (1986), and Uhl and Schneider (in preparation) made a prediction before attempting a list-learning task. Then, after completing the list-learning task and testing over the material on the list, the subjects were told that they would be doing another list-learning task and were asked to predict performance on this second list. Although first and second predictions do not differ in accuracy for grade-2 and grade-3 children, grade-4 children's predictions did improve with practice. Pressley and Ghatala (in press) provided complementary data. In their study, grade-1 and -2, grade-4 and -5, and grade-7 and -8 subjects predicted performance on a vocabulary test, took the test, and then predicted performance on a future test of comparable difficulty. Although there was no evidence of prediction improvement from first to second prediction at the grade-1 and -2 level, there was a strong trend toward improvement at the grade-4 and -5 level, and unambiguous improvement from first to second prediction at the grade-7 and -8 level.

More negatively, prediction improvement may be limited to tasks involving fairly simple materials. When Uhl and Schneider's subjects went through the prediction-learning-testing-prediction-learning-testing cycle with prose materials, there were no improvements in prediction with practice. Uhl and Schneider (in preparation) speculated that accurate awareness of the amount recalled on a test of prose content may be less certain than accurate awareness for list items, and thus, test monitoring during prose study and testing might not be sufficient to permit improvements in predictions about future prose learning. (It was obvious in Pressley & Ghatala's, in press, study with simpler materials that prior test monitoring and future test predictions were related.)

In addition to being able to predict overall performance better than preschoolers, grade-school children are also capable of predicting which items on a list are more likely to be remembered than other items (Kelly et al., 1976; Monroe & Lange, 1977; Worden & Sladewski-Awig, 1982). There are developmental shifts in accuracy of individual-item predictions, however. For example, Worden and Sladewski-Awig demonstrated that grade-2 children were more liberal than grade-6 children in their predictions. Thus, the younger children were more likely than the older children to predict memory of items that in fact were not remembered subsequently.

In summary, the most obvious improvement in performance prediction is the shift between preschool and the elementary-school years from great overconfidence in future performance to more reasonable expectations. There are also more subtle improvements during the elementary-school years, including increased use of awareness of past performance as a predictor of future performance and increased awareness of the relative recallability of particular pieces of information.

Monitoring When Information Is "On the Tip of the Tongue"

Wellman (1977a) studied the accuracy of children's feelings that they knew items, even when they could not recall them. He showed children pictures and asked them to name the object in each picture. For those objects that were not named, feeling-of-knowing judgments were elicited: The subjects were asked whether they knew the item well enough that they would recognize its name if they heard it. Then, a recognition test was given in which the name of the object was provided with the child required to select the item from a group of pictures. Feeling-of-knowing accuracy increased from kindergarten (youngest subjects in the study) to grade 3 (oldest subjects in the study). Wellman (1977a) also noted that only the grade-3 children registered the frustration that is typical of adults who have something on the tip of their tongue, but who cannot remember it. (See Brown and Lawton, 1977, for similar developmental trends in a study of children with learning difficulties.)

Cultice et al. (1983) presented 4- to 5-year-old children a simplified version of the task used by Wellman (1977a). The participants were asked to name children who were depicted on photos presented to them. The pictures included very familiar faces (i.e., children from their own preschool group), somewhat less familiar faces (i.e., children from another group in the preschool), and completely unfamiliar pictures. When the children could not name the person in the picture, they were quite capable of saying whether they would recognize the person when the name was provided. Thus, when feeling-of-knowing problems are simply structured and involve highly meaningful materials like faces, even preschoolers evidence the memory-monitoring competence tapped by the feeling-of-knowing task.

Knowledge of Recall Readiness

In Flavell et al.'s (1970) study of memory span, kindergarten, grade-1, grade-2, and grade-4 subjects provided recall readiness data. The subjects were asked to study the learning material long enough to be absolutely certain that they would be able to recall the entire list perfectly. There was clear developmental improvement in estimation of recall readiness. Kindergarten and grade-1 children were usually unable to recall the entire list correctly, although they believed that they would be able to do so. Recall readiness estimates of grade-2 and grade-4 subjects were considerably more accurate. Flavell et al. believed that the older children's more accurate assessments were due to their greater use of self-testing during study.

One of the problems with Flavell et al.'s (1970) study was that relatively short lists were used, ones corresponding to each child's memory span. Markman (1973) demonstrated conclusively that recall readiness assessment skills are typically overestimated when children learn materials that are not particularly challenging. More positively, even very young children can be taught self-testing strategies that permit them to make reasonably accurate recall readiness judgments during list learning. Brown and Barclay (1976) demonstrated that even children with learning disabilities (mental age = 8 years) can do so.

KNOWLEDGE OF WHICH ITEMS REQUIRE ADDITIONAL STUDY

Masur et al. (1973) required grade-1, grade-3, and college students to learn a list of pictures and then free recall them. After the first study and first recall trial, subjects were instructed to select half the pictures for additional study. Although grade-3 and college students tended to select items not recalled correctly on the first trial, grade-1 subjects did not seem to consider first-trial performance in making selection of items for additional processing. Similar findings were reported by Bisanz et al. (1978) for a paired-associate task. They found that grade-5 and college students were more likely than grade-1 or grade-3 students to select items not learned on a first trial.

It is somewhat puzzling that young grade-school children do not choose to allocate more study to items that they have not yet mastered? It does not seem likely that it is because they are unaware of which materials are not known. For instance, Pressley et al. (1987) and Pressley and Ghatala (in press) both showed that even grade-1 and -2 children are aware of which test items they are almost certainly answering correctly and which are probably answered incorrectly, albeit there is developmental improvement in these discriminations during the grade-school years. When processing differentially learnable text, even grade-2 children know which parts of text are easier to acquire than others (e.g., Danner, 1976). Apparently, knowing which information is known already or easier to learn and which information is unlikely to have been mastered is not sufficient to result in appropriate self-regulation (i.e., studying the items that have yet to be learned). See Kobasigawa and Dufresne (in press) for an exceptionally thorough and intelligent discussion of potential relationships between awareness of knowledge state and whether cognitive self-regulation occurs.

Some of the work of Ann Brown and her associates suggests that sophisticated selection of text material for additional study develops somewhat later than the grade-school years. An optimal strategy for restudy of text is to concentrate not on the most important ideas of the text (which will probably be recalled anyway) but rather to concentrate on ideas of intermediate importance. One source of difficulty for children is that they are not aware of the relative importance of different parts of complicated text (Brown & Smiley, 1977; Kurtz & Schneider, in press), even though they can differentiate important from less important information in short texts and simple, conventionally-structured stories (e.g., Denhiere & Le Ny, 1980; Hoppe-Graff & Schöler, 1980; Yussen et al., 1980). Brown, Smiley, and Lawton (1978) demonstrated that between ages 5 and college there is development in knowledge of parts of text not mastered during a first study-test cycle. Consistent with the hypothesis that children would not make effective use of additional study opportunity, Brown and Smiley (1978) demonstrated that grade-5 children's recall of text did not improve following five minutes of additional study. Grade-7, grade-8, and high-school students did benefit from the additional study time, with the total pattern of data suggesting that knowledge of text parts that were not yet mastered may have directed restudy at those age levels.

SUMMARY: MONITORING

The only evidence of monitoring in preschoolers was produced in a simplified feeling-of-knowing task. Although there are clear increases in monitoring skills during the grade-school years, additional developments occur during adolescence. Additional developmental data on monitoring are presented in Chapter 7. The data reviewed there are also consistent with the conclusion that effective monitoring occurs only in highly constrained situations during the early grade-school years and continues to develop well into adolescence.

Metamemory-Memory Relationships

One of the main motivations for research on metamemory has been the theoretical conviction that there are important relationships between knowing about memory and memory behaviors (e.g., Brown, 1978; Hagen, 1975). Such relationships have sometimes proven elusive, however. Why might there be occasions when a child possesses important pieces of metamemory (e.g., knowledge of how to execute categorization-organizational strategies and that their use improves recall), but does not use the knowledge (e.g., does not use categorization strategies to learn a categorizable list of items)? There are a lot of potential reasons (Flavell & Wellman, 1977; Weinert, 1984, 1986). For one, the learner might not be motivated to exert the effort necessary to use the strategy; the learner may be too tired to carry out the strategy; or there may not be sufficient time to use the procedure. If the list is so short that it can be learned without strategic effort, no strategy may be employed. If the list is so long that the child perceives that there is no hope of mastering it, the child may make no strategic efforts. Even if a child knows that a strategy facilitates performance and is willing to say so on a metamemory interview, he or she may still believe that pure effort represents the best strategy (Wellman, 1983). Perhaps it should not be surprising that metamemory-memory behavior correlations are far from perfect.

But are they inconsequential, as suggested by some reviewers (e.g., Cavanaugh & Perlmutter, 1982)? Our point of view is that one of the best ways to begin to come to terms with *all* of the available evidence is through meta-analytic procedures (e.g., Hedges & Olkin, 1985). Schneider (1985c) reported such an analysis of studies containing metamemory-memory relationship data. Following Glass, McGaw, and Smith (1981), he simply averaged the available correlation coefficients from the individual studies, reporting an overall correlation of 0.41.

Since that analysis, it has become clear that it is better to estimate an overall correlation by averaging over individual correlations that are weighted by the sample sizes that generated them (Hunter, Schmidt, & Jackson, 1982; Fricke & Treinies, 1985). Thus, a meta-analysis is summarized briefly here, with correlations weighted by sample sizes (as were variances). With the exception of this one change, this meta-analysis is procedurally identical to Schneider's (1985c) evaluation of the literature. The meta-analysis involves aggregation of conventional product-moment correlations. In a number of cases, this required calculation of the correlations from t, F, and χ^2 statistics. Those few studies that did not summarize data in sufficient detail to permit calculation of the correlation were dropped from the meta-analysis. When a publication contained several independent experiments, each experiment was treated as a separate study. When authors reported coefficients for several dependent variables, average correlations were calculated within the study following procedures outlined by Hunter et al. (1982).

Updating Schneider's (1985c) meta-analysis was also mandated by the enormous number of new publications containing estimates of metamemory-memory relationships. Schneider's (1985c) meta-analysis was based on 27 publications, which generated 47 correlations based on a total of 2231 subjects. The current meta-analysis is based on 60 publications providing 123 correlation coefficients based on data from 7097 subjects. Since much more data were available for this new meta-analysis, a more exact estimate of the overall correlation was expected.

The most important finding in this new meta-analysis was that the overall metamemory-memory correlation coefficient was 0.41, exactly the same value produced by Schneider (1985c). The standard deviation was reduced, however, from 0.18 to 0.14. The overall correlations as a function of grade and kind of study are summarized in Table 5.1. (Because some authors only reported correlations aggregated over age, there are fewer correlations for each age level than could have been the case with more complete reporting of data in the individual reports.)

In summary, there is no doubt that there is a statistical association between metamemory and memory. More pessimistic evaluations based on only a very small portion of the data base (e.g., Cavanaugh & Perlmutter, 1982) were in error. There are two problems (memory monitoring, organizational strategies) that have been studied in especially great detail, with metamemory-performance relationships obtained in both of these literatures. Even though caution is required in evaluating the age trends due to the small number of correlations contributing to some of the values reported in Table 5.1, the data are generally homogenous from grade 4 on. The correlations for memory monitoring are greater than the correlations for organizational strategies at the younger age levels. Although this meta-analysis provides a good sense of the overall quantitative relationships in the data, qualitative analyses of studies of metamemory-memory relationships are still revealing, making especially clear that some metamemory-performance relationships are more theoretically compelling than others. Not surprisingly, some metamemory-performance correlations are more likely to be obtained than are others. In addition, examination of significant metamemory-performance correlations makes obvious that some of these index situations where metamemory might play a causal role in directing processing, and through direction of processing, play a causal role in memory. Sometimes, it is apparent that such a causal sequence is unlikely. Four of the more visible questions that have been explored as part of the search for metamemory-performance correlations are considered in greater detail in the remainder of this section.

TABLE 5.1. Overall correlations between metamemory and memory, classified by kind of study and school grade of subjects (number of studies providing data in parentheses).

Type of study	School grade					
	K	1/2	3/4	5/6	7 +	Average
Memory monitoring	.39	.45	.35	.42	.59	.39
(lab tasks)	(5)	(7)	(10)	(8)	(2)	(16)
Memory monitoring	.24	–	.28	.49	.41	.44
(text processing)	(2)		(3)	(10)	(4)	(15)
Memory monitoring	–	.52	.37	.37	.28	.40
(training studies)		(4)	(10)	(10)	(1)	(13)
Organizational strategies	.12	.15	.41	.47	–	.33
(clustering)	(1)	(6)	(14)	(5)		(43)
Organizational strategies	–	.39	.32	–	–	.37
(training studies)		(10)	(19)			(36)

Relationships Between Prediction Accuracy and Memory Performance

People who are good information processors should have good memories. Presumably, proficient information processors also monitor their performances better than poor information processors. Thus, they should know more about their memory capacities and limitations and be better able to predict their memory performances than other people. Therefore, people who have good memories should predict memory more accurately than people with poor memories.

The first explicit test of the relationship between prediction accuracy and memory performance was conducted by Kelly et al. (1976) who obtained negative results. There was no obvious relationship between prediction accuracy and memory in their study. Ceiling effects might have played a part in this failure, however (Schneider, 1985c). Since prediction accuracy was generally very high at all age levels, it probably is not surprising that the correlations between prediction accuracy and memory performance were low (i.e., there was restricted range in the metamemory measure).

Follow-up investigations were more successful in establishing prediction accuracy-recall relationships. Levin et al. (1977) administered recall and recognition tasks to grade-1, grade-5, and college students and elicited performance predictions for both tasks. The authors hypothesized that higher prediction accuracy would be obtained for recall compared to recognition, arguing that recall tasks are more like the memory tasks that children and college students usually confront. As expected, there were correlations between prediction accuracy for recall at all age levels, but generally poor prediction accuracy for the recognition test. In general, the Levin et al. (1977) results were replicated by Yussen and Berman (1981) with grade-1, grade-3, and grade-5 subjects. In both studies, children tended to overestimate recall, with developmental increases in prediction accuracy with respect to recall (i.e., overestimations declined with increasing age). There was clear underestimation of recognition memory in both studies. In general, people do not realize how really good recognition memory can be!

Wippich (1981) found that even kindergarten children could provide reasonable predictions about their recall in everyday situations (i.e, shopping). Wippich found no relationship between prediction accuracy and recall in children's recall in the laboratory, however.

In summary, although there was some evidence of prediction accuracy-memory linkages in these studies, there was also clear data that prediction accuracy-performance relationships were task specific (e.g., obtained with recall but not recognition, more likely in "natural" situations with 5-year-olds).

Additional evidence of specificity has been obtained when there have been comparisons between performance prediction-memory relationships for categorizable versus noncategorizable lists. The earliest work on prediction of recall of categorizable and noncategorizable lists established that by the middle of the elementary-school years, there is clear understanding that categorizable lists can be learned more easily than noncategorizable lists (e.g., Moynahan, 1973; Yussen, Levin, Berman, & Palm, 1979). More recent studies (Hasselhorn, 1986; Schneider et al., 1987; Weinert et al., 1984) have focused on the differences in prediction accuracy for the two types of lists. In general, the performance prediction-memory correlations in these studies were positive, but not large (i.e., typically in the .10 to .30 range). There were developmental trends, with increasing correlations between prediction and performance with increasing age during the grade-school years. The correlations between predictions and performance were higher for the noncategorizable than for the categorizable lists. The lower correlations for the categorizable lists were due in part to general underestimation of the positive effect of list structure on memory.

A likely hypothesis is that metamemory-memory relationships are greater when memory tasks are more difficult. More difficult tasks require more explicitly controlled processing in order to produce high recall, with controlled processing presumably more likely to be initiated by metacognitively advanced learners (Borkowski, 1985; Pressley, 1985). That the prediction-performance correlations are lower for categorizable list recall than for recall of noncategorizable lists is consistent with this hypothesis, since noncategorizable lists are more difficult to learn. (For the same reason, so is the lower prediction-performance correlation for learning of noncategorizable materials compared to serial list learning.)

Relationships Between Knowing Which Items Require Additional Study and Memory Peformance

As discussed earlier in this chapter, Masur et al. (1973) required children to select items for additional study after an initial study-recall cycle. Metamemorial competency was presumed when subjects selected items not recalled on the previous trial. Although both grade-3 and college subjects made appropriate item selections, only college students' subsequent memories were affected by selection of appropriate items. There was adequate metamemory (i.e., knowing which items to select) and reliable memory improvement at the college level only. Brown (1978) offered an interesting explanation of this pattern of results. She argued that in focusing attention on the items that were not learned previously, children failed to process additionally the items that were recalled previously. These previously recalled items were not mastered so well that subsequent recall was certain without additional encoding effort. Thus, even though memory of previously unrecalled items may have increased on subsequent recall tests, recall of previously recalled items would have declined, resulting in little advantage for the child subjects who selected unrecalled items for additional study. Brown (1978) suggested that effective restudy in this situation requires complex coordinations that have only been partially mastered by young grade-school children, if they have been mastered at all.

In addition to consideration of allocation of effort during encoding, there have also been studies of selective effort allocation during retrieval. Wellman (1979) reanalyzed Wellman's (1977a) data. He investigated whether there were correlations between children's feeling-of-knowing judgments and the effort deployed to try to retrieve the word. There were at all three age levels in the study (kindergarten, grade 1, and grade 3), although the relationship between the strength of feeling-of-knowing judgments and effort increased with age. This finding is consistent with the conclusion that even very young children can sometimes use their knowledge of information availability to guide strategic efforts.

Relationships Between Metacognition and Text Processing

There are consistent correlational relationships between various types of metacognitive knowledge about text and various outcome measures that presumably reflect text processing, such as comprehension and recall of what was read (e.g., Forrest-Pressley & Waller, 1984; Jacobs & Paris, 1987; Körkel, 1987; Uhl, 1986). These correlations generally range from low to moderate (i.e., .10 to .50).

One of the more completely researched correlational relationships is between knowledge of the relative importance of information in text and recall of text. Even preschool children tend to remember more central information in text compared to less important information (e.g., Brown & Smiley, 1977, 1978; Brown et al., 1977; Christie & Schumacher, 1975; Denhiere, in press; Denhiere & Le Ny, 1980; Hoppe-Graff & Schöler, 1980; Young & Schumacher, 1983). These correlational relationships do little to convince that recall of higher-order information is due to metacognitively-directed, differential processing of that information, however. Perhaps the most convincing evidence on this point was provided by Brown and Smiley (1978) who inferred from recall patterns that seventh- and eighth-grade children directed their attention to the more important aspects of text when they were given additional study time. In contrast, fifth graders studied less selectively. In short, Brown and Smiley's (1978) evidence suggested that metacognitive control of text processing based on knowledge of relative importance of text knowledge occurs a number of years after correlations between recall and importance levels are present. In fact, a finding in many of the studies that established the correlational relation-

ship between importance of information and recall also established that their
youngest participants were not consciously aware of the relative importance of
text elements. This pattern of data simply does not add up to a convincing case
that knowlege of importance levels directs the text processing of children in the
early elementary grades, although it may do so later in development (Brown
& Smiley, 1978). (See Chapter 4 for additional commentary about mechanisms
that can mediate recall of more important compared to less important text information.)

Relationships Between Metamemory, Strategy Use, and Recall of Categorizable Materials

Salatas and Flavell's (1976b) study is a favorite citation for those who argue that
metamemory is not strongly related to memory behavior (e.g., Cavanaugh &
Perlmutter, 1982). This study dealt primarily with the ability of young children
(grade-1 students) to react sensitively to differences in instructional demands. Subjects in the experimental condition were instructed to do everything that they could
in order to remember a set of categorizable items. Control subjects were merely
instructed to look at the pictures; they were not even aware that their memory of the
materials would be tapped. After memory was tested, both experimental and control
subjects were given a metamemory quiz, consisting of two questions. The children
were asked whether lists containing categorizable items were easier to remember
than lists of noncategorizable items. As expected, the subjects in the experimental
group remembered more items than the control subjects. There was no systematic
relationship between metamemory and categorical strategy use, however. This
study offered no evidence that metamemory is a necessary prerequisite for use of
strategies in memory tasks.

The situational specificity of Salatas and Flavell's (1976b) result was made clear
by a study initiated by Harriet Salatas Waters (Andreassen & Waters, 1984). The
presentation of the items in the new study differed in one way from the presentation
of the items in the old study. Salatas and Flavell presented the list items on cards that
were placed in a four-row array. Each of these rows had a lid that had to be lifted in
order to expose the pictures. This setup made it possible for Salatas and Flavell to
record time used for looking at the pictures during the study phase, but it also made
it impossible for the subjects to look at the entire item set at once. Andreassen and
Waters (1984) believed that the application of the organizational strategy may have
been made unnecessarily difficult by this aspect of the procedure, and thus, they did
not use the lid in their replication study.

A second change or addition to the design was made with respect to assessment
of metamemory. In Salatas and Flavell (1976b), the metamemory interview always
followed the memory test. In the new experiment, half of the subjects answered the
metamemory items before the experiment and half answered them after the test.
Andreassen and Waters (1984) believed that metamemory questions before the
actual memory test would produce information about children's general, day-to-day

knowledge about memory. The answers to metamemory questions after completion of the recall task should more strongly reflect metamemory activated during the task that was just completed (e.g., Ericsson & Simon, 1980). The correlation between metamemory and organizational behaviors was $r = -.05$ for the interview-before subjects and $r = .39$ for the interview-after subjects. This latter correlation in particular contrasts with the results of Salatas and Flavell (1976b). The timing of the metamemory interview obviously has an important influence on whether metamemory-strategic behavior correlations are obtained, a result confirmed by Schneider's (1985c) meta-analysis. Stronger correlations between metamemory and memory were obtained when the metamemory interview followed the memory task than when it preceded it (overall $r = .54$ vs. overall $r = .25$).

What specific conclusions can be drawn from comparison of Salatas and Flavell (1976b) and Andreassen and Waters (1984)? It seems that minimal modification of the recall task resulted in children recognizing and/or using the categorical structure of the item set better. Furthermore, their findings show that specific knowledge about the effects of categorization is activated when grade-1 children do a memory task that can be mediated using categorization strategies. Such activation does not lead to long-term activation of the metacognitive knowledge, however. Andreassen and Waters repeated the memory task six weeks later. The categorization behaviors of children at the later date could not be predicted by their metamemory at the end of the first experiment.

Wimmer and Tornquist (1980) also produced clear correlations between knowledge of organizational strategies and their use in grade-1, grade-4, and high-school students, findings consistent with the data in the interview-after condition in Andreassen and Waters (1984), but inconsistent with Salatas and Flavell. Wimmer and Tornquist administered a warm-up task (memory span) that may very well have heightened awareness of their subjects about the difficulty of memory tasks and have alerted them to the utility of strategic efforts during memorization.

In Cavanaugh and Borkowski (1980), kindergarten, grade-1, grade-3, and grade-5 children completed all 14 subtests of Kreutzer et al.'s (1975) interview. Three different memory tasks were also administered, ones that benefit from use of various organizational strategies. When the data were aggregated across age groups, there were significant correlations between metamemory, strategic behaviors, and memory performances, although these were relatively low. When the data were analyzed according to developmental level, however, significant correlations between metamemory and strategy use and performance were only obtained with the oldest subjects. Task-specific subtests in the interview battery predicted strategic behaviors in children even when the aggregated metamemory scores failed to do so, however. Similar support for the predictive potential of task-specific metamemory items has been produced in other studies as well (e.g., Best and Ornstein, 1986; Cantor, Andreassen, and Waters, 1985).

In concluding that there are correlational relationships between knowledge about the efficacy of organizational strategies and memory behaviors, it must also be pointed out that samples of young grade-school children (e.g., grade-1) typically include very few subjects who know a lot about semantic organizational methods and the advantages associated with these strategies. For instance, Wimmer and Tornquist (1980) used the data of 24 grade-1 students, who were equally divided into a metamemory-before-memory-task and a metamemory-after-memory-task group. Adequate metamemory was obtained for half of the children in the before and after groups. From those, about half of the subjects in the before group also showed spontaneous sorting behavior, while not a single child in the after group used semantic organizational strategies. This means, that out of the 24 grade-1 children, there were only three subjects who possessed adequate knowledge of semantic organizational strategies and used semantic categorization. Sodian et al. (1986) obtained a statistically significant correlation ($r = .37$) among 6-year-olds between reported preference for sorting strategies and their use in a memory task. Nonetheless, perceptual sorting strategies were preferred over semantic-organizational strategies by this age group. The positive correlation reflects the fact that the few subjects who reported preference for semantic sorting in their metacognitive interview also used this strategy to a large extent.

Although relationships between metamemory about semantic organizational strategies, use of semantic organizational strategies, and memory performances can be obtained reliably with older children (Cavanaugh & Borkowski, 1980; Cos & Paris, 1979; Hasselhorn, 1986; Justice, 1985; Körkel, Schneider, Vogel, & Weinert, 1983; Schneider, 1986; Schneider et al., 1987; Weinert et al., 1984), it cannot be taken for granted that even these children clearly prefer semantic organization to alternative procedures (like rehearsal). For instance, Cox and Paris (1979) found preferences for rehearsal strategies in grade-4 students. Although Justice (1985) and Schneider (1986) noted tendencies at this same age level to favor semantic organization over rehearsal, nontrivial proportions of the children used rehearsal. More positively, by grade 6, students are more likely to provide across-the-board endorsement of semantic organization over rote rehearsal (e.g., Justice, 1985).

Finally, even though correlations between metamemory about organizational strategies and organizational strategy use are regularly obtained in contemporary research, we believe that much greater correlations between metamemory about strategies and memory-strategy use are likely if the focus in this research is broadened to reflect more completely the nature of strategy development. For instance, really proficient use of semantic organizational strategies also incorporates a self-testing component. Metamemory and strategic assessments that capture both use of semantic organization and self-testing should correlate more highly with each other and memory performance than measures based on semantic organization alone. See Schneider (1986) and Schneider et al. (1987) for preliminary evidence consistent with this point of view.

A typical feature of more recent studies is that they do not limit themselves to analyses of simple intercorrelations. In several studies (e.g., Kurtz et al., 1986; Schneider, 1986; Schneider et al., 1986; Weinert et al., 1984) multivariate regression analyses were used in order to determine the relative importance of metamemory components and other potential predictors (e.g., verbal intelligence, academic self-concept, attributional style) of semantic organizational strategy use and/or memory performances in tasks that can be mediated by semantic categorization. From about the third grade on, metamemory variables have emerged as significant predictors in these analyses (Kurtz et al., 1986; Schneider et al., 1986; Weinert et al., 1984). Task-specific metamemory is usually a better predictor than general metamemory measures. Metamemory predicts recall even when other factors are controlled statistically (e.g., Borkowski et al., 1983; Kurtz et al., 1982).

Research on the relationships between metamemory and memory behaviors and performances increasingly have tended to use even more sophisticated approaches than regression, including path and causal models. While most regression procedures do not require a theoretically specified sequence of predictors, causal modeling does. The basic causal model for analysis of the relationship between metamemory and memory generally assumes that metamemory theoretically precedes memory behaviors and performances. Thus, a child's knowledge about his memory ought to influence strategic behavior, and the amount of strategic behavior should predict memory performance. The models presented in the literature vary to the extent that they operate on observed versus "latent" variables (i.e., constructs in the latter case). Two versions of latent-variable models can be distinguished. Exploratory modeling emphasizes the construction of a potential model given the data on hand. Confirmatory approaches go farther, permitting tests of potential models that are specified in advance (e.g., Crano & Mendoza, 1987). Examples of exploratory analyses using the LVPLS (latent variable partial least square) computer program from Lohmöller (1984) can be found in Hasselhorn (1986), Hasselhorn and Körkel (1986), Körkel et al. (1983), Kurtz and Borkowski (1987), Kurtz et al. (1986), Schneider (1985b), and Schneider et al. (1986). Studies on the relationship of metamemory to memory using confirmatory LISREL (linear structural relationships; Jöreskog & Sörbom, 1984) modeling have been presented by Körkel (1987); Schneider, Körkel, and Weinert (1987b); as well as Weinert et al. (1984).

A study conducted by Fabricius and Hagen (1984) illustrates the possibilities for using path analyses with observed variables that were conceived of as a sequence of multiple regression analyses. Fabricius and Hagen assumed that metacognitive judgments about strategic use of categorical list structure during the initial session of their study would directly affect categorical strategy use and amount recalled in a categorical recall task presented a week later. There was a significant, direct path from first-session metacognitive judgments to use of the categorizing strategy. Use of the strategy positively influenced organization during recall, which positively affected amount recalled. While the path coefficients between metamemory and organization during recall and between metamemory and recall were positive, they were not statistically significant. Moreover, use of the sorting strategy did not directly affect recall.

Fabricius and Hagen (1984) limited their interpretations to the direct paths. It is possible to calculate the indirect paths, however, based on what is provided in the original report. For example, the indirect effect of metamemory on clustering during recall (which is mediated by use of the categorical organization strategy use during study) was greater than the direct path. The same was true of the indirect effect of metamemory on recall. In short, the contribution of metamemory was more obvious by consideration of both direct and indirect effects of metamemory on subsequent memory behaviors and performances. The advantage of path analyses is that such indirect effects can be calculated.

There is convincing evidence of relationships between metamemory, strategic behaviors, and memory from studies that used causal models with latent variables (Borkowski et al., 1983; Hasselhorn, 1986; Kurtz et al., 1982; Schneider, Körkel, & Weinert, 1987b; Weinert et al., 1984; Weinert, Schneider, & Knopf, in press). These analyses permit the conclusions that even relatively young elementary-school children possess knowledge about organizational strategies that has a direct influence on strategic behaviors, which increases the tendency to organize to-be-learned materials taxonomically. Metamemory has proven to be consistently predictive of strategic behaviors in these analyses even when general factors like intelligence are taken into account. It is a more powerful predictor of strategic behavior than theoretically related concepts like academic self-concept and causal attributional tendencies. On the other hand, the link between metamemory and recall is weaker than the link between metamemory and strategy use. Factors other than metacognitively directed strategy use can also influence recall level (e.g., speed of information processing). We emphasize in presenting these conclusions that they should not be considered general statements about strategy functioning, since virtually all of the relevant causal model analyses have involved study of metamemory as a predictor of semantic organizational strategies.

Summary

Quantitative averaging of metamory-memory performance correlations is a reasonable first step in understanding this data base. Meta-analyses makes clear that there are nontrivial quantitative associations between metamemory and memory. Qualitative review of the various metamemory-memory behavior problems makes obvious, however, that no single statistic could capture the diversity and richness of the findings. Sometimes there are associations between metamemory and memory behavior, and sometimes there are not. Some consistently positive associations are stronger than others. For instance, there are often stronger relationships between metamemory about a strategy and strategy use than between metamemory and memory, since strategy use directed by metamemory is only one of several determinants of performance (e.g., capacity, the nonstrategic knowledge base).

Metamemory about strategies is an extremely important type of metacognition, with its relevance to proficient memory behaviors taken up in much greater detail in the next two chapters. Presumably, such critical metamemory develops in part through monitoring processes, such as when people notice when a procedure they are using is improving performance (e.g., Pressley et al., 1984, 1985). That is one reason that monitoring will be considered in greater detail in the next two chapters, which are integrative discussions about the variety of factors that determine skilled memory.

6. Good Strategy Use: A General Model, A Specific Example, and Comments on How To Do Research on the Development of Strategy Proficiency

Up until this point, this book has been mostly about immature memory behaviors. We have focused on acquisition of individual components of memory competence (e.g., particular strategies) or, at most, on a few components in interaction (e.g., some strategies rely on certain aspects of the knowledge base). In contrast, this chapter begins with an overview of fully mature memory behaviors and the multicomponent articulation that characterizes truly sophisticated strategy use.

There are two motivations for presenting a portrait of refined memory behavior. First, explicit specification of the human memory potential makes obvious the immaturity of memory behaviors displayed by children, adolescents, and many adults. Second, it clarifies that most studies of memory development— ones that have focused on single acquisitions or acquisitions of only one or two components of competent memory behavior—are too narrow to capture memory functioning completely. Those who wish to plot naturalistic memory development must plan multidimensional research programs; those planning interventions to promote more mature memory behaviors must design treatments that address a variety of memory-relevant components in interaction.

Mature Strategy Functioning

What is reviewed here is a specific instantiation of a Good Strategy User Model (e.g., Borkowski, Carr, Rellinger, & Pressley, in press; Pressley, 1986; Pressley, Borkowski, & Johnson, 1987; Pressley, Borkowski, & Schneider, 1987; Pressley, Goodchild, Fleet, Zajchowski, & Evans, in press; Pressley, Johnson, & Symons,

1987) – a good *memory* strategy user model. In presenting it, we emphasize that it represents a hypothetical memorizing superperson. We also point out that in order to construct a coherent presentation about this type of complicated performer, it is necessary to do some simplification, and thus, good memory strategy use is taken up in a component-by-component fashion. Consideration of complex interactions between components is deferred until each is considered separately.

Strategies

Memory strategies are processes (or sequences of processes) that, when matched appropriately to a memory task, can facilitate performance. Earlier we discussed clustering and rehearsal strategies for learning categorizable lists. A well known encoding strategy is the pegword-mnemonic approach for acquiring information that must be recalled in order (e.g., the one based on the poem, "One is a bun, two is a shoe . . ."). Summarizing and imagery strategies can also be used to learn text containing arbitrary relationships.

A good memory strategy user possesses a variety of these memory strategies and used them consciously at one time, even though many of them now are used out of awareness (e.g., Baron, 1985, Chapter 3; Campione & Armbruster, 1985). The good strategy user has had many opportunities to use and practice strategies, and thus, their application in appropriate situations has become automatic and habitual. Strategies are always potentially conscious and controllable (e.g., Pressley, Forrest-Pressley, Elliott-Faust, & Miller, 1985), however. For instance, extension of familiar strategies to new tasks may be undertaken deliberately. By arguing that strategy functioning need not be deliberately controlled, we do not abandon the position that strategy use is always intentional in the sense of being goal directed, with memory improvement the goal in using memory strategies.

For example, making a shopping list is a memory strategy that most good memory strategy users would employ regularly. When the user becomes aware of the need for a good from the store, the item is added to a list that is always kept in the same place (e.g., beside the kitchen telephone). For many, this behavior is reflexive, done with little thought at all after years of experience with this approach. Making and using such a shopping list is controllable, however. A person could easily stop doing it or do it in a different fashion (e.g., recording the list on a microcomputer file). Consistent with the perspective that strategic behaviors began as conscious actions, there is usually a time in life when a conscious decision was made to keep shopping lists.

There are some distinctions that can be made about strategies that make more obvious how various memory techniques differ from one another. There are both external memory strategies (e.g., making shopping lists, putting a to-be-taken-to-school item near the door) and internal memory strategies (e.g., covert rehearsal and elaboration). Some memory strategies involve a mixture of external and internal factors, such as when a person arranges to-be-learned pictures in piles to facilitate the internal generation of meaningful stories that could be used to mediate recall of the pictures.

Some memory strategies can be used only in very, very specific situations in particular domains. These *task-* and *domain-limited strategies* are tricks for aiding memory of particular pieces of information. A number of these are described in an aptly-named volume by Slung (1985), *The Absent-Minded Professor's Memory Guide*. Slung's book includes chapters on how to remember particular historical, geographic, religious, linguistic, musical, and scientific contents. That these tricks are helpful only for certain tasks in particular domains can be appreciated by considering some familiar techniques for remembering specific musical content. The notes on the treble staff (E, G, B, D, F) can be encoded by memorizing the sentence, "*Every Good Boy Does Fine*." The notes in the treble staff spaces form a word— FACE. Memorizing the sentence, "*Good Boys Do Fine Always*," increases recall of the bass staff lines. Memory of bass staff spaces follows from, "*All Cows Eat Grass*." It seems a good bet that there are examples of *task-* and *domain-limited* strategies for virtually every domain, with these techniques often specific instantiations of more general procedures. That someone could know many specific tricks without abstracting or using the general memory techniques on which they are based (e.g., How many school children use the music-staff tricks, but do not understand or use first-letter mnemonics more generally?), however, mandates separating these procedures from approaches that are more general in their application.

There are a variety of *goal-limited memory strategies*. These can be applied to learn content across a variety of content areas, although particular strategies are suited to acquisition of material with particular structure (e.g., rehearsal facilitates learning of simple lists but not associations; forming images between paired items increases associative recall of one item given the other dramatically, but has little influence on free recall of pairs). The across-content applicability of goal-limited memory strategies can be appreciated by considering summarization (constructing summaries of text segment as reading proceeds along). This strategy can be applied with fictional and expository materials. Nonfictional content can range from recipes to history to mathematics. Learners who acquire a specific goal-limited memory strategy have a powerful tool at their disposal, for there is a great deal of evidence that rehearsal, elaboration, summarizing, and organizational techniques (among others) can improve memory tremendously (e.g., Garner, 1987; Ornstein & Naus, 1985; Pressley, Heisel, McCormick, & Nakamura, 1982; Rohwer, 1973).

Strategies that enhance memory are often used in concert with what we refer to as *general strategies*. These strategies do not aid memory themselves, but they support the profitable use of task-specific and goal-limited memory strategies. An important one is checking performance (i.e., monitoring) to determine if a memory strategy that is in use is achieving the current memory goal. Other general strategies include being generally attentive to the task at hand and trying to relate the current challenge to situations that have been encountered previously in order to acquire clues as to which strategy might be appropriate to use on a current task (e.g., Entwisle & Ramsden, 1983). Another is attending to the environment, specifically looking for clues as to how to proceed and which specific goal-limited strategies to use in a given situation.

The interaction between general strategies and more specific memory strategies can be understood through illustration. First of all, good strategy users are generally attentive to the material that they are going to read, and they approach challenging reading tasks with a set to be strategic (i.e., intending to use strategies to understand and remember material presented in text). Good strategy users also employ a number of more specific strategies for understanding and remembering text (e.g., Bereiter & Bird, 1985; Garner, 1987; Levin, 1982). They can rephrase or para-phrase text; they can backtrack and/or reread; they can search for cause-and-effect relationships; they can summarize; good strategy users can self-question; and, they can form mnemonics to encode what they perceive to be particularly hard-to-remember pieces of information. In order to know when these strategies are neces-sary, readers need to note which aspects of text are difficult to learn and when they are having problems understanding and encoding relationships specified in text— That is, they need to monitor their text learning (e.g., Markman, 1981). Good strategy users also monitor their use of strategies to determine if the procedures that have been elected are in fact permitting progress toward the goals of understanding and remembering text. If not, the good strategy user switches tactics (e.g., Baker & Brown, 1984). In short, adequate memory of text is accomplished through complex articulations of general strategies and goal-limited memory strategies. The use of all these strategies depends largely on a particular type of metacognition.

Metacognitive Knowledge About Specific Strategies
(Specific Strategy Knowledge)

One popular definition of metacognition is that it is, "... knowledge concerning one's own cognitive processes and products or anything related to them..." (Flavell, 1977, p. 232). Of course, strategies are processes and there are many pieces of information that a person could have about specific strategic processes. For instance, consider imagery techniques. One could recall a grade-6 teacher describ-ing an imagery strategy. A particular student might remember using imagery tech-niques in history or science class. The second author recalls vividly having to learn lists of tips about driving in driver education class and forming interactive images containing cues linked to each of the tips. Thus, memory of things to do before taking a long trip was accomplished by forming an image of a person looking at a map, while holding an oil dip stick in his hands, as windshield wiper fluid dripped on his shoe that was kicking the tire. Worse yet, he was being hit by water flying out of the radiator and one of the hoses. He came to realize during the course of high school that such images required effort and attention to create (a theme now explored in greater detail in his recent research; Pressley, Cariglia-Bull, Deane, & Schneider, 1987), and that they were worth nothing if they were not explicitly retrieved at test-ing (another theme explored in his research; Pressley & Levin, 1980; Pressley & MacFadyen, 1983). He also recognized, however, that when he did take the time and make the effort to create such images and used them at testing, that his learning and recall of lists of related items was more certain.

This general understanding of imagery-strategy utility, a piece of metacognitive knowledge about imagery strategies, evolved from many specific occasions when learning was enhanced through use of imagery. This type of information is important to acquire because persistent and consistent use of a memory strategy depends in part on people understanding that it aids memory (e.g., Black & Rollins, 1982; Borkowski, Levers, & Gruenenfelder, 1976; Cavanaugh & Borkowski, 1979; Kennedy & Miller, 1976; Lawson & Fuelop, 1980; Ringel & Springer, 1980). Other metacognitive knowledge is required for really general use of a strategy—transfer to situations not encountered before, but ones that benefit from application of the strategy. Generalization requires that learners understand when and where to use procedures (e.g., Duffy, Roehler, Sivan et al., 1987; Paris, Lipson, & Wixson, 1983; Pressley, Borkowski, & O'Sullivan, 1984, 1985; Roehler & Duffy, 1984).

The criticality of particular pieces of metacognitive information about strategies can be demonstrated easily using simple experimental designs, as was done in O'Sullivan and Pressley (1984). Those investigators hypothesized that embellishing strategy instruction by adding information about when and where to use the trained strategy (an imagery mnemonic strategy for vocabulary learning) would increase children's generalized use of the trained procedure. Students in grades 5 and 6 were presented two memory tasks during the experiment, both of which could be mediated profitably with the trained procedure. The first task was learning the products manufactured in particular cities, and the second was acquisition of Latin word definitions.

Control subjects learned both types of materials, but were provided no strategy instructions. In four other conditions, the subjects were taught to mediate the city-product task using the mnemonic imagery procedure, with the conditions varying in the amount of "when" and "where" information about strategy use. No subjects were instructed to use the strategy when the Latin task was presented. In general, transfer of the mnemonic imagery strategy from the city-product task to the Latin task was more likely given greater provision of when and where information during strategy instruction.

The good strategy user model assumes that every strategy that a person possesses can be accompanied by metacognitive knowledge, like when and where to use the strategy. People vary with respect to how much of this type of information they possess, although really good strategy users have a rich network of knowledge specifying the occasions when it is appropriate to use many of the strategic procedures that they know.

There are at least three ways that this type of information can be acquired (Pressley, Borkowski, & O'Sullivan, 1984). As was the case in O'Sullivan and Pressley (1984) and in many of the studies cited earlier that focused on strategy utility, an external agent (like a teacher or a parent) can provide the information to the child.

Alternatively, children can be left on their own to discover metacognitive information as they work with strategies. For instance, when people try two different strategies for accomplishing the same task (strategies that differ in potency), there is the opportunity to discover that one of the two strategies facilitates better the particular type of performance that was attempted with the two techniques (Pressley, Levin, &

Ghatala, 1988). Unfortunately, however, autonomous abstraction of metacognitive information about strategies is far from certain, with children less likely than adults to discover such information (Pressley, Levin, & Ghatala, 1984). It is also far from certain that children will use self-discovered metacognitive knowledge (Pressley, Ross, Levin, & Ghatala, 1984). Such failure to abstract and use important meta-cognitive information about strategies has prompted substantial research on a third method for increasing metacognitive knowledge.

Children can be taught metacognitive acquisition procedures. That is, they can be taught to monitor their use of strategies with an eye toward metacognitively important information such as how much a strategy enhances performance compared to alternative techniques. Ghatala and her associates have begun to study the effects produced by teaching simple metacognitive acquisition procedures (e.g., Ghatala, Levin, Pressley, & Goodwin, 1986; Ghatala, Levin, Pressley, & Lodico, 1985; Lodico, Ghatala, Levin, Pressley, & Bell, 1983), with these studies discussed more extensively in the next chapter. For the present, suffice to say that even 6- to 7-year-old children benefit from instructions to compare strategies with one another, to note which of two strategies is more powerful, and to use that information to guide future strategy use. On the other hand, such instruction with young grade-school children must be quite detailed, with explicit tuition to compare the strategies, note their relative potencies, and use the metacognitive information about relative potencies in decision making.

One point to stress in closing this subsection is that the study of specific strategy knowledge has just begun. In particular, almost nothing is known about how some potentially important categories of knowledge are acquired, such as understanding that a strategy is fun or burdensome to apply. There is little longitudinal study of the use of specific strategy knowledge, although there is an assumption that its initial deployment involves conscious analysis of a new task in order to identify elements that are specified in metacognitive knowledge about strategies possessed by the learner. For example, a learner who possesses strategies that are well matched to expository prose (e.g., summarization) might examine a new text to determine if it were truly expository, and once determining that it was, consciously summarize. Eventually, however, it is assumed that conscious and reflective matching of strategies to tasks vis-à-vis metacognitive knowledge about strategies gives way to automatic association of strategies to tasks. Studies need to be done to trace out explicitly the path from conscious to automatized use of metacognitive knowledge as a mediator of strategy use. Given the demonstrated potency of metacognitive information as a determinant of strategy use, this work is valuable as part of the validation of the good strategy user model and as part of pragmatic research designed to determine how to enhance general application of strategies that are taught.

Styles

Some people tend to reflect quite a bit before performing actions, and others are habitually impulsive (Baron, 1981, 1985; Messer, 1976). Some people confront academic challenges calmly; others are anxious given the slightest challenge (e.g.,

Tobias, 1977). In short, there are persistent and pervasive style differences between people. Of greatest concern here, a person's style can be an important factor mediating whether they use the metacognition about strategies that they possess in analyzing task variables in order to make strategy decisions.

Consider, for example, the habitually impulsive student. This is a person who has a "general bias to stop too soon when collecting evidence" (Baron, 1985, p. 157). Are such people, who react quickly and fail to take critical information into account (e.g., Messer, 1976), likely to make careful analyses of task situations, likely to search for task characteristics, and likely to match carefully the characteristics of new tasks to strategies as specified by specific strategy knowledge that they possess? Such analyses and matching takes time, and impulsive children often fail to delay their responding long enough for task analyses and metacognitively informed strategy planning to occur. Rapid and haphazard responding, which characterizes impulsivity, preclude the time-demanding processing that many academic and behavioral strategies require (Baron, 1985; Messer, 1976).

Habitually anxious people also exhibit behaviors that are inconsistent with good strategy use. It is well known that people can hold a limited amount of information in consciousness at any given time (e.g., Baddeley, 1986). It is also known that strategy planning and execution often demand a great deal of the limited amount of consciousness (i.e., short-term capacity) that a person has available (e.g., Case, 1985; Pressley, Cariglia-Bull, Deane, & Schneider, 1987). Unfortunately, anxious people functionally reduce their conscious capacity because they exert cognitive effort attending to signs of arousal and negative thoughts about themselves (Eysenck, 1979, Chapter 12; Sarason, 1972; Wine, 1971). Anxiety can, thus, have a negative effect on strategically mediated performance, especially for strategies that require a good deal of conscious capacity in order to acquire (Tobias, 1979).

More positively, there are styles that definitely can serve to facilitate strategy use and effectiveness. Reflective people think before they respond, and tend to study situations extensively and appropriately before acting. Habitually calm people do not waste scarce consciousness on irrelevant cognitions (like negative self-thoughts), keeping their heads and not permitting anxiety to distract and detract from the task at hand. Not surprisingly, reflection characterizes good strategy users.

Motivational Beliefs

People have beliefs about their current competencies and these play an important role in motivating good strategy use. Certain beliefs are considered to be particularly critical. One is the understanding that how well a person performs is largely a function of making an effort to use effective strategies (e.g., Clifford, 1984, 1986a, 1986b). Thus, the good memory strategy user believes that trying hard to memorize is not enough. Good memory only results from use of mental energy in the application of strategies appropriate to the material currently presented for mastery. Good memory strategy users have believed for some time that their personal memory competence can be increased a bit at a time by learning more effective strategies (cf., Dweck, 1987). When they were younger, they believed that they could become good memorizers and good learners by acquiring the skills and strategies possessed by mentally competent adults that they knew. In their view, there was nothing mysterious or unattainable about competence. These beliefs motivated the search for and mastery of the effective memory strategies that they now possess (cf., Markus & Nurius, 1986).

There are other beliefs that motivate behaviors, that are presumed to support good strategy use. For instance, good memory strategy users recognize that it is important to shield themselves from distractions as they perform important tasks (Kuhl, 1984, 1985; Heckhausen, 1982). This understanding presumably activates acquisition and use of attentional strategies, such as arranging for study time to occur in quiet environments that have few distractions. Good strategy users also understand that planning and execution of strategies takes time, but that it is time well spent (Baron, 1985, pp. 159–160). They probably believe that thinking is an enjoyable activity that pays off (e.g., Cacioppo & Petty, 1982). Good strategy users understood as students that the memory and learning strategies that they were acquiring in school were necessary (or at least helpful) in order to become an effective and competent member of society who is able to play a valued role. Believing that one's own cognitive efforts can really make a difference is an important motivator for the acquisition and use of strategies.

Just as important as supportive and appropriately motivating beliefs is the lack of dysfunctional and discouraging beliefs that would reduce interest in and the likelihood of memory strategy acquisition. Good memory strategy users definitely do not believe that memorizing ability is an innately determined and immutable ability that is determined solely by biological endowment or that memory is either "photographic" or it is not. They do not view themselves as helpless to discover ways of improving their lot, nor do they believe in effort alone (e.g., that going over and over material in order to "burn it in" is a good method).

In arguing here that good strategy users possess a host of global and specific beliefs about themselves that affect strategy use, we recognize that there is only a small data base that is directly relevant to the position that good strategy use is tied to motivational beliefs. The most relevant research efforts are the many demonstrations of increased use of strategies when people believe that use of strategies pays off (e.g., Black & Rollins, 1982; Borkowski et al. 1976; Cavanaugh & Borkowski, 1979; Kennedy & Miller, 1976; Lawson & Fuelop, 1980; Ringel & Springer, 1980). The reader may recall that these data were discussed earlier in this chapter in the subsection on metacognitive knowledge about strategies. In fact, all of the motivational beliefs discussed here qualify as metacognition because they refer to cognition about both thinking and cognitive tasks, although the lack of mention of this part of metacognition in Chapter 5 makes obvious that metacognitive theorists generally have neglected motivational beliefs. Some of the more specific beliefs are tied to specific strategies, and thus, qualify as specific strategy knowledge. Thus, the motivation associated with these beliefs is limited to the particular strategies to which they are attached. More global beliefs (e.g., good performance depends on effort used in the execution of appropriate strategies; I can become a good strategy user by learning the skills known and used by good learners) exert more general influences.

Undoubtedly, there will be more experimental data about the role of metacognitive beliefs in promoting good strategy use in the very near future. First of all, fairly complete theoretical statements about the role of metacognition and strategy use are now becoming available, with the work of Barbara McCombs, Jere Brophy, and John Nicholls especially notable for integrative completeness. McCombs (1986, 1987), Brophy (1985, 1986; Brophy & Kher, 1986), and Nicholls (in press) develop the ideas about motivational beliefs that are presented here in much more detail. See Borkowski, Carr, Rellinger, and Pressley (in press) as well. There are also encouraging research results. For instance, there is a growing data base confirming that getting students to attribute their strategically mediated good performances to the use of appropriate strategies increases continued use of strategies (e.g., Dweck & Elliott, 1983; Fowler & Peterson, 1981). Some of Borkowski's important, recent work on this problem is taken up in the next chapter. For the present, we emphasize the emerging interest of theoreticians and researchers in motivational determination of good strategy use.

Nonstrategic Knowledge Base

In addition to strategic procedures, metacognition about strategies, and other motivational beliefs, good strategy users know a great deal more. Their lifetime experiences have provided opportunities for acquisition of many specific facts (e.g., that the Japanese make good television sets) and many sets of related facts (e.g., the economic strengths and weaknesses of many parts of the world). They have organized and categorized knowledge that corresponds to the organized knowledge bases of many other people (e.g., that dolls, board games, and model trains are subsets of the larger set of toys). They know elaborate and generalized scripts that detail the temporal and spatial structures of recurring events in their lives. For example, their "taking a plane trip" script includes calling for reservations, buying the ticket before the trip, appearing at the airport an hour before flight time, checking in, waiting at the gate, boarding the plane. . . picking up luggage at baggage claim, departing the arrival airport. They have images and verbal descriptions of many important concepts. See any introductory cognitive psychology text (e.g., Anderson, 1985) for greater description of the various types of knowledge and representations of that knowledge that are stored in long-term memory.

This knowledge base can determine strategy use in a number of ways. First of all, a well-developed knowledge base permits some familiarity with some "new" to-be-learned content. In general, less strategic intervention is required with more familiar to-be-learned material. Thus, an experienced teacher entering a new school must learn a new set of routines. The teacher often has to learn when and how to take attendance and report it, where the recess- and cafeteria-duty rosters are placed, a percentage marking system used in the school, as well as a myriad of other specifics. Learning these "new" rules is easier for the experienced compared to the novice teacher because the experienced teacher already possesses a rich knowledge base about schools and school organization. This includes temporally organized schemas about the structure of the school day and the school year from the teacher's perspective. It includes specific knowledge about the type of paper work required of teachers as well as ways of accomplishing that paperwork. It includes knowledge of the laws governing teaching, employment in schools, and educational administration of students. The task faced by the experienced teacher is simply to adjust this knowledge base about schools to fit the current situation. This existing knowledge base guides the experienced teacher to expect particular events or classes of events to occur. When they happen, the prior knowledge base permits recognition of critical versus noncritical information. That is, details about the new school rules and structure are assimilated by the existing knowledge base.

To the extent that old knowledge is not perfect, experienced teachers can add to their knowledge of schools, a process referred to as accretion by Rumelhart (1980). Sometimes all that is required is fine-grained modification of existing knowledge, or fine tuning according to Rumelhart's analysis of knowledge change. If some aspect of the school is completely different from previous experience, it may be necessary to restructure (again, a term used by Rumelhart) some part of the knowledge base completely. For example, complete restructuring of knowledge about acceptable student dress might be required of a teacher moving from a conventional public school to a military school. Although the three mechanisms of accretion, fine tuning, and restructuring have most explicitly been developed with respect to schematized prior knowledge (Rumelhart, 1980), these types of changes probably occur for diverse types of prior knowledge representations. For example, categorizable information can be accreted (i.e., categories added), fine tuned (i.e., slight changes in particular categories to capture newly encountered contents), or completely restructured (i.e., reclassifying animals on the basis of indigenous geography rather than on the basis of genus and species considerations).

Summary of Good Use of Memory Strategies

Good memory strategy users are always looking for procedures to enhance performance. For many familiar tasks, there are automatic associations between memory goals and strategies. For the authors, these include writing out lists of items to be bought at the grocery store and mnemonically recoding the number-letter designation when one's car is parked in a multi-tiered garage (e.g., section 3-B can be remembered by imagining the *3 b*ears visiting the car). On other occasions, the good strategy user analyzes the task situation to determine if (s)he could recognize similarities between the current memory problem and previous academic memory experiences that were strategically mediated, and thus, generalize a previously acquired procedure to the new situation. If similarities are identified, that triggers strategies associated with previous, similar problems. Rather than just letting these strategies fire off in a helter skelter fashion, however, the good strategy user formulates a plan that sequences relevant strategies appropriately and includes monitoring of strategy use and execution. Once a person begins the sequence, performance is monitored to determine if progress is being made toward the goal. If not, the student might try harder or substitute other strategies until one is identified that provides progress toward the goal. Although this description of self-regulation is simplified, it captures the reflective, informed, and monitored use of memory strategies that characterizes good use of memory strategies. As such, this sketch of competent cognition is not controversial (e.g., Baker & Brown, 1984; Baron, 1985; Brown et al., 1983; Chi, 1985b; Frederiksen, 1984; Glaser, 1985; Rigney, 1980; Schoenfeld, 1985; Wagner & Sternberg, 1984), although the good strategy user model contains more explicit specification of its components than do many of the alternative descriptions of good thinking.

Use of memory strategies depends largely on appropriate beliefs and strategy knowledge according to the good strategy user model. The different types of strategies operate in conjunction with one another and with processing determined by style. That the operation of general strategies such as monitoring can change beliefs and strategy knowledge is also specified. Strategy use sometimes depends on the nonstrategic knowledge base; in turn, the nonstrategic knowledge base is often enriched by strategy functioning. Most strategy components are stored in long-term memory, but operate in short-term memory—thus, operations that occur in short-term memory can increase long-term knowledge. For example, use of a vocabulary-learning strategy sometimes increases long-term knowledge of particular words. When the learner monitors that long-term retention occurred, there may be increased recognition that the strategy is useful with the particular type of vocabulary that was acquired on this occasion—that is, a change in strategy knowledge.

The explicit selection and conscious execution and monitoring of strategies requires learner attention (Baddeley, 1986; Case, 1985; Kahnemann, 1973), especially during the early phases of strategy acquisition. Consider a child who is being taught to comprehend and remember text. The child can be asked to direct attention to relevant parts of text, to self-test, and to review. At first, execution and articulation of the strategies are clumsy. Awkward and conscious execution can consume most if not all of the child's attentional capacity, leaving little for other cognitive demands of reading (e.g., relating content that is being read to information that the learner already has stored). Fortunately, with practice, the amount of attention that is required to execute individual strategies and sequences of strategies decreases (Logan, 1985; Schneider, Dumais, & Shiffrin, 1984). Such automaticity frees attention for other activities. In short, much of good strategy use occurs automatically—out of consciousness. In fact, development of such automaticity for familiar tasks is an important goal of strategy education.

In summary, good memory strategy use is complicated since it involves the coordinated development and use of strategies, metacognition, and the nonstrategic knowledge base, all operating in the confines of limited capacity. (Hence the presentation of Chapters 2 through 5 on capacity, strategies, nonstrategic knowledge, and metacognition logically preceded the integration presented here and in the next chapter.) We emphasize that a global good strategy user is something of an idealized endstate. More optimistically, there is a good deal of evidence that children in fact do make substantial progress toward good strategy use. We turn our attention now to research on a particular group of strategies in order to illustrate this point.

The Development of Good Use of Elaboration Strategies

Children are often presented factual knowledge that they are expected to acquire. Sometimes the facts are listed out; sometimes they are presented in text. The memory strategies reviewed in this section can dramatically facilitate learning of factual information and knowledge of relationships between particular pieces of information. Such associative, factual knowledge plays a prominent role in the knowledge base. Because the knowledge base plays a large role in cognition and good strategy use in general (last section; Chi, 1985b; Pressley, Borkowski, & Schneider, 1987; Pressley, Goodchild, Fleet, Zajchowski, & Evans, in press), there is strong motivation to do all possible to increase both the amount and organization of associative knowledge (e.g., Anderson, 1983).

Introduction to Paired-Associate Elaboration

Until the last decade, almost all research on associative learning and associative strategies was conducted in the context of paired-associate learning. This paradigm has been used in developmental studies for most of this century (Vertes, 1913, 1931). Rohwer (1973) presented an extremely detailed task analysis of paired-associate learning. Review of that analysis provides a good introduction to the thinking of most researchers who are interested in various types of associative learning and approaches to elaboration.

During study, both pair members are usually presented simultaneously. At testing, only the stimulus is presented with the subject required to recall the paired response. Success at this task is more likely if subjects somehow associate the stimulus and response terms meaningfully as they study a pair. (In many studies, the stimuli and responses were not related in ways that were obvious at first glance.) Rohwer (1973) assumed that efficient learning of pairs was accomplished by generation of shared meaning between stimulus and response terms:

> . . .the hypothesis is that shared meanings are oriented in noun-pair learning by a process of generating an event that can serve as a common referent for the members of each pair. Hereafter, this process will be designated by the term *elaboration*. . . (p. 5).

Elaboration of paired associates specifically refers to joining of stimulus and response items into a common phrase or image. For instance, a verbal elaboration of the pair *cat-apple* could be, "The *cat* rolled the *apple* around." An imaginal elaboration might be an internal represention of a cat rolling the apple around, for example, an old yellow cat that one knew as a child playing with an apple that fell from the apple tree in the yard of the house that one grew up in. There has been anecdotal evidence for more than two millenia that creation of such elaborations improves memory (Yates, 1966), although systematic and programmatic study of paired-associate elaboration processes has been confined to the last 25 years (Pressley, 1977; Reese, 1977). Although an enormous amount of important information about memory development was generated within the paired-associate paradigm, researchers who are interested in associative elaboration strategies now consider processing of a variety of materials. Given the diversity of materials in studies of elaboration, it is not surprising that there are a number of different elaborative strategies.

Types of Elaborative Strategies

Two general categories of strategies (referred to here as transformational and non-transformational elaboration) emerge from inspection of the various elaborative techniques. Transformational strategies involve the introduction of relationships into to-be-learned material that are not always naturally connected to the materials. In contrast, nontransformational elaborations are additions to to-be-learned content that are naturally and meaningfully associated with the content. Brief consideration of various elaborative strategies will make this distinction more obvious and facilitate the discussion of the development of elaborative skills.

The best known transformational elaborations are the imagery mnemonics considered briefly in the last subsection. Although there are some developmental constraints on the construction of elaborative mnemonics (covered later), in general, the evidence is quite consistent that if a learner is exposed to or can form an imaginal or verbal transformational elaboration, learning of paired associations increases dramatically (e.g., Pressley, 1982; Rohwer, 1973). Such transformational mnemonic strategies have proven useful for learning more ecologically valid materials than paired associates. There is an enormous literature supporting the case that transformational mnemonics can be engineered to facilitate learning of vocabulary definitions (e.g., Pressley, Levin, & Delaney, 1982), with this claim extending across a number of populations, including mentally handicapped children (e.g., Mastropieri, Scruggs, & Levin, 1987; Pressley, Johnson, & Symons, 1987; Turnure & Lane, 1987). Acquisition of basic social studies facts (e.g., countries and their capitals, states and their products, presidents and their accomplishments) can be facilitated by mnemonic elaborative techniques, as can memorization of many pieces of scientific information (e.g., chemical reactions, parts of the skeletal and nervous systems, and mathematical equations). See Levin (1981a, 1983) and Higbee (1977, 1987) for examples. Many of these applications are specific instances of the keyword method, a procedure devised by Atkinson and Raugh (1975) and originally adapted to child learning by Pressley (1977; Pressley & Levin, 1978).

The keyword method is easily understood by considering a few examples. Suppose that as an English-speaking person you wish to remember that *der Spiegel* means mirror in German. First, note a sound association between the German word and a familiar word in English. For instance, the second author remembers vividly that during his childhood, winners on game shows were always given gift certificates for the Spiegel catalog. Then, form an image between this acoustically similar word (the keyword) and a mirror (the referent of the to-be-acquired foreign item). In this case, an image of someone holding a Spiegel catalog up to a mirror might do. Later, when *der Spiegel* is presented, the acoustic association to Spiegel catalog should come to mind, which would permit access to the interactive image which in turn permits retrieval of the meaning of *der Spiegel*. A second example can be culled from physics. Heisenberg proposed the uncertainty principle, which is that it is impossible to measure the position and velocity of an object at the same time. Perhaps heist could serve as a keyword for Heisenberg. Then imagine a robber leaving a scene of an accident wearing a pedometer that he has stolen. He is anxious to try out the captured instrument, but has trouble figuring out where he is on his escape route as he tries to measure his speed of walking.

Some of the most impressive applications of the transformational mnemonics have been provided with respect to memory of prose (McCormick & Levin, 1987, review that literature in detail). Consideration of a recently completed investigation makes obvious the power of this approach. Suppose that a person is required to learn a set of facts, perhaps biographical points about particular people. One common way of presenting such biographical information is in loosely structured prose. Consider the following text used by McCormick and Levin (1987) to present biographical information about a fictitious person named Charlene McKune (critical to-be-remembered content highlighted):

> Born and raised on a dairy *farm* where she helped take care of the cows, *Charlene McKune* has always been used to hard work. When she was a child, McKune enjoyed creating homes for her pets out of her toy *building blocks*. To earn extra money and because of her hatred for dirt of any kind, McKune began *washing cars* for her parents' friends. . . (p. 400).

Control subjects in McCormick's and Levin's research read this passage, with eventual recall of the name-biographical facts associations required.

There were elaborative transformations in three other conditions of their studies. In one of these three, the loosely connected passages were presented, with subjects instructed to use a keyword strategy to learn the content. Thus, for the illustrative passage, the subjects were provided the word *raccoon* as a keyword for Charlene McKune. They were told to imagine a pet *raccoon* outside a *farmhouse* jumping over a long row of *building blocks* with some kids *washing cars* nearby.

In the second transformational elaborative condition, subjects were presented the same biographical facts, but this time McCormick and Levin (1986) transformed the thematically loose passage into one in which a unifying theme tied the biographical facts together. For the Charlene McKune passage, the theme was "country":

> *Charlene McKune* spent much of her life living in the serenity of the remote countryside. Born and raised on a *farm*, McKune grew to love the peace and quiet of rural living. When she was a child, her father made her *building blocks* out of bits of wood on the farm, and McKune spent hours building "barns" and "silos" with these blocks. To earn extra money, McKune began *washing cars* — and sometimes tractors — for the neighboring farmers (p. 400).*

---

*If McCormick and Levin had started with just the name and biographical facts and generated the country-thematic passage given here, they would have been engaging in a nontransformational elaborative strategy, since they would have been generating linking prose that would be semantically consistent with the biographical facts — that is, a farm logically is in the country, the building blocks logically would have been made of scrap wood from the farm, as a farm child it would make sense that she would construct barns and silos, and washing both cars and tractors would seem to be reasonable for a farm youngster trying to start a vehicle-washing service. Because these relationships do not map directly on to the facts as presented in the loosely structured passage, McCormick and Levin's passage is a transformational

The third elaborative condition involved presentation of both the thematic passage and the mnemonic.

McCormick and Levin (1986) had hypothesized that people would be able to remember which facts went together better when the facts were embedded in the thematic passage. That is, they would recall that whoever it was that lived on the farm had building blocks and washed cars. The thematic passage provided no link to the name of the individual, however, and thus, it was hypothesized that recall of the person who went with each set of biographical facts might be difficult even given the thematic passage. The special strength of the keyword images is that they provide interlinkages for the biographical facts and a link from the biographical points to the name of the person. In general, the results reported by McCormick and Levin (1986) to date confirm that the keyword approach provides greater overall learning than the thematic approach, and specifically facilitates acquisition of fact-name associations. Consistent with predictions as well, the thematic passages improve memory of which pieces of biography go together. This work is important for its implications about how prose content should be structured in order to improve *memory* of prose. Passages highlighting integrative themes have a lot going for them relative to passages that do not (more about this later when studies of precise elaboration are considered). In addition, there are occasions when keyword approaches can be reasonable adjuncts even for memory-facilitating, thematically integrative prose.

Short of completely transforming some given prose (i.e., by rewriting it as McCormick & Levin, 1986, did), there are a number of nontransformational elaborative techniques that can be used with prose that facilitate performance. For instance, many readers construct images representing the content of text that they are reading (e.g., Denis, 1987). Text can be presented with questions that require the learner to go beyond the information presented in the material in order to provide an adequate answer (e.g., Pressley, McDaniel, Turnure, Wood, & Ahmad, 1987). People can be taught to pose questions to themselves (and to look for answers to those questions) as they process text (e.g., Wong, 1985); they can be taught questioning strategies to facilitate inference formation (e.g., Elliott-Faust & Pressley, 1986; Hansen & Pearson, 1983). All of the strategies in this paragraph involve going beyond the information given in the to-be-learned content, but doing so in a way that involves introduction of relationships that are naturally and meaningfully consistent with the content that is being studied.

Both transformational and nontransformational elaborative strategies have been studied developmentally. There are clear developmental increases in noninstructed use of these procedures; there are also clear developmental differences in the adequacy of elaborative strategy use following instruction. In this section of the chapter, we review some of the most important developmental findings, ones that make clear

---

elaboration, particularly because there is deletion of content that did not fit the transformational "country" theme. In making this point, we also appreciate that this example makes clear that the boundary between transformational and nontransformational elaborations is sometimes a fuzzy one.

that the road to good elaborative strategy use is a slow one. There is far too much literature on the development of elaboration to provide a comprehensive overview. Instead, we present important developmental conclusions that are relevant to the good strategy user model, briefly mention some of the more important studies that support the conclusion, and then discuss in detail some particularly pertinent results that support each of the main conclusions that are presented.

Development of Elaboration Skills

1. *There is greater use of elaborative strategies (without instruction to do so) with development. There are especially impressive increases from late childhood to late adolescence.* The empirical tipoff that there was increased use of elaboration among older adolescents was provided by Rohwer and Bean (1973). They noted that in all of their experiments, grade-school children benefited from instructions to construct transformational elaborations when learning paired associates; in contrast, this instruction only worked some of the time with samples of older adolescents. The most sensible explanation of instructional failure when it occurred with 11th- and 12th-grade students was that they were already elaborating, and thus, the instruction failed to promote cognitive activity over and above what the older adolescents were already doing. This explanation seemed sensible given that it was well known by 1973 that university students would elaboratively mediate paired nonsense syllables and other materials as they tried to learn them (e.g., Prytulak, 1971; Underwood & Schulz, 1960).

Pressley and Levin (1977a) provided some more direct support for Rohwer and Bean's (1973) developmental interpretation. They interviewed students in grades 5, 7, and 9 about their strategy use during paired-associate learning. There was a clear increase with age in the proportion of children reporting use of elaboration, although at no developmental level did even a majority of students report elaborating most of the pairings that they were trying to learn. One of the most striking aspects of the results reported by Pressley and Levin (1977a) was that classifications of children with respect to strategy use was much more predictive of associative learning performance than age. For example, the associative learning of fifth-grade elaborators was almost as good as the associative learning of ninth-grade elaborators. Both of these groups outperformed fifth- and ninth-grade students who relied on rehearsal. Again, there was only a slight cued recall difference between fifth- and ninth-grade rehearsers.

Others have also generated data consistent with the strategic development position advanced by Rohwer and Bean (e.g., Kemler & Jusczyk, 1975; Kennedy & Suzuki, 1977; Waters, 1982). Beuhring and Kee (1987a, 1987b) have recently reported a set of results that provides especially strong support for Rohwer and Bean's (1973) hypothesis. They included samples of 10- to 11-year-old children and 16- to 18-year-old adolescents. The subjects were presented two lists of 36 unrelated noun pairs. They were given each pair one time for 15 seconds and were told to learn it so they could recall the second pair member given the first. The subjects were also required to verbalize their thoughts while they studied. The researchers were extremely careful not to prompt the subjects about the types of strategies that could be used to learn the word pairs. It was explained explicitly that the purpose of the study was to find out what people really did to learn this material. There were several indicators that the subjects were faithful to the instructions, including high ratings of confidence that they had in fact reported all of the elaborations as they were occurring.

The verbalized strategies were classified into three categories: rehearsal, elaboration, and other associative strategies:

Rehearsal was defined as the repetition of a noun pair with or without a conjunction (e.g., The CATTLE and the BAY) and Elaboration was defined as the description of a direct interaction between the members of a noun pair (e.g., The CATTLE swam in the BAY). Strategies that provided associations other than a direct interaction were grouped together in a category of Other Associative Strategies (e.g., identifying an attribute the nouns shared in common such as color or shape; indicating that the pair members were owned by the same person; forming an interaction between the stimulus and a new, intermediate, response that would cue the actual response because of some preexisting association with it) (pp. 260–261).

The mean number of each type of mediator reported at each age level is recorded in Figure 6.1. There was a dramatic decrease with increasing age in the mean number of rehearsals that were reported. There was concomitant increase in the number of elaborations and other associative strategies. In short, these data supported Rohwer and Bean's (1973) hypothesis that the use of elaborative strategies increased with age. In addition, regression analyses were conducted in which the number of elaborations reported, the number of other associative strategies reported, and the age of subjects were entered (in that order) as predictors of paired-associate memory. Number of elaborations accounted for 42% of cued recall; number of

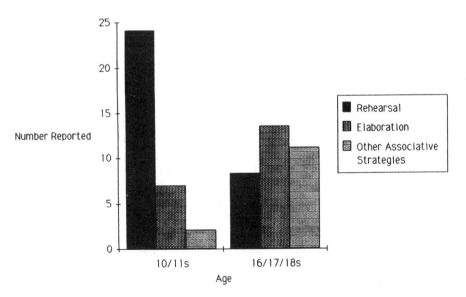

FIGURE 6.1. Mean number of mediators (maximum = 36) reported at each age level in Beuhring & Kee (1987a, 1987b).

associative strategies accounted for another 29% of the performance variability; age accounted for less than 4% of the remaining performance. Beuhring and Kee (1987a, 1987b) concluded that nearly all of the developmental increase in recall could be accounted for by the developmental increase in elaborative strategy use.

In short, there is a good deal of evidence that elaborative activity increases during adolescence. It is noteworthy that compared to some of the other strategies reviewed earlier in this book (e.g., cumulative rehearsal), elaboration is a late development. It is also notable that elaboration is not universally applied by university-age adults, either during paired-associate learning as in Beuhring and Kee (1987a, 1987b) or during learning of other materials with associative structure. For instance, in recent studies of vocabulary learning, Pressley and Ahmad (1986), Pressley (1987), and Pressley, Levin, and Ghatala (1988) reported that university students used keyword-elaborative strategies between 20 and 30% percent of the time (specific value varied slightly from condition to condition). A number of subjects reported no use of elaboration for vocabulary learning, relying exclusively on rehearsal. There is plenty of room for additional development of elaborative competence, even in good adult learners like those enrolled in a university. It is clear from these data that if good elaborative strategy use is to occur, it cannot be left to naturalistic development.

2. Some elaborative strategies can be carried out by older but not younger children. A great deal of research effort was expended in the last 15 years toward determining when children can generate transformational imagery strategies. Much of this work was done using paired-associate materials, with the relevant experiments including conditions in which the subjects were instructed to construct interactive images to learn the pairings and control conditions in which subjects were left to their own devices to learn the associations. Most of this work was stimulated in part by Rohwer's (1973) developmental elaboration hypothesis (see Pressley, 1982), that with increasing age less and less explicit cuing would be required to activate elaboration in children. Support was found for this hypothesis in the case of transformational imaginal elaboration.

In most of these studies, ability to construct transformational elaborative images was inferred if there was greater stimulus-cued recall of responses in a condition in which children were provided transformational imagery instructions than in a control condition in which subjects were not provided imagery directions. Although there is evidence that even 4-year-olds can generate imagery mnemonics for paired associates (e.g., Bender & Levin, 1976), a lot of prompting and environmental support is required (e.g., pairs are presented as toys rather than as words). Less prompting and support is required with increasing age, with development of imagery generation skill continuing until the end the of the elementary-school years (e.g., Danner & Taylor, 1973; Kemler & Jusczyk, 1975; Pressley & Levin, 1977b).

Development of elaborative imagery skill has also been explored in the context of vocabulary learning, with researchers studying an imagery version of the keyword method. Pressley and Levin (1978) specifically proposed a developmental model of imagery skills as a function of environmental support for generation of elaborative images. Consider the Spanish word, *carta*, which means *letter*. Suppose that a child learner is presented the word, its definition, an English keyword (e.g., cart), and a direction to use the keyword method to learn the word. To carry out the elaboration instruction, the child learner must retrieve from long-term memory images of a letter and a cart, and then must construct a semantic relationship that links a letter and a cart as well as an image to represent the relationship. The information-processing load is reduced considerably if the learner is presented the word, a key-word, and its definition, with pictures of the keyword and definition referents provided as well. Compared to the purely verbal presentation, the child learner given the pictures of the keyword and definition referents does not need to retrieve images for these two items.

Pressley and Levin (1978) hypothesized that whether young children could exe-cute an imagery-elaborative strategy would be tied to the amount of processing required to construct the imagery mediator. This hypothesis arose from supporting work that established that functional short-term memory (i.e., consciousness) is more limited in younger children than in older children and adults (e.g., Case, 1985, Chapter 13; Dempster, 1981). Thus, they expected that children would be able to execute the keyword strategy given pictorial support before they would be able to execute the strategy if they were provided only verbal materials.

Pressley and Levin (1978) included grade-2 and grade-6 children as subjects. In three conditions of the study, children were given keyword instructions. In one of these conditions, the subjects were also presented pictures completely representing a complete mnemonic image (e.g., a picture of a large postal letter in a cart). In the second condition, pictorial support for imagery generation was provided. In the third, there was no pictorial support, with only verbal presentations of the vocabu-lary and keywords. There were also two control conditions, one in which the defini-tions were presented as pictures and one in which the vocabulary and meanings were presented verbally only. The results of this experiment are presented in Figure 6.2. Interacting pictures promoted learning of the vocabulary at both grade levels. There was also significant facilitation at both grade levels due to the keyword instruction when picture support was provided. In contrast, although the keyword instruction facilitated the performance of sixth graders when they were provided the materials verbally only, no comparable facilitation was obtained at the grade-2 level. These data generally supported Pressley and Levin's (1978) hypothesis that grade-2 chil-dren could generate elaborative images given an instruction to do so, if they were provided support that promoted generation of the images. Grade-6 children do not require pictorial support for them to construct keyword-mnemonic images.

Pressley and his associates continue to study the development of children's abili-ties to construct imaginal elaborations. Given the contemporary prominence of theories relating the development of children's cognitive performances to the development of short-term memory (e.g., Case, 1985), there is renewed interest in determining whether children's ability to generate images is tied to how much infor-mation a child can hold in consciousness at any one time—whether imagery-generation skill in children is tied to *functional* short-term memory differences between children, with functional short-term memory a product of short-term

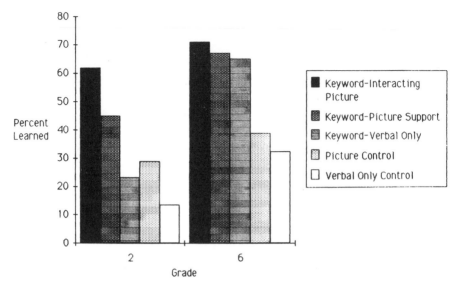

FIGURE 6.2. Mean percent learned as a function of grade level and condition in Pressley & Levin (1978).

storage determined by biological factors, management of that biologically determined capacity, and the learner's knowledge base (Case, 1978; Chi, 1978).

Pressley, Cariglia-Bull, Deane, and Schneider (1987) studied in detail the relationships between children's use of a nontransformational imagery strategy and functional short-term memory differences (as assessed by a battery of measures administered as part of the experiment), differences in general verbal competence (Peabody scores), and differences in age. Their hypothesis was that functional short-term memory would be highly predictive of sentence learning when children were using an imagery strategy to code sentences, but would not be so predictive of learning when children learned any way that they wanted. Six- to 13-year-old children were presented 20 sentences to learn, ones referring to very concrete events that were amenable to imagery encoding (e.g., The angry bird shouted at the white dog; The fat boy ran with the gray balloon; The policeman painted the circus tent on a windy day; The pirate dropped the gold key in the middle of the jungle). Subjects in the imagery condition were told to make a picture in their head for each sentence. The instructions stressed that the images should represent the meaning of the sentence content as closely as possible. Control subjects were simply instructed to try hard.

Consistent with data generated by Levin, Bender, and Pressley (1979), there was a clear developmental effect in that the imagery instructions significantly promoted sentence learning for the older half of the sample (grades 4, 5, 6), but there was only a slight trend for the younger half of the sample (grades 1, 2, 3). The sentence learning data are presented in Figure 6.3. Much more interesting, children with higher

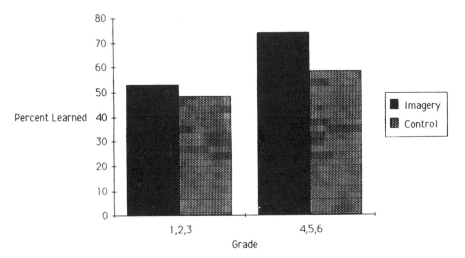

FIGURE 6.3. Mean percent learned as a function of grade level and condition in Pressley, Cariglia-Bull, Deane, & Schneider (1987).

functional short-term memory scores were more successful in the imagery condition than were children who were less able to hold a number of items in consciousness at one time (zero-order correlation = .71). The potency of short-term memory as a predictor in the imagery condition was especially clear given that it was a significant predictor even with age and verbal competence in the regression equation. LISREL analyses made clear that even the predictability of sentence learning from verbal competence was mediated in the imagery condition in part by the influence of verbal competence on functional short-term memory. In contrast, the relationship between short-term memory and sentence learning was much less pronounced in the control condition (zero-order correlation = .40). With age entered into the regression equation, neither verbal competence nor short-term memory differences between children were additionally predictive of sentence learning in the control condition. In short, all of the analyses in Pressley, Cariglia-Bull, Deane and Schneider (1987) were consistent with the conclusion that imagery-generation competence in children is tied to functional short-term capacity. Kee and Davies (in press) have presented complementary evidence that elaboration is short-term capacity demanding for children, with decreasing capacity required to execute elaboration strategies with increasing age during adoloscence. We expect a great deal of additional research on the developmental relationship between use of elaboration and functional capacity given the clear relevance of this work to a variety of theoretical perspectives.

Because of the enormous general interest in the development of imagery skills during the 1970s and 1980s (e.g., Bruner et al., 1966; Kosslyn, 1980; Piaget & Inhelder, 1971), the development of imaginal elaboration received much more attention than the development of verbal elaboration skills. The identification of clear developmental trends in imagery generation fueled interest in imagery addition-ally—It became clear that imagery generation was more certain with primary-grade children with to-be-learned materials presented pictorially compared to verbally, with paired items that had obvious semantic relationships compared to nonobvious relationships, and when materials were presented relatively slowly. In contrast, by the end of the grade-school years, children can generate elaborative images given purely verbal presentations, given materials that are arbitrarily related, and given fairly rapid presentation of to-be-learned materials.

From a pragmatic perspective, it is unfortunate that more attention has not been given to children's verbal elaboration under instruction, because there is very con-vincing evidence that some verbal elaboration skills are developed far in advance of imagery elaboration. Even nursery school children's learning of paired associates can be improved easily by very brief instructions to them to construct meaningful sentences linking paired items (e.g., Levin, McCabe, & Bender, 1975; Milgram, 1967).

The potency of verbal elaboration instruction relative to imagery elaboration instruction for young grade-school children can be appreciated by comparing the results of a study reported by Pressley, Levin, and McCormick (1980) (summarized in Figure 6.4) with the results of Pressley and Levin (1978) (Figure 6.2). Grade-2 and Grade-5 children were presented the same vocabulary to learn that children in Pressley and Levin (1978) studied. Subjects in the verbal elaboration condition were simply told to make up a meaningful sentence containing the keyword and the mean-ing for each vocabulary word as it was presented (e.g., The mailman carried the let-ter in his cart). Control subjects were given the same instruction as control subjects in Pressley and Levin (1978). At both age levels the keyword instruction had a large and dramatic effect on children's learning of the vocabulary words. The ease and potency of verbal elaboration instruction with young grade-school children makes it an appealing alternative to imagery elaboration instruction during the primary grade-school years.

A good deal of developmental work on a variety of elaborative strategies is antici-pated in the coming years. One motivation for this work is that new and potentially very powerful strategies are being proposed and developed. For instance, Bransford and his associates have argued that memory for seemingly arbitrary relationships in text can be improved by providing elaborations that make clear the significance of the relationship stated in text (i.e., precise elaborations, following their terminol-ogy). Bransford and colleagues have conducted a number of studies (e.g., Bransford et al., 1982; Owings, Petersen, Bransford, Morris, & Stein, 1980; Stein, Littlefield, Bransford, & Persampieri, 1984) in which subjects (both children and adults) have been presented a series of mutually interfering sentences that specified relationships that are not obviously meaningful at first glance (base sentences, again following the terminology employed in Bransford's publications). For example, three base sen-tences used in these studies were the following:

The hungry man got into the car.
The strong man helped the woman.
The brave man ran into the house.

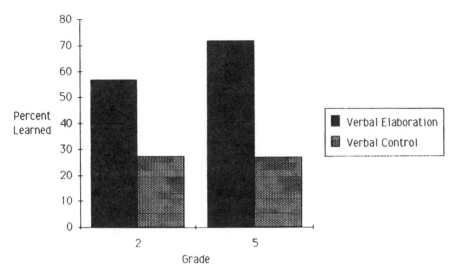

FIGURE 6.4. Mean percent learned as a function of grade level and condition in Pressley, Levin, & McCormick (1980).

These base sentences can be expanded with precise elaborations:

The hungry man got into the car to go to the restaurant.
The strong man helped the woman carry the heavy packages.
The brave man ran into the house to save the baby from the fire.

What are the effects of precise elaborations on learning? Pressley, McDaniel, Turnure, Wood, and Ahmad (1987) investigated in detail the effects of providing precise elaborations to adults. The results were complicated. When learning was incidental (i.e., subjects were not aware as they processed sentences that they would be required to recall them later), there was a small positive effect on adult learning, a result compatible with Bransford and his associates' own data (e.g. Stein & Bransford, 1979; Stein et al., 1984). In contrast, when learning was intentional, subjects who studied only the base sentences actually outperformed subjects given the precisely elaborated sentences. Supplementary analyses determined that during intentional learning, adults generated many and very effective elaborations of their own as they read base sentences. The most important data in the experiment were in conditions in which subjects were instructed to generate their own elaborations for base sentences by responding to "Why?" questions (e.g., Why did the hungry man get into the car? Why did the strong man help the woman? Why did the brave man run into the house?). Answering why questions promoted both incidental and intentional learning, and to a large extent. The results of the Pressley, McDaniel et al. (1987) studies are summarized in Figure 6.5.

These adult results suggested that questioning was an elaborative technique that should be explored in greater detail, especially given the prominent and natural role of questioning during classroom learning (e.g., Redfield & Rousseau, 1981; Winne,

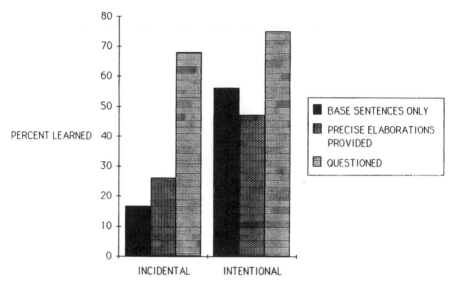

FIGURE 6.5. Mean percent learned under incidental versus intentional instructions as a function of elaboration condition in Pressley, McDaniel, Turnure, Wood, & Ahmad (1987).

1979). Wood, Pressley, and Winne (1988) provided such a test. Children in grades 4 through 8 were presented sentences to learn with the learning goal strongly emphasized (i.e., learning was intentional), sentences similar to those used in Bransford's studies. In one condition of the experiment the subjects were presented only base sentences with an instruction to try hard to learn the sentences. In a second condition the subjects were provided precisely elaborated sentences and were told to try hard to remember them. In the third condition, base sentences were presented and the participants were required to answer why questions. In the fourth condition, the base sentences were presented and the subjects were asked to construct nontransformational images representing the content of each of the sentences. Thus, Wood et al. (1988) replicated the three elaboration conditions in Pressley, McDaniel et al. (1987) and included an imagery condition as well.

The results were somewhat different for the younger compared to the older participants in the study. The data are summarized in Figure 6.6 by splitting the sample at the median age into a younger (mean age = 9 yrs, 9 mos) and into an older group (mean age = 12 yrs, 4 mos). At the younger age level, the percentage learned in the questioned and imagery conditions significantly exceeded the percentage learned in the base sentence condition ($p < .01$ for this and all significant comparisons in this study). Provision of precise elaborations produced nonsignificantly more learning than presentation of base sentences only, and nonsignificantly less learning than occurred in either the questioned or imagery condition. At the older age level, provision of precise elaborations, questioning, and generation of images all produced greater learning than occurred in the base sentences only condition. In addition,

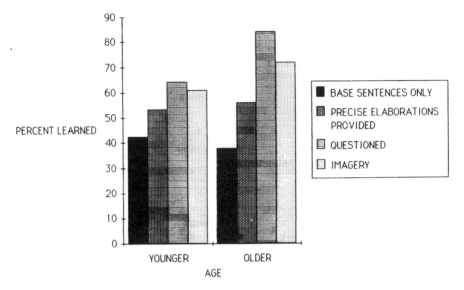

PERCENT LEARNED

BASE SENTENCES ONLY

PRECISE ELABORATIONS PROVIDED

QUESTIONED

IMAGERY

YOUNGER   OLDER

AGE

FIGURE 6.6. Mean percent learned as a function of age and elaboration condition in Wood, Pressley, & Winne (1988).

answering why questions produced greater learning than simply receiving precise elaborations. In short, these results provide support for the hypothesis that both elaborations produced by questioning and nontransformational images promote learning of arbitrary content in children between 9 and 14 years of age.

The results obtained in Wood et al. (1988) are encouraging in that questioning produced striking learning gains, but they are somewhat limited in that the materials used in the Bransford studies are somewhat artificial. Given the limited development of children's knowledge about many topics, they are often presented information to learn that would seem somewhat arbitrary on first inspection. Thus, there is motivation to study the questioning and precise elaboration strategies with materials that have greater ecologic validity. As this book is being written, Wood, Pressley, and Winne are conducting such a test, with children learning passages about Canadian wild animals.

In summary, it is apparent from this brief review of examples that there are more elaborative strategies that can be taught profitably to older grade-school children than there are strategies that can be taught to children in the primary grades. Although even very young children can be taught to use verbal elaboration to learn paired associates and verbal versions of mnemonic techniques like the keyword method, both nontransformational and transformational imagery strategies are more likely to be executed by older compared to younger grade-school children. The gains produced by the questioning strategy investigated by Wood et al. (1988) were more impressive with their older sample than with the younger sample, with answering why questions unambiguously promoting acquisition relative to the precise elaboration-provided condition at the older but not the younger age level.

An encouraging note with respect to the younger children, however, is that as more is learned about the mechanisms that mediate developmental susceptibility to elaborative-strategy instruction (e.g., short-term memory factors), it should be easier to design materials so that young children are more likely to be able to carry out complicated elaborative strategies. For instance, providing picture supports during vocabulary learning increases the likelihood that children as young as 7 years of age can carry out keyword-mnemonic strategies (Pressley & Levin, 1978); providing certain types of pictorial supports encourages formation of nontransformational images during prose learning (Digdon, Pressley, & Levin, 1985; Guttmann, Levin, & Pressley, 1977; Ledger & Ryan, 1985; Miller & Pressley, 1987; Pressley & Miller, 1987).

It must also be remembered that even on those occasions when young children cannot generate their own elaborative mediators, there is always an alternative instructional strategy. The children can be provided mediators, such as interactive mnemonic pictures (transformational elaborations), pictures that represent prose exactly (nontransformational pictures), and precise elaborations. There is impressive evidence that provision of elaborations often promotes young children's learning substantially. For instance, Pressley, Samuel, Hershey, Bishop, and Dickinson (1981) asked kindergarten and nursery-school children to learn 10 Spanish vocabulary words. The children were either left to their own devices as they studied each word for 12 seconds, or they were provided keyword-mnemonic pictures for each word (e.g., picture of a duck with a pot on its head for *pato-duck*). Learning was much better in the mnemonic-picture condition compared to the control condition, with the results displayed in Figure 6.7. Suffice to say in closing this subsection that there are many demonstrations of impressive learning gains associated with the provision of elaborations both to normal and special child populations (e.g., Levin, 1982, 1985a, 1985b; Mastropieri et al., 1987; Pressley, 1977; Pressley & Miller, 1987; Taylor & Turnure, 1979; Turnure & Lane, 1987).

3. *Older children are more likely than younger children to retrieve and use elaborative mediators that they have created.* Constructing a mediator at study does little good if it is not used at test time. Pressley and Levin (1980) hypothesized that there might be important developmental improvements in retrieval of elaborative mediators. They asked grade-1 and grade-6 students to learn 18 paired associates. The subjects were asked to construct interactive images in two of the three conditions of the study. The third condition was a control treatment in which subjects were instructed simply "to try hard to remember that _____ and _____ go together."

At testing, one of the two groups of imagery subjects (hereafter, imagery + retrieval condition) were explicitly instructed to retrieve the elaborative mediators that they had constructed. Subjects in this cells were instructed to: "Think back to the picture you made of the (test stimulus) doing something. What went with *(test stimulus)*?" Subjects in the simple imagery condition were not prompted to use the

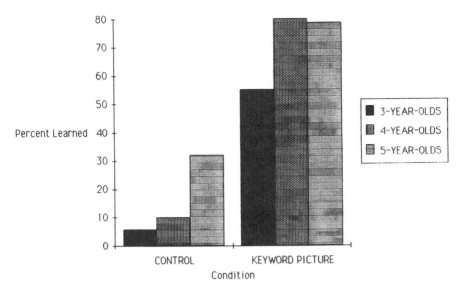

FIGURE 6.7. Mean percent learned as a function of condition and age in Pressley, Samuel, Hershey, Bishop, & Dickinson (1981).

imagery mediators at testing. As each test item was presented, these subjects were told: "Try hard to remember what word was presented with _____. What went with _____?" Control subjects received this same instruction at testing.

What was very clear from examining the data (presented in Figure 6.8) was that the retrieval instruction was necessary for the imagery instruction to promote associative recall effectively with the grade-1 children but not with the grade-6 subjects. That is, the grade-1 subjects did not retrieve the mnemonic mediators without a prompt to do so; the explicit retrieval prompt to use the imagery mediators at testing was not necessary with the grade-6 children.

Pressley and MacFadyen (1983) continued the study of the development of elaborative mediator retrieval. They hypothesized that one reason that *provided* mnemonic pictures were powerful with children as young as 5 to 6 years of age was that the mnemonic pictures might establish a trace so strong that it would be elicited at testing without the necessity of a retrieval prompt. On the other hand, it still seemed possible that retrieval deficiencies might occur with provision of mnemonic pictures, perhaps at a still younger age level. Thus, Pressley and MacFadyen (1983) presented kindergarten and nursery-school children the same 18 paired associates used by Pressley and Levin (1980). The difference in this study was that the pairs were presented as pictures in this experiment (separated pictures in the control condition and interactive mnemonic pictures in the two mnemonic picture conditions) compared to the verbal only presentations in Pressley and Levin (1980).

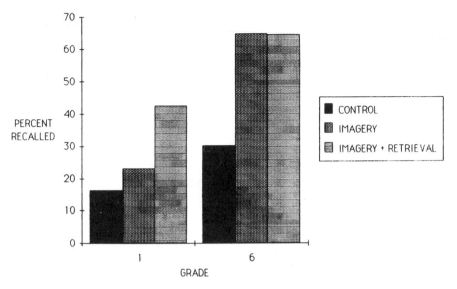

FIGURE 6.8. Mean percent learned as a function of grade and condition in Pressley & Levin (1980).

The results of the experiment are depicted in Figure 6.9. At the kindergarten level, there was significantly better recall in both the mnemonic picture + retrieval and retrieval conditions compared to the control condition, indicating that the kindergarten subjects did not have a retrieval deficiency with respect to the elaborative mediators. In contrast, at the nursery-school level the provision of the mnemonic picture at study had no effect unless there was also a retrieval instruction at testing (i.e., there was a retrieval deficiency in the nursery-school data). Moreover, in a supplementary study, Pressley and MacFadyen (1983) replicated the retrieval deficiency at the nursery-school level, so that confidence is high that such a deficiency does exist at that level.

Although retrieval deficiencies have been studied prominently in many other memory situations (e.g., Kobasigawa, 1977), there is a lack of such study in the elaboration literature, despite the fact that good use of elaboration strategies is highly dependent on both study and testing behaviors. In addition to the work of Pressley and Levin (1980) and Pressley and MacFadyen (1983), see Turnure (1985) for especially persuasive data substantiating the need for additional study of elaborative study and testing interactions.

4. *There is a developmental increase in the propensity to transfer elaborative strategies.* The study by O'Sullivan and Pressley (1984) that was described earlier also included a sample of adults. Although instruction provided to the children in the study had to contain a lot of specific strategy information (when and where to use the strategy) in order to produce general use of the keyword method (i.e., transfer),

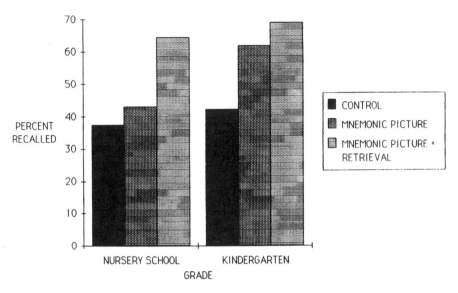

FigURE 6.9. Mean percent learned as a function of grade and condition in Pressley & Mac-Fadyen (1983).

19- to 20-year-old subjects transferred the strategy without explicit provision of specific strategy information. One interpretation of this result is that university students are more likely than children to derive specific strategy information on their own as they practice using a strategy, a result supported by some other research conducted by Pressley and his colleagues and discussed in the next chapter (e.g., Pressley, Levin, & Ghatala, 1984). See Pressley and Ahmad (1986) for another example of transfer of an elaborative strategy by university students following instruction that was not embellished with specific strategy information.

Pressley and Dennis-Rounds (1980) were the first to propose that there might be striking changes during adolescence in the propensity to transfer elaborative strategies. Their hypothesis was stimulated in part by the development of "spontaneous" elaborative strategy use during adolescence, with Pressley and Dennis-Rounds hypothesizing that much of the "spontaneous" strategy use by adolescents was probably transfer of elaborative strategies that the teenagers had encountered in other contexts.

Pressley and Dennis-Rounds' subjects performed two associative tasks, the first learning of cities and their associated products and the second the acquisition of Latin definition linkages. There were three conditions in the study that are relevant to the current discussion (this study is taken up in greater detail in the next chapter). Subjects in two of these three conditions were taught to use the mnemonic-keyword method to mediate city-product learning. Control subjects were left to their own devices to learn the cities and their products. The critical manipulation with respect to transfer occurred before the Latin words were presented. The subjects who were given control instructions for city-product learning were also given control instructions for Latin learning, as was one of the two groups that were given keyword instruction for the city-product task (hereafter, those in the keyword no-transfer instruction condition). Subjects in the other keyword condition received additional keyword training before presentation of the Latin words (keyword complete reinstruction condition). They were taught explicitly how to apply the keyword method with Latin words. Transfer would be apparent in this design if performance of no-transfer instruction subjects exceeded the performance of control subjects on the Latin task. The more performance in the no-transfer instruction condition resembled performance in the complete reinstruction condition, the greater the transfer.

The most critical data in the study are presented in Figure 6.10. There was no evidence of transfer among 10- to 13-year-old subjects—the no-transfer instruction and control means were virtually identical. Consistent with the perspective that propensity to transfer increases during the adolescent years, there was significant transfer among 16- to 19-years-olds. That is, complete reinstruction in the keyword method was not necessary to induce keyword method use on the Latin task. On the other hand, performance in the no-transfer instruction condition was far below performance in the complete reinstruction condition at both age levels, indicating that spontaneous transfer was far from complete. Thus, although these data support the case that transfer of elaborative strategy use increases during the adolescent years, it is apparent that transfer is far from perfect during middle to late adolescence.

5. *With advancing age, coordination of elaboration strategies and the knowledge base becomes more proficient.* The first study of this development was conducted by Pressley and Levin (1977b). They presented lists of paired associates to 7- and 8-year-olds and 10- to 12-year-olds. The to-be-learned pairs included ones that could be elaborated easily and quickly (based on an extensive pilot investigation) with readily available relationships in the knowledge base. For instance, the pair *needle-balloon* can be elaborated as a *needle popping a balloon* and *towel-plate* can be elaborated as a *dish towel used to dry a plate*. The list also included pairs that were not so readily elaborated (e.g., *lamp-key, button-comb,* and *bird-watch*).

The subjects in Pressley and Levin (1977b) either were instructed to construct transformational images to learn the pairs (imagery condition), or they were permitted to study the pairs any way that they wanted (control condition). Half of the subjects were presented the pairs at a relatively rapid rate (i.e., 6 secs), with the remaining subjects receiving the pairs at a slower rate (12 secs). The main hypothesis in the study was that even if younger subjects could benefit from imagery instructions with easy-to-relate pairs and/or when the pairs were presented at a relatively slow rate, they might have greater difficulty using the strategy with hard-to-relate pairs and/or when the pairs were presented rapidly. Consistent with expectations, the older children benefited from the imagery-elaboration instruction for both easy and difficult pairs, regardless of the rate of presentation of the materials. Statistically significant facilitation due to imagery use was obtained with the younger children as well, except when the difficult pairs were presented at a rapid rate.

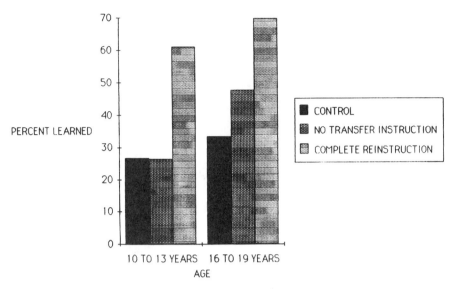

FIGURE 6.10. Mean percent learned on the transfer task as a function of age and transfer instruction in Pressley & Dennis-Rounds (1980).

Elaboration of difficult pairs required a search of the knowledge base that could not be completed in six seconds by the younger subjects. Older subjects could search the knowledge base at that faster rate.

Rohwer, Rabinowitz, and Dronkers (1982) provided additional data substantiating the dependence of mnemonic strategy use on the knowledge base and substantiating developmental shifts in the accessibility and use of the knowledge base in the service of elaborative strategy use. In fact, in some cases it seems that accessibility is so automatic that conscious use of an elaborative strategy is unnecessary. Eleven- and 17-year-olds were presented one of two types of paired associates to remember, ones closely related in the knowledge base (e.g., ranch-cowboy) and ones not so closely related (e.g., ranch-floor). Subjects were presented the pairs and were provided either an instruction to learn them by generating verbal elaborations (little stories joining the pairs) or a no-strategy control instruction.

The elaboration instruction failed to improve performance on closely related pairs at either age level. Rohwer et al.'s (1982) preferred interpretation of this finding was that both the children and the adolescents automatically accessed elaborations given closely related pairs. In contrast, there was a clear developmental difference with the not-so-closely related pairs. The elaboration instruction improved 11-year-olds' learning of unrelated pairs, but had no effect on the 17-year-olds. The generally high performance at the 17-year-old level was interpreted as evidence that these adolescents were probably elaborating the not-so-closely related pairs without an instruction to do so; the elaboration versus control difference at the younger age level was interpreted as evidence that the younger children did not spontaneously elaborate the not-so-closely related pairs. Such a developmental shift is generally consistent with the conclusion drawn earlier that there are significant increases in use of elaboration strategies during the adolescent years. The more critical outcome for the present discussion was the differential effectiveness of the elaboration instruction with closely related compared to not-so-closely related pairs at the 11-year-old level. Very closely related materials seemed to be elaborated automatically at that age level in the Rohwer et al. (1982) study; the fifth graders did not seem to elect the elaboration strategy on their own given the not-so-closely related pairs. See Waters (1982) as well for additional data substantiating that uninstructed use of elaboration strategies depends in part on the knowledge base. It is clear from Rohwer et al. (1982), Waters (1982), and Pressley and Levin (1977b) that knowledge base factors are critical determinants of spontaneous use of elaboration strategies and use of elaboration strategies under instruction and that complete understanding of the development of elaborative competence requires consideration of nonstrategic knowledge.

6. *Metacognition about elaboration strategies increases with development.* The very first study of metamemory tapped children's developing knowledge about the usefulness of elaboration as a memory strategy. Kreutzer et al. (1975) showed seven pictures of objects to their child subjects, using the following interview to elicit perceptions about the potency of elaboration:

The other day I showed these pictures to other boys and girls your age. I asked one girl to learn them so that she could tell me what they were later when she couldn't see them any more. And I showed the same pictures to another girl, but also told her a story about the pictures [E put down each picture as its depicted object was mentioned] (to-be-learned objects italicized):
A man gets up out of *bed*, and gets dressed, putting on his best *tie* and *shoes*. Then he sits down at the *table* for breakfast. After breakfast he takes his *dog* for a walk. Then he puts on his *hat* and gets into his *car* and drives to work.
I told the girl who heard this story that she was supposed to learn the pictures so she could tell me what they were later when she couldn't see the pictures. She didn't have to tell me the story, just the pictures. Do you think the story made it easier or harder for the girl to remember the pictures? Which girl do you think learned the most? Why? (p. 11)

The most important result was that there was a clear developmental increase in understanding that verbal elaboration facilitates learning. Kindergarten subjects chose the elaboration strategy as more effective 50% of the time (i.e., at chance level). In contrast, all grade-3 subjects and 85% of the grade-5 subjects selected elaboration as more potent; 70% of the grade-3 and 80% of the grade-5 subjects could also offer appropriate explanations for their selection of the elaboration strategy as more potent.

Beuhring and Kee (1987a, 1987b) provided additional data about the development of metacognition about elaboration strategies. They included three items that tapped understanding of elaborative utility:

Elaboration-rehearsal. Asked the student to judge the relative ease of learning three lists composed of the same noun pairs connected either by a conjunction, a locational preposition, or an interactive preposition (the MOP and/by/in the PAN, the JACKET and/by/in the BAG, the WATCH and/by/in the ROBE, the NICKEL and/by/in the SNAKE). Empirically the first two are equivalent to rote rehearsal and the third is equivalent to elaboration (Begg & Young, 1977). Consequently this item assessed knowledge that interactions provided an association that would aid cued-recall memory and side by side relationships did not.

Elaboration-structural. Asked students to judge the relative ease with which they could learn three lists of noun pairs for which the most readily implied association was either phonetic (goat-coat, money-honey, cart-heart, dirt-skirt), orthographic (phone-purse, coin-coat, rose-radio, horse-hose), or an elaborated interaction (bug-garden, coin-purse, bee-rose, water-plant). This item assessed awareness of implied association and knowledge that meaningful interactions would aid cued-recall more than the less specific letter or rhyme associations (see Paivio, 1971; Rohwer, 1973).

Elaboration-shared attribute. Asked the student to judge the relative ease of learning three lists of noun pairs for which the most readily implied association was either an attribute they shared in common (wire-thread, milk-snow, buzzer-trumpet, key-penny), a realistic interaction (scissors-pants, horse-corn, towel-glass, pencil-napkin), or an interaction that was very unlikely to occur (ball-jar, lion-sweater, teeth-chair, needle-sponge). This item assessed both awareness of the implied associations and knowledge that pair-specific interactions would aid cued-recall more than general associations whether the interactions were plausible or not (see Rohwer, 1973).

The main conclusions that emerged from the responses to the items was that the 17-year-olds understood efficacy of elaboration more than did the 11-year-olds. Nonetheless, there were some 17-year-olds who did not recognize the utility of semantic elaborations relative to the alternative strategies. Perhaps most striking, the responses to the elaboration-shared attribute item made clear that the preponderance of 17-year-olds believed that general associations are better than pair-specific elaborations. When the data collected by Beuhring amd Kee (1987a, 1987b) are combined with those obtained by Kreutzer et al. (1975), it is clear that development of knowledge about the superiority of elaboration develops over a very long period of time and is still incomplete by late adolescence.

It is somewhat surprising that study of the naturalistic development of metacognitive knowledge about elaboration strategies has been limited to study of awareness of strategy utility. It is disturbing given the criticality of when and where information for general use of strategies. More positively, there is a good deal of recent interest in delineating what adults know about elaboration and especially imagery (e.g., Denis & Carfantan, 1985; Paivio & Harshman, 1983).

A recent study by Katz (1987) is especially revealing about adults' knowledge of when to use imagery. Katz presented adult subjects with descriptions of 22 tasks, some of which required use of imagery (or at least were facilitated by imagery) and others of which did not. Nonimagery tasks included language usage, spelling, and rating words on a good-bad dimension; imagery tasks included spatial relations, memory for designs, and production of autobiographical memories. Both adults who were classified as high imagers (i.e., those who reported using imagery a lot) and low imagers were able to discriminate between tasks that required imagery and those that did not.

Given demonstrations that the addition of when and where information to instruction increases children's use of elaborative strategies, and given that such explicit instruction of when and where information does not seem as critical to adults (e.g., O'Sullivan & Pressley, 1984), it seems likely that there are important developmental differences in the possession of when and where information about elaborative strategies that one already knows. Undoubtedly, there are also individual differences in the acquisition of such information when learning and practicing new elaborative strategies. The developmental study of when and where information should be a high priority.

SUMMARY

There is clear development of the good use of elaborative strategies. Adolescents are more likely to use elaboration spontaneously than are children. Although older grade-school children can be taught many elaboration strategies, they do not transfer those strategies as readily as adolescents. Even though young grade-school students can execute some elaborative strategies, they are less likely than older children to use the elaborations that were constructed to mediate later performance. Adolescents possess more metacognitive information about elaboration strategies than do children. In short, there are many and important developments that have already been documented.

What is striking, however, following almost 20 years of developmental research on elaboration, is how much remains to be learned. First of all, development has been mapped out much more extensively for learning of paired-associate elaboration and for keyword-mnemonic mediation of vocabulary learning than for other elaborative techniques. There are fairly small developmental literatures concerning nontransformational imaginal elaborations of text (although there are a number of investigations on this strategy conducted at single age levels; Levin, 1976; Pressley & Miller, 1987), elaborative summaries of text, or pegword mnemonics.

In addition, not all aspects of good strategy have been covered in detail. We already noted the lack of research on the development of knowledge about where and when to use elaboration strategies that one possesses. There is little literature relating cognitive styles to the development of elaborative strategy use. Borkowski and his colleagues have begun a program of research on this problem, however. They have determined that impulsive children profit from instructions to use elaborative techniques and that impulsive style factors are probably not as important in determining long-term strategy use as metacognitive factors (e.g., Borkowski et al., 1983) — More about this reseach in the next chapter. The role of motivational beliefs in stimulating and/or undermining the use of elaborative strategies at different developmental levels has not been studied either, although Borkowski and his associates have started to work on this problem. They have succeeded in showing that maintenance of trained elaborative strategies is more likely if training includes a reattribution component — when children are led to understand that their improved performance following strategy instruction is due to use of the strategy (Reid & Borkowski, 1985). Again, more about this research will be presented in the next chapter. All things considered, however, there are important components of good strategy use that need to be addressed in future work on elaboration. This is despite the fact that the development of elaborative strategies has been studied more extensively than the development of many other strategies.

It should be apparent by this point that many developmental functions were identified in this work on elaboration. In addition, it became clearer during the course of this research as to how to collect data that were really revealing about good elaborative strategy use. We believe that these insights about methodology are generally relevant to the study of good strategy use and thus, conclude this chapter with a review of procedures that promote clear and complete knowledge of strategy deployment.

How to Collect Data on Good Strategy Use

The journals are filled with articles about memory development and memory strategy use. Many of these studies are convincing and informative, and others are less so. Our purpose in this section is to provide some guidelines that would increase the proportion of articles about memory strategy development that fall in the former category. We recognize that some of these recommendations may seem obvious to many readers, but present them because we encounter many reports by researchers who have not internalized the suggestions reviewed here.

Conduct Programmatic Research

Because good strategy use is complex, and its development even more complicated, compelling data on good strategy use require programmatic research. For instance, the many developmental functions associated with elaborative strategy use that were reviewed in the last section were produced by researchers who made long-term commitments to understanding elaboration and its effects. The best work in memory development has been produced by researchers who have conducted many experiments tapping different questions surrounding the use of the particular strategies in which they were interested. Names like Ackerman, Belmont, Bjorklund, Borkowski, Brown, Butterfield, Flavell, Kobasigawa, Levin, Moely, Ornstein, and Rohwer come to mind. The impressive bodies of data produced by these workers make obvious that there is a lot to be said for persistent and cumulative work on particular strategies.

One obvious benefit of programmatic research is that the researcher gains experimental savvy as experience with a strategy increases. This permits ever more sophisticated studies of a technique. In addition, programmatic efforts permit exact and constructive replications of the most important effects produced by a strategy. No single study can provide telling evidence about which of its significant effects are wheat and which are chaff. Only replications across materials, settings, and populations can do that. Thus, we strongly advocate programmatic research on strategies, believing that only programmatic efforts can produce data that cover the many dimensions of good strategy use.

In making this recommendation, we have vivid memories of many consulting editor's reports from journals, evaluations generated in response to our own work, to the work of colleagues who have shared correspondence with us, and to the work of other researchers whose work we have refereed (and thus, have access to evaluations generated by other reviewers). A common criticism of programmatic efforts is that the researchers are not really breaking new ground, that they are doing work that is simply "paradigmatic," and that reports in well-researched areas often do not open up enough new questions. Such evaluations are bothersome because they do not reflect an appreciation of the need for exhaustive programmatic efforts. On the other hand, they make clear that there is often a fine line between cumulative research that advances understanding about an important strategy and "beating a dead horse." Researchers who go the programmatic route should give some thought to the lyrics of the old Burt Bacharch tune, "Knowing when to leave." Although the time comes when the enormous talents of a programmatic researcher should be redirected to a new strategy or area of memory functioning, we believe, however, that researchers should not rush away from a strategy or paradigm that they know well until they have produced studies addressing a number of aspects of good strategy use and its development. Knowing when to leave can be very hard to determine.

Conduct Studies Both of Naturalistic Strategy Use and Strategy Use Under Instruction

Motivating questions in developmental research on memory strategies include (a) What strategies do children use and when do they use them?, and (b) What strategies can children use and when can they use them? The "a" questions tap children's naturalistic performance; the "b" questions tap their competence to use strategies. The "a" questions are resolved by studies in which observations are made when children are presented a memory task but are left to their own devices to learn to-be-remembered materials. The "b" questions can be studied by instructing children to use a strategy and comparing performance with uninstructed controls. Both naturalistic and instructed use of strategies are important to study, with each tapping unique information about cognitive development.

All of the memory strategies that have been studied intensely from a developmental perspective have been studied in both naturalistic-observational and instructional studies, often by the same investigators. For instance, research on cumulative rehearsal (e.g., Ornstein & Naus, 1978), categorization (e.g., Moely, 1977), and elaboration (e.g., Pressley, 1982) come to mind.

In addition to providing comprehensive information about theoretical issues surrounding cognitive development, combined naturalistic-instructional study provides a great deal of information for those interested in memory interventions. The observational work makes clear whether children are using efficient or inefficient strategies, and thus, makes obvious which children do not need instruction about efficient strategies since they use them already. Instructional research promotes understanding of which children are capable of executing a procedure and learning to deploy it proficiently.

Include Manipulations Checks

Subjects in memory strategy research do not always do as they are told. Sometimes they are obstinate, and other times they simply do not understand directions. For instance, a brief instruction to use a mnemonic strategy like the keyword method often elicits something else, such as free association to the to-be-learned vocabulary or attempts to relate the vocabulary to cognates in the subject's native language. Every effort must be made to make certain that subjects know exactly what to do.

At a minimum, subjects should be required to report or demonstrate to the experimenter how they are going about the assigned memory task, with corrective feedback from the experimenter when subjects are not following the directions as intended. There is also a well-developed think-aloud technology (Ericsson & Simon, 1983) that can be employed in many studies. Post-experimental reports and demonstrations of strategy use are sometimes helpful. Although we recognize the many potential problems of on-line and post-experimental reports (see Chapter 5), our experience suggests that much can be gained from them, especially if subjects are impressed with the fact that they should report as accurately and honestly as possible. In addition, it is often possible to obtain objective validation of the reports. For instance, there is a substantial body of data confirming that post-test reports of elaborative mediation are strongly related to more objective measures of performance such as memory (e.g., Pressley, 1987; Pressley & Ahmad, 1986; Pressley, Levin, Digdon, Bryant, & Ray, 1983; Pressley, Levin, Kuiper, Bryant, & Michener, 1982).

Include Dependent Variables That Should be Affected by Use of the Strategy and Ones That Should Not Be Affected

It is almost always a good thing to include multiple dependent measures. In memory development research, memory performance and strategy execution measures are often variables expected to reflect operation of a memory strategy. When children are observed cumulatively rehearsing to-be-recalled serial lists of items, confidence that the rehearsal strategy was actually executed as it has been defined in the memory literature is increased if there is improved recall relative to when the children did not use the strategy. Failure to see improvement in recall might suggest that the children were going through the motions of cumulative rehearsal, but were not doing so intentionally, and hence, not paying much attention to the serial items as they were overtly processed. Improved recall without observation of cumulative rehearsal could be mediated by a variety of other mechanisms (e.g., the children were using a pegword mnemonic approach). Clearly, the conclusion that a sample of children was using cumulative rehearsal, and this mechanism increased recall, is best supported by recall and cumulative rehearsal strategy covariation.

Why include dependent variables that are not supposed to be affected by the strategy? It is a matter of discriminant validation (e.g., Campbell & Fiske, 1959). For instance, one explanation of elaborative mnemonic benefits that has been presented to us is that mnemonics are fun or novel compared to the methods naturally used by people, and thus, improved learning given elaboration instructions simply reflects gains produced by increased motivation when mnemonics are used. By collecting a variety of measures, this hypothesis can be easily tested, and contrasted with the alternative hypothesis that elaboration effects are really quite specific. Most researchers interested in elaboration believe that methods like the keyword method are effective because they strengthen the associative linkages between vocabulary and their definitions, but do not do much else. If the general motivational hypothesis were true, both associative and nonassociative aspects of vocabulary learning should be increased by keyword-mnemonic instruction.

Pressley et al. (1982) provided telling data on this question, demonstrating strong keyword-instructional effects when subjects were required to match vocabulary meanings (an associative task) and negligible mnemonic-instructional effects when subjects were asked to perform nonassociative free recall of definitions presented during study (i.e., without the vocabulary presented at testing). Such a pattern of significant and nonsignificant effects provides a convincing case against those who would try to explain elaborative-mnemonic effects as little more than artifacts of differential motivation between elaborative and other conditions.

Include "Benchmark" Replications in New Experiments

After a strategy has been studied awhile, certain "classic" effects emerge. For instance, providing keyword-mnemonic pictures to children always improves associative learning compared to when children try to use their own strategies to learn vocabulary (e.g., Pressley, 1982). Teaching nonrehearsing 8-year-olds to rehearse cumulatively as they process a serial list of items always improves serial recall (e.g., Ornstein & Naus, 1978). Manipulations that produce well-replicated effects such as these can be included in studies that are more centrally concerned with new hypotheses. If the researcher once again replicates the classic effect, confidence is bolstered in the more novel findings of the study. Perchance the classic effect is not replicated, there is a red flag that something is amiss. The researcher is alerted to look for other factors that may be different between the strategies and situations currently being studied and the strategies and situations studied by others who produced the classic effect.

Contrast the Effects Produced by the Strategy With the Effects Produced by Many Different Control Conditions

Different control conditions achieve different purposes. Instructional research on elaboration has included rehearsal control conditions designed to preclude efficient processing (i.e., subjects are instructed to say paired words or vocabulary and their meanings over and over) and no-strategy control conditions designed to mirror learning as it naturally occurs (i.e., subjects do what they want). In addition, elaborative methods like the keyword method have been contrasted with a variety of semantic-context procedures (e.g., making sentences using the vocabulary words correctly, constructing semantic maps that locate the new vocabulary in a network of related words) presumed by vocabulary learning theorists to enhance performance (e.g., Levin et al., 1984). In general, elaborative strategies like the keyword method have proven potent relative to all control conditions studied to date (Pressley, Levin, & McDaniel, 1987). When a technique is tested against a variety of alternative procedures, including ones that have either proven potent in the past or are presumed potent by practitioners, it is hard to argue that instructional experimental tests of the method have been with "straw men" controls.

Summary

There are many things that can be done to make research better. In making our recommendations, we recognize that memory development research is already expensive, certainly relative to research on adult memory. Simple multiple-age replications of conditions increase the costs. There is often a need for pilot testing to avoid ceiling and floor effects at all age levels and to determine that measurements are really tapping what they are intended to measure (and doing so at all age levels!). Nonetheless, the best, most informative, and most believable research on good strategy use and memory development in general has had this labor-intensive quality to it.

We would be remiss in closing this chapter if we did not note one other important methodological difference that distinguishes high quality work from research that is less than it may appear to be. Good scientists are extremely candid about what is "in" their data and what is not "in" their data. They limit their conclusions to ones that are unambiguously justified by their manipulations and outcomes. Ambiguities are dealt with in subsequent experiments aimed at resolving them. Unfortunately, not all researchers conform to this behavioral pattern. Like all other areas of research, there are scientists who identify with memory development who attempt to make the most out of very modest manipulations and findings. It is often possible to construct a fantastic and interesting tale when one does not feel constrained by the available data. One pattern that we have discerned is the production of a single experiment on a problem (perhaps involving only two conditions), followed by a large number of book chapters or invited journal "thought" pieces that review the modest study and its results in every possible light, often to the exclusion of more telling and systematic work by other scientists.

Thus, the first recommendation made in this section about conducting programmatic research seems to suggest a consumer guideline. Readers of research and those who attempt to devise applications based on research should consider carefully whether the authors of a particular study are year-in, year-out contributors to the archival literature or individuals who prefer the one-shot approach. The scientists who are conducting a lot of experiments that make sense as packages are the ones to consider most seriously.

7. Is Good Strategy Use Possible?

How much truth and how much theory is there to the description of good strategy use provided in the last chapter? Are there really people who know many strategies and have a lot of strategy knowledge? Unfortunately, there are no large-scale, process-sensitive direct observations of learning and memorization across a variety of ecologically valid domains to provide the answers to these questions, despite a great deal of interest in ecologically valid, self-regulated learning (e.g., Bandura, 1977, 1982, 1986; Meichenbaum, 1977; Pressley, Borkowski, & Schneider, 1987). More positively, there are data that permit the conclusion that some people regulate their learning better than other people do.

Interview studies about self-regulated learning in the real world are being conducted, and these are suggestive that some generally competent strategy use occurs. One of the best of these was reported by Zimmerman and Pons (1986), who interviewed high-school sophomores. Half of the participants were doing well in school and half were doing poorly. These students were probed about their studying in the classroom, at home, when doing writing assignments outside of class, when preparing for tests, and when they were unmotivated. Studying in these situations was tapped by having students respond to meaningful scenarios such as the following:

Most teachers give tests at the end of the marking periods, and these tests greatly determine report card grades. Do you have any particular method for preparing for this type of test in English or history? (p. 617)

These probes elicited rich responses from the students, with many general, goal-specific and domain-specific strategies cited. For instance, students reported checking and recording what they did not know (i.e., a form of monitoring), organizing and transforming to-be-learned materials (e.g., making outlines), goal-setting and planning ahead (e.g., formulating a two-week study plan), seeking information (e.g., going to the library), taking notes, structuring their environments to be conducive to study, self-rewarding themselves for doing well, rehearsing, seeking social assistance (e.g., asking a knowledgable friend for help), and reviewing texts and notes. The most striking finding in the study, however, was that the high- and low-achieving students differed greatly in their reported use of self-regulating strategies. The differences in strategy use between ability groups were most notable with respect to seeking information, monitoring, and organizing and transforming. Nonetheless, with the exception of checking their work, high-ability students reported more use of every strategy than did the lower-ability participants. Using discriminant analyses, it was possible to predict achievement grouping (high or low) on the basis of strategy use data alone. In short, Zimmerman and Pons' (1986) data suggest that some adolescents use strategies extensively and that there are substantial associations between achievement and reported strategy use.

One of the most extensive interview studies of classroom learning ever conducted was recently completed by William Rohwer, John Thomas, and their colleagues at the Far West Laboratory for Educational Research. Students enrolled in junior high school, senior high school, and university social sciences classes served as subjects in the study. The courses that the students were taking were analyzed with respect to the demands that were placed on students and the supports that were provided to students to assist them in completing requirements. Study activities used by students were tapped with a questionnaire that included probes about how students selected important information to study, what they did to comprehend lecture and reading material, how they went about trying to memorize important content, and approaches they used to integrate material within or across informational sources.

The most revealing analyses of the Far West data for the present discussion were conducted by Christopoulos, Rohwer, and Thomas (1987). They found that simple rehearsal and nonselective restudy decreased with increasing age level. With increasing age, there was more reporting of self-initiated extra processing of information that was anticipated to present comprehension or memory difficulties. There was also increasing self-initiated investigation, identification, and allocation of attention to material that was likely to be presented on a test. Selective notetaking increased with age, too. Consistent with the data presented in the last chapter, there was increased elaboration, reorganization, contrasting, integration, and summarization of newly encountered information.

Christopoulos et al. (1987) also documented that with increasing age, however, courses place greater demands on students with diminishing supports, an argument that was bolstered by analyses of this large data set by Strage, Tyler, Rohwer, and Thomas (1987). Thus, Christopoulos et al. (1987) argued that much of the developmental increase in strategy use might be in reaction to changing environmental demands. Nonetheless, despite the pressures applied to university students by their class work, they often engage in less than optimally efficient processing, with some students using very good strategies and others relying predominantly on less efficient routines.

The Zimmerman and Pons (1986) and Far West data are consistent with other reports of strategy use by adolescents, reports in which very direct measures of strategy use have been employed (Pressley, Levin, & Bryant, 1983). There are a number of sophisticated memory strategies that have been observed in some adolescents but not others. Individual differences in observed and reported use of strategies are almost always correlated with learning and achievement. Consider three examples: (1) Barclay (1979) reported that a minority of high-school students used "cumulative rehearsal and fast finish" to learn a serial list of single items (i.e., cumulatively rehearsing early items in a list combined with rapid processing of the final list items) — a strategy that positively affects performance compared to cumulative rehearsal, an approach more typical of high-school students. (2) In studies of adolescent associative learning discussed in the last chapter (Beuhring & Kee, 1987a, 1987b; Kemler & Juscyk, 1975; Pressley & Levin, 1977a), only some adolescents used elaborative strategies (e.g., constructing interactive images or meaningful sentences containing the to-be-associated items). Invariably, those adolescents who elaborated learned more associations than did those who did not elaborate. (See Chapter 6.) (3) Brown and Smiley (1978) demonstrated that not all high-school students use underlining and note-taking strategies when trying to learn text; students who do use these techniques learn more from text than students not employing these techniques. In short, by late adolescence there are students who are appropriately strategic in at least some demanding memory situations.

The research to date does not permit the conclusion, however, that anyone develops into the good strategy user described in the last chapter. It is not known whether there are people who are appropriately strategic across demanding situations. Would the same students who use the cumulative-rehearsal, fast-finish strategy for serial list learning be the ones who would use associative elaboration for pair learning and/or take notes during reading of text? It is not known whether there are people who consistently monitor when learning and thinking are going well and when they are going poorly, with strategies continued or changed contingent on performance successes and failures. The resolutions of these issues require intensive within-person investigations. It can be concluded based on the extant data, however, that even very capable adults (e.g., university students) often fail to behave like good strategy users. Some of the most telling data have been provided in studies of monitoring by adults and in investigations of strategy transfer.

Monitoring and Failures of Monitoring

Are people aware of how well learning, comprehension, and memorizing are proceeding? Consistent with the conclusion that people are aware of their performance levels, there are demonstrations with simple materials (e.g., paired associates, sentences) that people can predict which items will be remembered on a post-test. Two demonstrations of this effect were provided by Lovelace (1984). In one of his experiments, university students studied paired associates, and in the other study, adults tried to learn sentences of the form, "The adjective noun verbed the adjective noun." During study the subjects rated on a 1 to 5 scale how sure they were that they would recall the item on a test later. The main finding was that there were monotonic relationships in both experiments, such that items that were rated as more likely to be recalled were in fact better recalled on the post-test. What findings like these reflect is that materials with some characteristics are more learnable than materials with other characteristics, and people have some knowledge about characteristics that positively influence learning and those that make learning difficult. Predictions of future recallability can be based on knowledge of these characteristics. The ability to predict differential learnability of simple materials seems to hold throughout the adult lifespan (Lovelace & Marsh, 1984; Rabinowitz, Ackerman, Craik, & Hinchley, 1982).

Even children can make accurate estimates of the recallability of simple materials based on some materials characteristics. For instance, children understand that lists containing members of the same category are more likely to be remembered than lists containing items that are not readily grouped into categories, and they realize that highly associated paired associates are more memorable than unrelated pairings (Dufresne & Kobasigawa, 1987; Kreutzer et al., 1975; Moynahan, 1976; Tenney, 1975). Despite widespread ability to predict differential learnability of some simple materials, there is less awareness of performance when adults are learning more complicated materials and when they are using strategies that differ in potency.

Monitoring of Comprehension and Learning of Text

According to the good strategy user model, good learners should monitor their progress as they are memorizing, reading, or carrying out any activity. Such monitoring presumably would produce awareness of cognitive progress that permits decisions about strategy use. Specifically, capable learners should notice whether they are comprehending and remembering text. When miscomprehension is detected, reading would be adjusted accordingly. At a minimum, good strategy users would reread. They should also begin to read more carefully and use strategies that had not been called on previously. When they monitor that they are understanding and remembering material, they should be likely to stick with the reading strategies that they have been applying. In short, monitoring is presumed to provide information about ongoing processing, information that is a form of metacognition, and in turn, this metacognition has been assumed to orchestrate subsequent reading.

Despite the intuitive appeal of this good strategy user description of mature reading (e.g., Baker & Brown, 1984), evidence is accumulating that skilled readers (e.g., university students) often fail to monitor completely their comprehension and learning as they read text. Some of the most compelling data on this point have been provided by Glenberg, Epstein, and their colleagues (e.g., Glenberg & Epstein, 1985, 1987; Epstein, Glenberg, & Bradley, 1984; Glenberg, Wilkinson, & Epstein, 1982; Glenberg, Sanocki, Epstein, & Morris, 1986).

For instance, university students in Glenberg and Epstein (1985, 1987) read a series of one-paragraph essays on unrelated topics. For each paragraph, the subjects rated their confidence that they would be able to use what was learned in the text to draw correct inferences about the central theme of the text. Then, an inference for each paragraph was presented with the subject's task to determine if the inference followed from what had been read previously. The most important result was that the correlations between confidence ratings and performance on the inference verification task were very low. Generalizing across experiments within Glenberg and Epstein (1985, 1987) and Glenberg et al. (1986), the correlations were essentially zero, a result inconsistent with the assumption that adults monitor their comprehension. Even in those cases where awareness exceeded zero, it did not do so by much (e.g., Glenberg & Epstein, 1987). Nonetheless, Glenberg and Epstein's observations are consistent with those of others who have examined whether university students can discriminate between the parts of text that they have learned during reading and the parts that were not learned (Maki & Berry, 1984). Even the most optimistic of these estimates, however, suggest that the correlation between awareness and learning is not greater than approximately .30.

Pressley, Snyder, Levin, Murray, and Ghatala (1987) examined a different aspect of text monitoring, focusing on whether university students could monitor how ready they were for a test over an entire chapter of material. Pressley et al. were interested in the students' *perceived readiness for examination performance* (PREP for short) after they read text. In all three of the experiments that they reported, students read chapters from university-level textbooks and took objective examinations following reading. The participants estimated how well they would do on the post-test either before they read the chapter or after reading it. The accuracy of the before-reading estimate was assumed to reflect reader's awareness of their usual performance level following a single reading. The accuracy of the post-reading estimate was assumed to reflect awareness of usual performance plus awareness of learning of the particular chapter as it was read. That monitoring occurred during reading could reasonably be inferred if and only if there was more accurate estimation of performance following reading than before reading. On the positive side, post-reading estimations were consistently more accurate than before-reading estimations. On the negative side, these before-to-after improvements were very small.

Given these monitoring problems experienced by adults, it is not surprising that children are also less than expert in monitoring of their prose processing. For instance, Ghatala, Levin, Foorman, and Pressley (in press) had grade-4 children read a social studies article in preparation for a fill-in-the-blank test over the article's content. In the condition of the study that tapped children's naturalistic regulation of study, the children were permitted to read the article as many times as they wished with the demand that they should not stop reading until they knew that they could achieve 100% performance on the completion test. A reward was promised if they in fact achieved mastery. The failure to monitor was clear. The subjects stopped when they were able to answer 49% of the questions on average. After they stopped studying (but before they took the test), the subjects were asked to predict how many items they would get right on the upcoming test. Children's monitoring failures were striking, with most subjects overestimating what their performance would be.

The paradigm used most frequently to evaluate text monitoring in children was developed by Markman (e.g., 1977, 1979), with greater attention to monitoring of children's comprehension than to their learning of prose content. In Markman's paradigm, children are presented short prose pieces that either are internally consistent or contain inconsistencies. For example, consider the following story used by Zabrucky and Ratner (1986) that contains a contradiction (highlighted in italics):

Paul finally had a day off from work. He decided that he would go to the lake for just the afternoon. Paul packed up his car and headed towards the lake. When he got to the lake, he saw that he was the only one there. The water in the lake was very clear and blue. Paul found a place to sit near the lake and he leaned against the tree. He watched the clouds in the sky and after a while he fell asleep. All of a sudden, a noise woke him up. *Paul caught a big fish with his fishing pole.* Afterwards he opened up his picnic basket and ate a sandwich. *Paul was sad that he forgot to pack his fishing pole* (p. 1406).

A consistent version of this passage can be constructed simply by replacing the last sentence of the inconsistent version with "Paul was happy that he remembered to pack his fishing pole."

The dependent variable that concerned Markman (1977, 1979) was whether children would report problems in text. She reasoned that detection indicated that the children were monitoring whether they were comprehending text—whether their understanding of each new piece of information was consistent with their understanding of information presented previously. This type of monitoring is assumed by Markman and others (e.g., Baker & Brown, 1984) to be important in self-regulation of strategies during reading. When students monitor that there are comprehension problems, they are in a position to initiate strategies to resolve the difficulties. For instance, they might look back at discrepant information or construct bridging inferences to explain why the incompatible pieces of information coexist in the same passage (i.e., use fix-up strategies).

The observation that motivated a great deal of research on comprehension monitoring was that young grade-school children (e.g., 8-year-olds) often fail to detect glaring inconsistencies in prose (e.g., Markman, 1985; Wagoner, 1983). Not surprisingly, they often fail as well to use the fix-up and rereading strategies that are presumably called into play by monitoring (e.g., Garner & Anderson, 1982; Markman, 1979; Wagoner, 1983). More positively, there are developmental improvements in monitoring.

An especially thorough investigation by Zabrucky and Ratner (1986) illustrates the developmental trends in error detection. Twenty grade-3 and 20 grade-6 children read eight short stories like the sample presented earlier. Four of the stories were consistent and four contained inconsistencies. Grade-6 children were more likely to detect problems than were grade-3 children. This held both when subjects were asked a general question about consistency (Did the story make sense?) and when subjects were asked follow-up questions that specified the inconsistent sentences explicitly. For instance, for the inconsistent "Paul" story presented earlier, subjects were asked, "The story said that *Paul was sad that he forgot his fishing pole* and that *Paul caught a big fish with his fishing pole*. Does that make sense? (p. 1407)"

The striking developmental trend on error detection was not paralleled completely, however, by developmental trends for the use of strategies presumably regulated by error detection that occurs as a function of comprehension monitoring. In particular, at both grade-3 and grade-6 levels, subjects spent more time reading inconsistent sentences than matched consistent sentences, with this effect about the same size at the two grade levels. Consistent with the developmental trend for verbal reports of inconsistencies, both grade-3 and grade-6 students evidenced lookbacks when reading inconsistent passages, with more lookbacks at the grade-6 level. Finally, there was little use of inferential fix-up strategies at either age level. Within-age correlational analyses of errors and reading strategies complemented the between-age analyses. In general, there were only weak relationships between verbal reports of errors and use of strategies presumably regulated by comprehension monitoring.

What is going on here? A likely possibility is that monitoring occurs and directs rereading, but that children cannot articulate the errors that they have detected. This speculation is supported by reports that young children manifest nonverbal signs of error detection (e.g., they look perplexed) well before they can verbally report errors (e.g., Beal & Flavell, 1982; Flavell et al., 1981; Patterson, Cosgrove, & O'Brien, 1982). Regardless of the exact explanation of the low interrelations obtained by Zabrucky and Ratner (1986), what is more striking is that even their grade-6 subjects often failed to report errors, often failed to reread when they should have, and almost never made bridging inferences to try to reconcile discrepancies. What is more—Zabrucky and Ratner's (1986) data are not isolated—Such failures by older grade-school children have been observed repeatedly (Wagoner, 1983).

Moreover, adults often pass over problems in text. For instance, university students in Baker and Anderson (1982) missed one-third of the inconsistencies in textbook material; Glenberg et al. (1982) observed even more dismal performance, although with more complicated texts. Even more shocking, adults sometimes fail to detect grotesque inconsistencies in trivially easy texts. Elliott-Faust (1984) presented four simple passages to university students. These passages were modeled after ones designed by Markman (1979) for use with young grade-school children. Some were internally consistent and some were inconsistent. Here is an inconsistent passage that was used in the study (inconsistency indicated by italics):

There are many different kinds of snakes. Some snakes are eight feet long and very fat. Some snakes are only six inches long and very skinny. Some snakes have a poisonous bite, but some snakes are harmless and even help us. The garter snake, for example, helps us by keeping bad insects away from our gardens. Garter snakes eat these insects. They find the insects by listening for them. The insects make a special noise. *Garter snakes do not have ears. They cannot hear the insects. They can hear the sounds of the insects.* That is how they are able to find the insects (Elliott-Faust, p. 223).

The adults who listened to the stories were told that they were helping develop nature stories that would be presented to children in a research study. The adults were told that their task was to evaluate how easy the stories would be to understand. The experimenter told them, "I want you to listen carefully to each story. I am interested in your comments as to how clear each passage is, whether you found it easy to understand, whether it made sense, etc. I am also interested in your suggestions regarding how I might change the passages to make them easier to understand (p. 62)."

After hearing each passage, the subject was interviewed about the story. There were a number of opportunities to report inconsistencies, with each passage heard twice. Nonetheless, inconsistencies were often missed by subjects. It is hard to make a case that comprehension and comprehension monitoring are adequate in adults in light of data like these.

Thus far, we have highlighted some especially striking failures by both children and adults to monitor comprehension and learning of prose. Regardless of the type of text studied or the dependent variable employed to assess monitoring, it was apparent that monitoring is far short of what it could be. Readers cannot spot glaring inconsistencies in text; they do not know which parts of text have been learned and which they have failed to master; they are not aware of how much of the information in texts has been acquired. Nonetheless, in constructing this case, we ignored one of the most optimistic pieces of data in the literature supporting the case that at least some children monitor text comprehension, with monitoring guiding rereading and restudy.

Owings et al. (1980) presented grade-5 children with sets of sentences to learn, an easy-to-learn set containing sentences that were congruent with the child's prior knowledge (e.g., *The hungry boy ate the hamburger*) and a hard-to-learn set containing incongruent sentences (e.g., *The sleepy boy ate the hamburger*). After study, high achieving students were able to rate the relative difficulty of the two sets correctly, whereas low achievers could not do so. Moreover, the high achievers studied differentially in reaction to their perceptions of differential learnability. The high achievers studied the hard-to-learn sentences longer than the easy-to-learn sentences, with the low achievers studying the two types of sentences for the same amount of time. The authors concluded that the high achieving students were spontaneously monitoring during study, but that the low achievers were not doing so. Thus, these data suggest that even some children can monitor their prose learning while they study.

Why then did we ignore these data until this point? As it turns out, the participants in Owings et al. (1980) had had previous experience with the types of materials used in the experiment in that they had participated in a pilot study. Their perceptions of differential learnability could have been developed during the studying and testing that occurred in the earlier session, and thus, the Owings et al. (1980) data were difficult, if not impossible, to evaluate with respect to whether monitoring occurs during study. A recent follow-up by Ghatala, Pressley, Levin and their colleagues (Hunter-Blanks, Ghatala, Pressley, & Levin, in press) restudied the situation that concerned Owings et al., producing data that suggests that monitoring during study may in fact occur with the type of sentences used by Owings et al. (1980).

Hunter-Blanks et al. (in press) presented university students with a set of sentences to learn, half of which were very easy to acquire because they were precisely elaborated with an explanation that made clear why the particular actor would have carried out the action (Chapter 6). The remaining half of the sentences were difficult to learn because they were imprecisely elaborated, that is, completed with an elaboration that was semantically consistent with the rest of the sentence but did not make clear the significance of the relationship specified in the sentence. For instance, a precise elaboration for the sentence THE HUNGRY MAN GOT IN THE CAR would be TO GO TO A RESTAURANT; an imprecise elaboration would be TO TAKE A RIDE. The latter elaboration is imprecise because it does not make clear why it is a hungry man compared to a tall man or a tired man who got into the car.

In the portions of the Hunter-Blanks et al. (in press) experiment that are relevant here, subjects' perceptions of how many sentences of each type would be recalled were tapped either before they studied the sentences or after they studied the sentences. On both occasions subjects indicated incorrectly that they would recall both types of sentences equally well. Of course, this finding is reminiscent of the outcomes in the Glenberg studies and other experiments covered previously in this chapter. But there were some additional data collected after study that were completely out of synchrony with the hypothesis that people do not monitor as they study. The subjects in fact reported that they had picked up that the imprecise sentences were harder than the precise sentences as they studied them, and they had adjusted study accordingly, spending more time and strategic effort on the imprecise sentences! They believed that their compensation would offset the differential learnability, and thus predicted equal recall of the precise and imprecise sentences.

Hunter-Blanks et al.'s (in press) finding makes clear that future studies of monitoring during study need to take measures both of expected recall and perceived differences in learnability. Most of the research has focused on the former, whereas the latter may very well be the more telling with respect to whether people actually do monitor while studying and whether they make decisions to study some material versus other material or in one fashion versus another as they read. For the time being, however, we feel that the outcomes reported in the literature and interpreted as monitoring failures should be considered as red flags that people often experience difficulty monitoring text. One reason that we are reluctant to compromise this conclusion in light of the Hunter-Blanks et al. (in press) and Owings et al. (1980) results is that those studies involved highly unusual text material. Very rarely is real-world text as arbitrary as imprecise sentences are, and we sense that salient text arbitrariness is a feature that makes difficulty of text learning especially obvious. A second reason that we favor the conclusion that people have problems with text monitoring is that such monitoring failures are not isolated, a point that becomes more obvious in the next subsection.

Monitoring Memory Strategy Utility

People often fail as well to monitor the potency of strategies that they are using. The most extensive and analytical research on this problem has been carried out by Pressley, Levin, Ghatala and their associates, with their work stimulated largely by an earlier observation made by Shaughnessy (1981). In Shaughnessy's experiments, adults studied word pairs, using either a rote rehearsal or an imagery strategy. The criterion task was free recall of the pairs. Although the subjects remembered many more imagery than rehearsal pairs, they were not aware of the differential potency of these strategies as they used them—They gave identical ratings of recallability for items studied using imagery and those studied using rehearsal. This failure to notice the differential potency of the two strategies contrasted with accurate within-condition ratings of the relative recallability of pairs (i.e., Shaughnessy's data were nonetheless consistent with observations like those of Lovelace, 1984, reviewed earlier). Shaughnessy concluded that his university subjects were not monitoring the utility of the strategies they were being instructed to use.

Pressley, Levin, and Ghatala (1984) were intrigued by Shaughnessy's report and conducted an intensive examination of monitoring during strategy use. They required university students to learn foreign vocabulary items, with half of the words studied using the very effective keyword method (Chapter 6) and the remaining items studied using a less effective rote rehearsal procedure. In the parts of the experiments that are relevant here, participants were interviewed about the strategies and were asked to express a preference for one strategy over the other, with data collected either before subjects had an opportunity to study using the strategies (these subjects had had the techniques described to them) or after they studied using the strategies. The most important results consistent with the conclusion that monitoring did not occur during study were (1) that subjects did not have a preference for the keyword strategy even after study, (2) that they did not realize that learning was better with the keyword strategy even after study, and (3) that there were no dramatic shifts in awareness of strategy utility going from before study to after study.

It is not surprising, in light of the adult data, that children also fail to monitor the efficacy of strategies as they use them to study (e.g., Ghatala et al., 1985; Ghatala et al., 1986). Discussion of these research efforts are deferred until the next section because of their greater relevance to the topic of overcoming monitoring failures.

How to Improve Monitoring

So far it sounds very forlorn—Monitoring is simply not very good. The only exception seems to be for simple materials, especially when they possess characteristics that dramatically affect their learnability. There is a more positive side, however. It is possible to improve people's awareness of how much they have learned and what they have learned, at least in some situations.

TESTING

Giving people tests over what they have studied increases their knowledge of which content and how much content has been mastered. This occurs during simple list-learning and associative learning tasks (e.g., King, Zechmeister, & Shaughnessy, 1980; Lovelace, 1984; Thompson & Barnett, 1985) and during more complex tasks such as prose learning (e.g., Glenberg et al., 1986; Pressley, Snyder, Levin, Murray, & Ghatala, 1987). See Herrmann, Grubs, Sigmundi, and Grueneich (1986) for an especially thorough examination of this point. They compared before- and after-test evaluations of performance for 10 different tasks. There was evidence for at least some improvement in predictability for all tasks, with very striking improvements on some.

This "testing" effect can be appreciated by constrasting some of the failures to monitor discussed previously with the improved monitoring that occurs when a testing opportunity is introduced. For instance, Glenberg et al. (1986) have explored the effects of a practice test on prediction of future test performance. Subjects read one-paragraph passages. The practice test consisted of one dichotomous item for each passage. The item included an idea stated in the passage and one that was not stated in the passage, with the subject's task to select the one that had been covered. Then, readers rated the confidence that they would perform well on the actual test covering the passage. This actual test consisted of three types of items, ones identical to the practice items, ones containing items related to the ideas in the practice items, and ones containing ideas unrelated to the ones composing the practice items. Prediction of performance on items identical to the pretest items was fairly good (mean r ranged from .55 to .57 across experiments). Prediction of performance on related items was not as accurate (mean r across experiments ranged from .12 to .30), although these values were significantly above the zero correlations typically observed when predicting without the benefit of a pretest. Unfortunately, however, experience with the practice test did little to improve prediction of performance on test items that were unrelated to the practice test items with these correlations being close to zero.

More striking positive results were obtained by Pressley, Snyder, Levin, Murray, and Ghatala (1987). As discussed earlier, they observed that their adult subjects were only slightly better at predicting their post-test performance following reading than before reading. They also demonstrated, however, that subjects were reasonably well informed about how they did on the test after they took it. Thus, in the third experiment reported in the article, Pressley, Snyder, Levin, Murray, and Ghatala (1987) included conditions in which subjects took practice tests following reading but before the actual test. These practice tests were in the form of adjunct questions included in the text. Predictions when the text included the adjunct-question practice tests were quite accurate following reading, with the results of the study summarized in Figure 7.1. Subjects who processed the adjunct questions while they read were as accurate in their estimations of performance as subjects who made their estimations following the actual test. This is an impressive result compared to Glenberg et al.'s (1986) finding, since there was no overlap in items on the pretest and post-test. Pretests in the form of adjunct questions have great potential for informing learners about their mastery of material that they have read.

Testing can also make apparent the relative potencies of strategies. Just as Pressley, Levin, and Ghatala (1984) determined that adults did not monitor the differential utility of strategies as they used them, they also determined that testing opportunities made relative potency obvious. When they required learners to study vocabulary using the keyword method for half the items and rote rehearsal for the remaining items, and then required learners to take a test on all of the vocabulary that were studied, the subjects had a clear preference for the keyword method following the test. They had definite awareness that they had learned more keyworded than rehearsed items and indicated that this was the basis for their keyword-method preference. Particularly potent evidence that relative strategy knowledge was

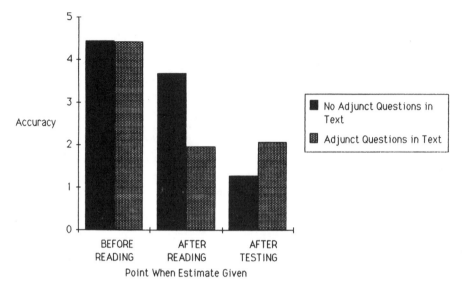

FIGURE 7.1. Accuracy of performance estimates as a function of when the estimate was provided in Pressley, Snyder, Levin, Murray, & Ghatala (1987). (Greater accuracy indexed by lower scores.)

gained during testing was generated in conditions in which the experimenter misinformed subjects, telling them that the rehearsal strategy was better. When subjects expressed preferences for strategies before trying them or after studying (but before testing), they were very much influenced by the experimenter's recommendation that rehearsal was the better procedure. After taking the test, however, virtually all subjects rejected the rehearsal strategy recommendation. In fact, some participants were very indignant about the experimenter's suggestion, indicating that he did not know what he was talking about!

Although tests certainly increase adults' knowledge of relative strategy potency to the point that they weigh this knowledge more than an experimenter's recommendation about differential strategy effects, testing effects that facilitate choice of efficient strategies are not as certain with children. Pressley, Levin, and Ghatala's (1984) study also included 11- to 13-year-old children. Although children did figure out that the keyword method was better than rehearsal as a function of taking a test, they did not perceive the difference produced by the two strategies to be as great as adults perceived it to be. In addition, based on the strategy-utility knowledge gained through testing, children did not resist the experimenter's suggestion that rehearsal should be preferred over the keyword method. This latter result suggested that children do not always use strategy utility information that they acquire on tests following strategy use, an hypothesis that was taken up in a follow-up study.

Pressley, Ross, Levin, and Ghatala (1984) hypothesized that children may need prompting in order to use metacognitive information that they acquire during a test over materials learned by different strategies. In all conditions of the experiment, 10- to 13-year-olds were told that they would be learning English vocabulary words that they did not know already. They were also told about the mnemonic keyword method and a semantic-context method for learning vocabulary. The keyword method was new to these children, but the context method was one they had experienced previously—making up meaningful sentences containing the vocabulary words. Control subjects were asked to express a preference for one strategy over the other after having the task and strategies described. Subjects in a second condition practiced learning vocabulary using the two strategies, followed by a test on the vocabulary that were studied. Practice subjects were then asked to express a preference for one strategy over the other for use in learning additional vocabulary. A third condition was identical to the practice condition except that before subjects in this condition made their strategy selections they were prompted to think back to the test and consider how they did with keyworded versus context-studied items. The hypothesis was that if children do not spontaneously use relative strategy utility information that they acquired during testing in order to make strategy selections, then keyword strategy selections would be more likely in this practice plus prompt condition than in the practice condition. The fourth condition was identical to the practice condition except that before making strategy selections, practice plus feedback subjects were given explicit feedback about the number of keyword and semantic-context items they got correct on the list. Consistent with the hypothesis that motivated the experiment, the percentage of practice subjects (42%) who preferred the keyword method did not differ significantly from the percentage of control subjects (35%) who preferred the keyword method. In contrast, 89% of the practice plus prompt and 89% of the practice plus feedback subjects selected the keyword strategy. Also, consistent with the motivating hypothesis for the study, some practice subjects (77% of them) realized that the keyword method produced better recall—But only half of these subjects selected the keyword technique for use on a future list. In contrast, of the 84% of practice plus prompt subjects who knew that the keyword method was better, 93% selected it. In short, the prompt worked.

The Pressley, Levin, and Ghatala (1984) and Pressley, Ross, Levin, and Ghatala (1984) data suggest that testing following strategy use can have an impact on children's continued use of strategies, although more prompting is required than with adults. In drawing this conclusion, we caution that this testing effect was established with children 10 years of age and older. More recent experiments by Pressley, Levin, and Ghatala (Ghatala et al., 1985, 1986) indicate that children younger than 10 years of age are less accurately aware of how well they perform on tests. In addition, they are less likely to use past test performance spontaneously as a predictor of future performance (Pressley & Ghatala, in press)—which seems necessary in order to use information about past performance as a guide to selection of strategies for future use. These observations make obvious why the successful monitoring training packages with children, which are reviewed in the next section, always include explicit information to note how well performance is proceeding and to make use of this type of information in making future strategy selections.

Although children do not efficiently or completely monitor the effectiveness of strategies they are using and do not routinely use strategy utility information that they derive from strategy use, they can be trained to do so. Elizabeth Ghatala has been the principal investigator in a series of studies (conducted in collaboration with Joel Levin and Michael Pressley) that have addressed the issues that surround training children to monitor their use of strategies (Ghatala et al., 1985; Lodico et al., 1983). The most recent investigation in this series illustrates the procedures used in these experiments and represents well the conclusions that can justifiably be drawn from this type of research.

Children from 7- to 8½-years of age (total $n = 180$) participated in Ghatala et al., (1986). The children were presented three 8-item paired-associate lists for study. Before studying these lists, 36 of the children received a 3-component training that had been shown by Lodico et al. (1983) to improve monitoring of strategy efficacy. They were taught (1) to assess their performance with different types of strategies, (2) to attribute differences in performance to use of different strategies, and (3) to use information gained from assessment and attribution to guide selection of the best strategy for a task. At the beginning of the training, the children were told that there are many ways to play games and that some ways are better than others. They were also told that in order to play a game well, they must choose a method that allows them to do better. The children then were provided two examples. The first involved drawing a circle, with the participants trying two different methods, one drawing freehand and the other using a circular cookie cutter to trace the circle. The children were then asked to decide which of the methods worked better (assessment component) and were encouraged to figure out why one method was superior to the other (attribution component). They were then asked which method they would use if they were asked to draw another circle and wanted to do as well as they could (selection component). Feedback was provided, and the few children who had difficulty repeated the circle game. At the conclusion of the game the children were told that "keeping track of how you are doing when you are playing a game helps you to choose the best way to play." The second example required memorization of a set of letters initially presented in random order. The children studied the letters and tried to recall them. Following this, the children were prompted to rearrange the letters so as to spell their names (each child received a different set of letters), with recall requested once the rearranged letters were removed. Then, children were asked to assess when they had remembered more letters, to attribute the differential performance to the way the letters were arranged, and to decide how they would want the letters presented if they were to replay the game. Again, children were reminded at the end of the task that it is good to monitor performance, to make attributions about why they perform better in one condition versus another, and to use assessment and attribution information in making future study decisions.

In addition to the 36 children who received the complete 3-component training, there were three other conditions (each with 18 subjects in them) that received less than complete training. Participants in the 2-component condition were taught to make assessments and attributions, but they were not instructed to apply the knowledge gained from the assessment and attribution processes in making strategy selections. The participants in the 1-component condition were taught to make rule assessments but were not provided tuition in making attributions or in linking assessments to subsequent selections. The 0-component selection condition was actually a placebo condition. These children received a strategy-affect monitoring training intervention devised by Ghatala et al. (1985). These subjects were trained to monitor how much fun they had while playing the circle and letter games, and to select the method that was more fun. This condition was a good control for the strategy-utility training conditions because it requires reflection on and making judgments about strategic behavior. Thus, whatever performance differences emerged in the other strategy-utility-monitoring training conditions relative to the 0-component condition could be attributed to the strategy utility components of training and not to monitoring training per se.

Following training, subjects in the 3-, 2-, 1-, and 0-component conditions were told that they would be playing another game that involved remembering pairs of words. They were told to do their best to remember as many word pairs as they could. The children were then given two 8-item paired associate lists. On one list they were instructed to use a strategy that is moderately helpful for young children studying paired associates, repetition of the pairs as they were presented. On the other list, they were required to use a strategy that impedes performance, searching for letters that match in the paired words. (Order of strategy practice was appropriately counterbalanced.) Then, subjects were given a third paired-associate list and were told that they were to learn as many pairs as possible. The children were asked to choose one of the two practiced strategies for use on the third list. The children were also asked to justify their choices by selecting one of three explanations for their selection, either strategy utility (i.e., it helps me to remember), affect (i.e., it is fun to use), or effort (i.e., it is easy to use).

The most important result was that selection of the more effective repetition strategy for the third list was a linear function of the number of components that had been included in monitoring training. Eighty-nine percent of 3-component subjects selected repetition, with 61%, 50%, and 44% of the 2-, 1-, and 0-component subjects doing so respectively. Among the 3-component children who selected repetition, 88% selected the strategy-utility reason for doing so. Again, whether subjects who selected repetition did so on the basis of relative strategy utility was a decreasing linear function of the number of training components. Sixty-four percent of the 2-component, 33% of the 1-component, and 25% of the 0-component subjects who selected repetition did so on the basis of strategy utility.

In addition to the conditions in which subjects were trained to monitor, Ghatala et al. (1986) also included conditions in which assessment, attribution, and selection information was provided to subjects after they tried the two strategies on the first two paired-associate lists. These information-provided conditions varied as to the number of components of information that were provided, just as the monitoring training conditions varied with either 3, 2, 1, or 0 components of information generated by the subjects. Thus, 3-component, information-provided subjects were told:

Let's see which time you remembered more pairs. You remembered more pairs the [first, second] time when you learned these pairs (pointing to the appropriate list). You used the repeating method that time. It must have helped you remember better (attribution). The repeating method would be a good one to use again if you wanted to remember as many pairs as possible (selection) (p. 82). (Parenthetical comments added here.)

Two-component, information-provided subjects heard only the assessment and attribution portions of the above remarks. One-component subjects were provided assessment information only, and zero-component subjects received no feedback at this point.

Both 3- and 2-component-provided conditions produced preponderant selection of repetition (94% in both conditions). In contrast, only 44% of either 1-component or 0-component subjects selected rehearsal. Ninety-four percent of the repetition selectors in the 3-component treatment justified their selection on the basis of strategy effects on memory, with 76%, 12%, and 25% of the repetition selectors doing so in the 2-component, 1-component, and 0-component conditions respectively.

What Ghatala's research has established is that even children 7- to 8-years of age can be taught to monitor the relative efficacy of strategies that they are using and to use utility information gained from monitoring in making future strategy selections. It is impressive that 3-component monitoring-trained subjects were as likely to select repetition as 3-component-information-provided subjects— who were all but told directly before they made their strategy selection that they should choose the repetition method. On the other hand, in order for monitoring training to be effective, it had to be very explicit, including directions to compare performances with the two strategies and assess which was better, to attribute the differences in performance obtained with different strategies to use of the strategies, and to select strategies for use in the future on the basis of how the strategies had worked in the past.

Impressive gains in monitoring can be produced with young children by providing training that is well matched to the requirements of the task. That was the case in Ghatala et al. (1986) who first analyzed the strategy monitoring task into assessment, attribution, and selection components and then taught these to children. This same tactic of performing a thorough task analysis followed by training matched to the analysis was taken by Elliott-Faust and Pressley (1986) who sought to improve children's comprehension monitoring as assessed in the Markman (e.g., 1977, 1979) error detection task.

As discussed earlier in this chapter, young children often accept prose that contains direct contradictions as fully comprehensible. Markman (1979) hypothesized that children may overlook inconsistencies of this type because they do not activate and compare contradictory text segments to assess whether the various parts of texts are internally consistent. This analysis of comprehension monitoring suggests that training comparison processing should improve comprehension monitoring in children. To evaluate this hypothesis, Elliott-Faust and Pressley (1986) included conditions in which comparison processing was trained.

One of the conditions involved training the 8-year-old subjects in the study to compare the two most recently encountered sentences. This was termed local comparison training since it involved teaching subjects to make comparisons in a restricted area of the text. In a second comparison-training condition, subjects were taught local comparison along with more wholistic comparison—to compare the meaning of the most recently encountered sentences to the meaning of the entire passage. Because the inconsistent sentences were contiguous in the passages, it seemed possible a priori that local comparison alone might be sufficient to produce improved comprehension monitoring. On the other hand the more complete meaningful processing in the local + wholistic comparison condition provided more extensive analysis of the text and its meaning and thus, might produce more cues that made obvious the inconsistency in the text. The comparison training was carried out with five practice passages, with subjects performing the comparison processing overtly at first, followed by gradual experimenter-guided internalization of the comparison activity by the subjects.

Performances in the comparison-trained conditions were contrasted with four "control" procedures. The most demanding of these was one in which subjects were given explicit instructions as to what it meant for something not to make sense. In particular, they were told that passages that contained contradictory sentences are passages that do not make sense. This "appropriate standard of comparison" control condition was similar to the condition in which Markman's subjects detected the most inconsistencies (Markman & Gorin, 1981). In general, performances in comparison conditions were high relative to the control conditions, with error detection in the local + wholistic cell particularly striking and significantly better than in any of the controls. In short, it proved possible to improve comprehension monitoring by teaching processes that are critical to monitoring but not performed spontaneously by children.

In conclusion, the failures of children to make comparisons (e.g., of text segments with one another, of strategies with one another) results in poor naturalistic monitoring. More optimistically, comparison skills can be developed in young children through instruction. Ghatala et al. (1986) trained children to compare strategies with one another during the assessment phase of their treatment, and Elliott-Faust and Pressley (1986) taught their subjects to compare recently encountered information with earlier text content. We view these comparison strategies as prime examples of the metacognitive acquisition procedures that were discussed in the last chapter—Comparison is a strategy that is explicitly geared to the generation of metacognitive information, such as utility information about strategies and information about whether comprehension is proceeding as it should. In closing, we must emphasize that even though it is sometimes challenging to get children to execute a procedure like comparison at all, maintenance and generalization of this type of strategy requires even more extensive intervention than what has been discussed so far. Thus, we will return to the Ghatala et al. (1986) and Elliott-Faust and Pressley (1986) studies in the next section, which is concerned with problems of strategy durability, problems that reinforce the impression that good strategy use is a scarce commodity.

Continued Use of Memory Skills Following Instruction

Good strategy users should use the strategies that they learn both durably and appropriately. They should continue to use the strategies for the tasks encountered during training of the techniques (i.e., *maintain* strategies). They should stretch the strategies to new tasks that benefit from their application (i.e., *generalize* strategies). Yet, maintenance failures sometimes occur and generalization failures are epidemic in the strategy instructional literature (e.g., Brown et al., 1983). This conclusion holds for normal and special populations, for children and adults, and for intellectual and nonintellectual tasks (Adams, 1987; Borkowski, 1985; Belmont, Butterfield, & Ferretti, 1982; Gick & Holyoak, 1980, 1983; Hayes & Simon, 1977; Reed, Ernst, & Banjeri, 1974).

A few examples make obvious the nature and severity of these difficulties. Some of the best known generalization failures by adults were reported in the problem-solving literature by Gick and Holyoak (1980, 1983). Their studies make clear that even sophisticated learners like university students often fail to transfer strategies that they have acquired—even when the problems are incredibly similar to ones encountered previously as part of training. For example, in some of Gick and Holyoak's work, adults have been presented a problem about a general who wishes to capture a fortress in the middle of a country. There are many roads to the fortress. All are mined, however, so that while small groups of men can pass over them safely, an entire army would detonate them. A full scale, frontal attack is impossible. The strategic solution to the problem of conquering the fort is to divide the army, send small groups on the individual roads, eventually converging simultaneously at the fort.

What is amazing is that after learning the solution to the "general" problem, adult subjects often fail to solve a problem like the following:

Suppose you are a doctor faced with a patient who has a malignant tumor in the stomach. It is impossible to operate on the patient, but unless the tumor is destroyed the patient will die. There is a kind of ray that can be used to destroy the tumor. If the rays reach the tumor all at once at a sufficiently high intensity, the healthy tissues that the ray passes through on the way to the tumor will also be destroyed. At lower intensities the rays are harmless to healthy tissue, but they will not affect the tumor either. What type of procedure might be used to destroy the tumor with the rays, and at the same time avoid destroying the healthy tissue (p. 3, Gick & Holyoak, 1983).

We trust that many readers realized that this problem can be solved with an analog of the "divide-and-conquer" strategy used by the general, that is, to employ separate, low intensity rays that converge at the location of the tumor. Based on Gick and Holyoak's findings, however, we know that not all readers of this volume solved this problem! That many university students and intelligent people like our readership do not automatically transfer the divide-and-conquer strategy in a close generalization task makes clear that transfer should never be assumed to be an automatic byproduct of learning a strategy. Fortunately, there are ways to increase durable use of strategies, with two approaches taken up in the remainder of this section.

Hints at the Time That the Strategy Should Be Used

Even when people do not transfer a strategy "spontaneously," there is a bright side. It is often possible to get them to use the technique by giving them hints to deploy it. For instance, Gick and Holyoak (1980) were able to increase the likelihood that subjects would solve the radiation problem by telling them that "one of the stories you read before will give you a hint for the solution of this problem." With the hint to look for a hint in the general story, 92% of the subjects produced the ray dispersion solution; without it, only 20% of the subjects solved the problem.

Partially motivated by the Gick and Holyoak results, Pressley and his associates have explored the effects of hinting on use of monitoring and encoding strategies. Although the results with adults have not always been as dramatic as the ones reported by Gick and Holyoak (1980), there have been consistent benefits (e.g., Pressley & Ahmad, 1986). With children, hints have generally proven to be powerful facilitators of children's continued use of strategies.

For instance, earlier in this chapter we discussed Pressley, Ross, Levin, and Ghatala's (1984) demonstration that 10- to 13-year-old children were more likely to make use of strategy utility information that they had gained through strategy practice if they were given a mild prompt to do so. Following such a hint, most children selected the more powerful keyword strategy for vocabulary learning over a less powerful semantic-context approach.

Ghatala et al., (1986) also established the importance of hinting in maintaining young children's use of monitoring skills. In addition to the first session of the study that was discussed earlier, there was a second session for 3-component monitoring-trained, 0-component monitoring-trained, 3-component information-provided, and 0-component information-provided subjects. Subjects in these conditions were reminded at the beginning of the second session that they had played a memory game during the previous visit with the goal of remembering as much as possible. Then, half of the subjects in the 3-component monitoring-trained condition were given the following hint: "Last time you learned to do some things to help you choose the method that works better. Do those things as we play the game today." Half of the 3-component information-provided subjects were given a comparable hint: "Last time you were told some things to help you to choose the method that works better. Remember those things as we play the game today." Of course, these hints were designed to activate the strategy-monitoring training/information from the first session.

Then all of the subjects who participated in this second session were given two additional paired-associate lists to study and recall. For one of the lists the subjects were instructed to use the repetition strategy that they had been taught during the previous session. For the other list they were told to use a sentence-elaboration strategy (i.e., to make up sentences to link each of the paired items), which is much more powerful than repetition. (The order of strategies was counterbalanced within conditions.) Following the test trial on the second list, strategy selections were elicited and an interview was conducted about the basis for strategy selections.

The greatest selection of the more potent elaboration strategy occurred with 3-component monitoring-trained subjects who were given a hint. Eighty-five percent of these subjects selected elaboration with 80% of those doing so justifying the choice on the basis of memory. In contrast, only 67% of the 3-component monitoring-trained subjects selected elaboration, with only 42% of these subjects justifying their choices on the basis of memory. Considering that elaboration would have been selected 50% of the time by using a coin flip, this 67% figure is not particularly impressive. In addition, the strategy selections and rationales of 3-component monitoring-trained subjects who were *not* given a hint did not differ from 0-component monitoring-trained subjects or information-provided subjects. Thus, only 3-component monitoring-trained subjects given a hint manifested any evidence of maintenance of the monitoring strategies taught during the first session.

That younger children are more dependent on hints than older children was demonstrated in Pressley and Dennis-Rounds' (1980) experiment, part of which was discussed in Chapter 6. The younger sample were enrolled in grades 5 and 6; the older sample were students in grades 11 and 12. There was no evidence at the younger age level of spontaneous transfer of the keyword strategy from one associative task (learning city-product pairs) to another associative task (learning Latin words). The older subjects did transfer the keyword strategy somewhat. Although not discussed previously, the experiment also included a condition in which subjects who had received keyword training for the city-product task were given a hint to use the keyword strategy for Latin learning. When subjects in this condition were presented the Latin task, they were told to "use a technique that is like the one you used to learn the cities and what they are known for." Providing the hint was sufficient to boost the performance of the 10- to 13-year-old subjects over the level of younger control performance. That is, the hint produced "transfer" of the keyword strategy from the city-product to the Latin task for the 10- to 13-year-olds. There was no significant hint effect at the older age level, presumably because the older subjects transferred the keyword strategy without a prompt to do so. In concluding that older subjects transferred spontaneously and that younger subjects did so given a hint, we also emphasize that at both age levels Latin learning was greatest (and by a good margin) when there was complete reinstruction in how to use the keyword method to learn Latin vocabulary. Hinting apparently did not lead to the complete and consistent strategy application that occurs in response to direct and detailed instructions in strategy use. Complete transfer of a strategy apparently requires more powerful mechanisms, some of which will be taken up later.

Even though hinting may not lead to complete transfer, we believe that it deserves much additional study, however, because it is assumed to be an important mechanism of cognitive growth in several contemporary theories of cognitive change. The most important of these is Vygotsky's (e.g., 1978) hypothesis that mature thought develops in social contexts, a point of view shared by many others (e.g., Feuerstein, 1980; Hinde, Perret-Clermont, & Stevenson-Hinde, 1985). According to this perspective, children first experience sophisticated processing in interpersonal situations, with more mature thinkers (i.e., parents, teachers, other children) guiding their cognition, often providing hints as to how the children should proceed when they cannot manage on their own. One tenet of Vygotskian theory is that an important individual difference dimension distinguishing more competent from less competent children is the amount of prompting that they require in order to manifest a new cognitive skill given the same starting competence, with data beginning to accumulate in support of this hypothesis (e.g., Campione & Brown, 1984; Campione, Brown, Ferrara, Jones, & Steinberg, 1985; Day & Hall, 1987; Ferrara, Brown, & Campione, 1986).

Of course, this same theme of progressive prompting for decreasingly competent children has been detailed with respect to developmental level and memory (Pressley, 1982; Rohwer, 1973; Waters & Andreassen, 1983; Chapter 6, this volume). Recent theoretical and empirical work suggests, however, that hinting can play a role in the development of memory and skill even in adults. Schank (1982) made the case that reminding is at the heart of cognitive change, with the good thinker continuously being reminded of knowledge in long-term memory that is relevant to current thinking, knowledge that could promote understanding of a current situation. Good thinkers consistently and intentionally remind themselves. Even more relevant here is Ross' (1984) work on the transfer of newly acquired cognitive skills. He found that when the generalization situation contained elements that could remind adult learners of the training of a skill, adults noticed the reminders and were affected by the presence of these hints. Ross explicitly develops the case that contextual hints play a key role in the naturalistic development of skill—a theoretical position that harkens back to association by similarity explanations of transfer (e.g., Thorndike, & Woodworth, 1901; Woodworth & Schlosberg, 1954). All too unfortunately, however, children often do not receive hints to use strategies or hints that are explicit enough.

Training for Transfer

What can be done to increase the likelihood of strategy maintenance when environmental prompts are not provided or are too subtle? There are many recommendations about how to train strategies so that they transfer. There are many articles filled with recommendations about how to train for transfer (e.g., Deshler, Alley, Warner, & Schumaker, 1981; Deshler, Schumaker, & Lenz, 1984; Deshler, Schumaker, Lenz, & Ellis, 1984; Ellis, 1986; Ryan, Weed, & Short, 1986), recommendations that follow from detailed task analyses of what transfer entails. One of the more complete task analyses of the different types of transfer was provided by Salomon and Globerson (1987). In singling out their framework to begin this discussion of training for transfer, we emphasize that Salomon and Globerson's perspective is consistent with many other points of view, including the good strategy user model with which we identify (Chapter 6; Pressley, Borkowski, & Schneider, 1987).

Sometimes transfer is "data driven"—A strategy is elicited automatically by environmental cues. This can be expected for strategies that have been used and practiced to the point of automaticity. One important characteristic of automatic transfer is that the thinker uses little short-term capacity (attention or consciousness, depending on your theoretical terminological preference!). In fact, such strategy use often seems to occur completely out of consciousness. For instance, one strategy that author M. P. has used consistently for years has been to place an object that he wants to transport from home to office by the door leading to his garage, so that he could not leave in the morning without tripping over the object. Lately M. P. has begun to use this same strategy when he is "on the road" (e.g., attending a convention). He places the handouts that he must remember in the morning by the door of the hotel room before tucking in for the night. The most important point here is that this transfer occurred without any deliberation, and in fact, the "put-near-the-door" strategy gets executed all of the time without him thinking about it.

Automatic transfer of strategies deserves a lot more research attention, for automatic, appropriate functioning is a very desirable endstate. About all that we know about the development of automaticity is that it is linked to strategy practice, and even this relationship to practice has not been studied in especially great detail (Adams, 1987; Schneider et al., 1984). One reason for this neglect of automatic strategy use is the belief by some that automatic, unconscious use of procedures is not really strategic—strategic functioning is presumed to require conscious attention to procedural application (e.g., Paris et al., 1985). Our perspective, presented in the definition of strategy use detailed in Chapter 3, is that strategy use need only be potentially controllable and intentional in the sense that it is directed at the accomplishment of particular cognitive goals. This definition captures data-driven use and transfer of cognitive procedures, and as such, more adequately deals with the range of activities that are commonly considered to be strategic.

The second type of transfer considered by Salomon and Globerson (1987) is definitely strategic by all definitions of strategy in that it involves explicitly conscious use of cognitive processes. Salomon and Globerson (1987) provided a thorough analysis of such mindful transfer. The mindful strategy user is fully aware of the current goal and deliberately seeks a way to do it efficiently. Part of the process may involve conscious inhibition of task-inappropriate or task-inefficient strategies that were used in the past. For instance, when confronted with an associative learning task, a person can consciously decide simply not to repeat the paired items over and over, recalling that in the past such efforts required a lot of energy and yielded little gain (e.g., Pressley, Levin, & Ghatala, 1984). A student can decide not to write down the first thing that comes to mind when composing an essay, realizing that this "natural response" was inefficient in the past.

Once inefficient strategies have been suppressed, the search for more efficient strategies can begin. This normally involves close examination of the memory task with an eye toward identification of subtle features that might provide clues as to the selection of a strategy that is well matched to the task. The person thinks of alternatives and considers each, relying on the metacognitive knowledge that is coded with each strategy to guide selection and deployment. In short, "mindful" transfer and use of cognitive procedures requires great cognitive effort deployed in very particular ways.

The two-sided portrait of competent transfer (automatic and mindful) described by Salomon and Globerson (1987) is completely consistent with the good strategy user conception of efficient strategy deployment. There are occasions when strategies are "fired off" as automatic reactions to situations, and other occasions when strategy execution only follows deliberation. We believe that the good strategy user model is more explicit with respect to the most important mechanism mediating transfer, and in a fashion that is completely consistent with historically prominent analyses of transfer.

Although Salomon and Globerson (1987) acknowledge "metacognitive guidance" as a key ingredient to deliberate strategy selection, the good strategy user model details the nature of the metacognition that is crucial to strategy transfer. The good strategy user not only knows strategies but also knows a lot about situations that are associated with effective use of those strategies. This strategy knowledge can be used to guide matching of strategies to tasks. Readers familiar with early 20th-century experimental psychology will recognize this point of view as a conscious and cognitive version of "identical elements" theory (e.g., Thorndike & Wood-worth, 1901). The identical elements position was that use of a skill on a current task depends on the person recognizing similarities of the present situation to attributes that define occasions when it is appropriate to use the skill in question.

Thus, a student can "know" a strategy in that they can execute the procedure, but understand little about when and where to use it. This is not a desirable state. In contrast, a metacognitively mature thinker will recognize the attributes of situations that permit the strategy to be used profitably. Only this type of metacognitively mature person would be expected to transfer the strategy. Mindful transfer is mediated by conscious analyses of situations and comparisons with strategy knowledge; automatic transfer might begin after many trials of conscious strategy transfer. With experience, the critical attributes that define situations that call for use of a strategy might be readily perceived (e.g., Gibson, 1969). In addition, as a function of experience in transferring a strategy, it would be expected that strategy knowledge would be more detailed in ways that would make it easier to assess whether a current situation calls for a strategy. It would also be expected that with use, strategy knowledge would be more accessible and would be more tightly tied to the strategy. Thus, even if a learner encodes the teacher's explanation that a comprehension strategy can be employed whenever the child is reading a conventional fictional story, initial transfer of the strategy might be clumsy. Confronted with a new story, the child might recall that there is "something" that she was taught to do when reading short fiction, but require a few minutes before the exact procedure would be recalled. With practice, the sight of a story title would automatically and quickly lead to recall and application of the skill.

Given that strategy knowledge may be able to account for both mindful and automatic transfer, it is not surprising that much research on ways to facilitate transfer has focused on embellishing strategy knowledge, although all of the research to date is about mindful transfer (e.g., O'Sullivan & Pressley, 1984). The promise of embellished strategy instruction as a way to promote transfer has especially captured the interest of special educators. These people face many populations who have severe learning problems that cannot be remedied by conventional instruction. More optimistically, both retarded and learning-disabled children often respond to strategy instruction, in that they can carry out many cognitive strategies that are taught to them (Campione, Nitsch, Bray, & Brown, 1982; Ceci, 1986, 1987; Ellis, 1979). It must be pointed out, however, that the amount and detail of instruction required to execute a strategy often exceeds the amount and detail of instruction required by normal learners (Day & Hall, 1987), and that transfer is even less likely with slow learners than with normal children (e.g., Campione & Brown, 1984). That special populations can execute skills but do not seem to generalize them easily has prompted a lot of thinking by the special educator community about how to design strategy instruction that is most likely to generalize.

Deshler and his associates at the University of Kansas (e.g., Deshler et al., 1981; Ellis & Lenz, 1987) have particularly led these efforts, putting together a set of recommendations based on research results, experimenter and teacher intuitions, and theoretical convictions. In short, Deshler and his associates advocate extremely direct and explicit strategy instruction. Their recommendations include fully explaining strategies, including each step of the procedures. In addition, Deshler espouses modeling of strategies by a variety of teachers in a variety of settings with conditions varied greatly over the course of instruction. The advantages of using the strategy should be fully explained, with students required to assess their own gains as a function of strategy use. The subjects need to rehearse the strategy explicitly and extensively. Students should be taught to use general monitoring and checking strategies in conjunction with other procedures. They should be taught to employ motivational procedures, like use of self-coping statements (e.g., "I can handle this") and use of self-reinforcement (e.g., "I'm doing well here"). These motivational components are included because of the belief by many children who experience learning difficulties that they really do not have the ability to carry out academic tasks (Ryan et al., 1986). Students should also be told explicitly to try to generalize strategies. They should be cued that trained strategies are relevant to future, real-world demands and that they should try to adapt the skills that they are learning to these new situations (cf., Hatano, 1982). Finally, the child has to be transited from the highly structured instructional environment to a world where the cues to use strategies are much less explicit and precise. Gradual loosening of control with the learner slowly assuming self-direction of his thinking is more likely to result in continued use of trained procedures than would an abrupt shift from a highly controlled instructional environment to unstructured settings (e.g., Schumaker, Deshler, & Ellis, 1986).

We believe that the many instructional recommendations made by Deshler and his associates make sense, and they are consistent with other suggestions that have been made following thorough analyses of the development of educationally relevant skills (e.g., Brown et al., 1983; Kendall & Braswell, 1985; Pressley, Goodchild, Fleet, Zajchowski, & Evans, in press). We also believe, however, that the Kansas suggestions may not go far enough. Borkowski, Carr, and Pressley (1987) in particular detailed ways to improve the likelihood of generalization by instructing learners in ways specifically consistent with the good strategy user model. Their suggestions included providing explicit and specific information about when and where to use strategies as part of instruction, rather than requiring learners to abstract such metacognition from experiences in multiple settings. Although diverse experiences with strategies would be sufficient for some learners to figure out when to use procedures that they learned, others would probably not develop metacognitive knowledge that would be adequate to direct future use of strategies. Worse yet, some of the time students would probably abstract errant information.

Studies that are particularly relevant to consider in this context were conducted by O'Sullivan and Pressley (1984), ones that were discussed in part in Chapter 6. In their experiments, children in grades 5 and 6 learned the keyword method in the context of a task requiring acquisition of city-product pairs (i.e., the products produced in particular cities). Most relevant here, subjects in an "experience" condition practiced using the technique with other types of materials, including two that could be learned better with the keyword procedure (e.g., acquisition of men and their profession associations, memorization of foods and countries that produce them) and one task that could not be mediated effectively with the strategy (i.e., verbatim recall of prose). In contrast, subjects in an elaborated instruction condition practiced the keyword strategy with the same tasks, but with the experimenter explaining the attributes of the situations that signalled that use of the strategy was appropriate. When the children in the experience and elaborated instruction conditions were presented a task not encountered during training but one that could be mediated using the keyword technique (i.e., learning of Latin vocabulary definitions), transfer of the keyword method was evident in the elaborated instruction but not in the experience condition. Requiring children to discover strategy knowledge on their own is much less certain to lead to durable strategy use than directly providing strategy knowledge to them as part of instruction.

In addition to developing the case that children often require explicit instruction about when to use particular strategies, Borkowski et al. (1987) also developed in detail the argument that explicit efforts must be made to get students to attribute to strategy use the performance gains derived from appropriate strategy application. While the Kansas group goes far in making the case that students need to be impressed that effort is an important determinant of achievement (especially Ellis, 1986), Borkowski et al. (1987) believe that students must come to realize that the key to success is effort directed through appropriate strategies. The natural tendency of many problem learners to believe that low performance is their fate because of innate deficiencies in themselves (e.g., Ryan et al., 1986) must be supplanted with an understanding that they are capable of deploying and executing strategies that can produce high performance.

In support of this claim, Reid and Borkowski (1985) reported a study in which hyperactive, underachieving 7- to 10-year-olds were taught some memory strategies. What varied between conditions was whether subjects were taught to attribute their capable memory performance following strategy training to use of the strategies. When such an effort-channeled-through-strategies attribution was part of training, greater strategy maintenance (two weeks and nine months later) and strategy generalization were observed. See Licht and Kistner (1986) for additional arguments that effort attributional and strategy training should be combined.

Although much has been written about all the components and embellishments that should be included in good strategy training, there has been little evaluation of whether the en masse implementation of these recommendations really benefits performance as proposed. Perhaps even more disturbing, many of the components that are included in these packages of recommendations have not been tested in well-controlled experiments that permit the inference that the component is really critical to transfer; virtually none of the components have been subjected to extensive and exhaustive investigation. Studies like O'Sullivan and Pressley (1984) and Reid and Borkowski (1985) are unique in providing rigorous, true experimental evaluation of components. More such work is sorely needed, even though it is often very expensive. A detailed consideration of one such study by Barbara Moely and her colleagues makes the time- and resource-intensive nature of this type of work obvious, but also makes clear that such research is worth it.

Leal, Crays, and Moely (1985) wanted to determine if 8-year-olds could be taught the self-monitoring presumed to be so critical to good strategy use—including transfer of the monitoring skill to untrained problems. In particular, they studied whether children could be taught to test themselves to determine if additional study were necessary before they were ready for a criterion test. In two of the three conditions of the study, subjects were told that self-testing was useful for evaluating task performance. The subjects were required to practice self-testing with three practice items. The participants studied these items, looked away, tried to recall them, and then checked to determine that their recall was correct. The experimenter explained that if all items had not been recalled that this would be an indication that not all of the items had been learned and additional study was necessary. The trained children were reminded at the beginning of each of 12 practice trials about the self-testing strategy and about how self-testing aids performance.

The two training conditions differed in that in one condition subjects performed all 12 practice trials on one task—free recall of lists of items for half of the subjects in this condition and serial recall of lists of items for the remaining participants in the condition. In the second training condition subjects practiced on both free and serial recall tasks, doing each for half of the practice trials. Leal et al. (1985) hypothesized that practicing self-monitoring with more than one task would promote generalization of the strategy relative to practice with one task, by increasing the child's awareness that the strategy could be applied to more than one situation. In particular, Leal et al. (1985) expected that general use of self-monitoring would be greatest with the two-task training, but some generalization would occur even with one-task training (e.g., Belmont, Butterfield, & Borkowski, 1978) relative to the third condition in the study, a control condition. Control children were also given 12 trials of practice, with half of the trials requiring serial recall and half requiring free recall. In contrast to the trained subjects, controls were never provided any information about how to study, although they were encouraged to do well and were given consistent praise for their efforts.

One week following the 12 training/control practice trials, subjects were administered tasks to determine if the self-monitoring strategy would be maintained in the absence of a verbal prompt to use the strategy. That is, subjects were given free and serial recall tasks. There was evidence of equal maintenance in the two trained conditions for both free and serial recall in that there was greater use of self-monitoring and greater recall in both of the trained conditions relative to the control condition. In addition, subjects were given three generalization tasks. In one, the children were required to learn the locations of stores on a blueprint of a shopping mall. In the second task, children were required to learn to spell sets of three six-letter nonsense words. The third task was a variation of paired-associate learning. There was evidence of one-week generalization of self-monitoring in all three of these tasks in that more time was spent self-testing in the trained conditions than in the control condition. Again, however, there appeared to be equivalent generalization in the one- and two-task training conditions.

In short, Leal et al. (1985) failed to find any compelling difference between training with one task and training with two—a finding that seems to fly in the face of recommendations by Deshler et al. (1981) and others that training with multiple tasks promotes durable use of strategies. As careful and thorough as Leal et al. (1985) were, however, it must be emphasized that their evaluation was limited to a comparison of training with one task versus two and to training of only self-testing. Much more careful work on transfer following practice on multiple tasks is required before a definitive conclusion would be justified, although the result obtained by Leal et al. (1985) is consistent with the transfer failure in O'Sullivan and Pressley's (1984) experience condition discussed earlier in this subsection. More well-controlled studies like Leal et al. (1985) and O'Sullivan and Pressley (1984) are the most certain route to a definitive conclusion about the training with multiple tasks issue.

In closing this subsection, we recognize that we have recommended here two very different approaches to evaluation of strategy instruction—both evaluation of training packages and component analyses. There is an urgent need to evaluate packages of "best bet" components because such packages are being developed for immediate dissemination (e.g., Schumaker et al., 1986). Complete understanding of instruction, however, requires identification of the really active ingredients in these packages. It may be that only a very few of the components have really striking effects on generalization. Although those providing packaged instruction may be able to get a "feel" for the active versus inert ingredients in their training, only carefully controlled comparative experiments can provide definite "thumbs up" or "thumbs down" evaluative information about a component. This type of analytic work in turn permits the more potent parts of instruction to be highlighted in the design of future instructional units. Thus, the evaluation of packages and components are complementary activities, not mutually exclusive or antagonistic ones.

Challenges to the Teaching of Good Strategy Use?

The evidence reviewed in this chapter thus far makes clear that really good strategy use is a rare commodity even among adults, let alone children. We have documented so far that monitoring, which is presumably absolutely critical to good strategy use, is often defective. There are also many demonstrations of transfer failures. These imply that people either do not possess the strategy knowledge necessary to recognize when a strategy should be deployed, or that they do not access and use the strategy knowledge that they have. In short, this chapter has had a pretty somber tone.

There is good reason to suspect, however, that it might be possible to increase good strategy use through instruction. There are many strategies that children can execute following brief and simple instruction (Pressley, Heisel, McCormick, & Nakamura, 1982). Given these skills, one hypothesis for explaining children's failures to use strategies on occasions when they could be deployed profitably is that children may be receiving little strategy instruction. In fact, that is the case. There is little evidence of classroom teaching of reading strategies (e.g., Durkin, 1979), writing strategies (e.g., Applebee, 1984, 1986), mathematical strategies (e.g., Thompson, 1985), and particularly relevant here, memory strategies (Moely, Hart et al., 1986; Moely, Leal et al., 1986).

Why so little teaching of memory strategies? – or any others for that matter? We believe the reason is that the comprehensive strategy instruction that would be necessary to get people to the point of generally good strategy use is very difficult to do, despite the fact that getting children to execute individual strategies is not very hard. We review in this section some of the obstacles to strategy instruction. We also review our perceptions as to how these obstacles might be overcome, for we remain optimistic that there is a cognitive revolution in instruction that is beginning and that strategy teaching should play a prominent role in cognitive reformulation of instruction. For even more detailed and extensive coverage of problems associated with implementation of cognitive strategy instruction, see Pressley, Goodchild, Fleet, Zajchowski, and Evans (in press).

1. *There are many, many strategies to learn.* Efficient list memorization requires different strategies than does associative learning; prose learning can involve a host of strategies, depending on the prose learning goal. Material that must be remembered in order should be approached differently than material that can be learned without consideration of order. On the other hand, there are not so many memory strategies that people should not be able to acquire them given years of instruction. Since it is easy for children to execute many memory strategies when they are provided fairly simple instructions about how to do so, it seems reasonable to expect that children could learn many memorization procedures – if they were only taught these skills (Moely, Hart et al., 1986). Given the potency of many memory strategies, it seems like the time is right for attempting an instructional experiment in which a number of strategies are taught to children over a period of time. It should become obvious in the context of such research whether the number of memory strategies is simply overwhelming or whether there are a managable number of techniques that can be conveyed as part of instruction.

2. *Teachers do not think in information-processing terms.* Very little time is spent during teacher education in developing awareness and understanding of information-processing skills. In fact, many teachers probably only get exposure to information processing as one small part of a survey course in educational psychology. It is easy to understand why teachers do not use information-processing inter-

ventions extensively. More positively, entire textbooks dedicated to the cognitive perspective are beginning to appear (e.g., Gagné, 1985) and excellent summaries of how to teach strategies are available (e.g., Devine, 1987). A number of special issues of professional journals have been published (e.g., April 1986 *Educational Leadership*), detailing how strategy instruction can be implemented in classrooms. Also, given the dependency of teachers on teacher's guides that accompany textbooks (e.g., Clark & Elmore, 1979; Duffy, Roehler, & Putnam, 1987; Durkin, 1979), there are opportunities to modify teacher's behaviors on a large scale by modifying the content of these guides. In short, there is plenty of reason to believe that even if teachers do not understand information-processing now, they are more likely to understand it in the future with substantial support from professional sources for implementing cognitive strategy instruction including the teaching of strategies aimed at improving memory.

3. *It takes a lot of effort for general, durable use of strategies to occur.* Transfer difficulties following brief instruction are the most frequently discussed instantiation of this problem. Consistent and efficient use of strategies require that learners be given opportunities to practice procedures until they have been executed fluently and without great cognitive effort. Teachers need to arrange opportunities for students to practice the skills in a variety of situations, with explicit efforts made to make certain that students acquire critical strategy information such as when and where to use a procedure. Although there are a variety of means for teaching strategies, Pressley, Cariglia-Bull, and Snyder (1987) developed the case that only more complete instructional techniques are likely to produce durable and general use of strategies. Only these more complete approaches promote complete understanding of strategies.

One approach favored by Pressley, Cariglia-Bull, and Snyder (1987) is direct explanation (e.g., Roehler & Duffy, 1984). The teacher who uses this approach explains strategies thoroughly, providing explicit and detailed information about how to carry out processing, about the effects produced by strategies, as well as information about when and where to use procedures. Direct explanation includes concrete examples, modeling, and practice. As part of teacher-guided practice, explanations to individual children are tailored to the difficulties that the students are experiencing. For an excellent example of research on direct explanation (as well as an example of educational research at its very best), see Duffy, Roehler, Sivan et al. (1987).

The second approach to teaching favored by Pressley, Cariglia-Bull, and Snyder (1987) is the reciprocal teaching approach developed by Palincsar and Brown (1984). Teachers and students take turns executing strategies that are being taught with instruction occurring in true dialogue. Strategic processes are made very overt, with plenty of exposure to modeling of strategies and opportunities to practice techniques over the course of a number of lessons. Children discover and teachers convey strategy-utility information as well as information about when and where to use particular strategies. Teachers using reciprocal instruction assume more responsibility for strategy implementation early in instruction, gradually transferring control over to the student. See Palincsar (1986) for extensive description of the implementation of reciprocal instruction.

When teachers are confronted with classrooms of pupils varying in abilities and motivations, the implementation of such complete and sensitive teaching is often difficult. The diagnosis demands are high for both direct explanation and reciprocal instruction, and so are the instructional-tailoring demands. On the other hand, "expert" teachers (e.g., Berliner, 1986) seem to be able to carry out such demands automatically. Given that serious research on direct explanation and reciprocal instruction has just begun, but that there is a flurry of work in progress on these two approaches, it seems reasonable to expect that there will be an enormous increase in the next few years in understanding how to implement these approaches effectively.

4. *Teachers can only make decisions based on objective evaluations if such evaluations have been done and are generally available.* Unfortunately, only a few of the many potentially educationally relevant strategies have been tested extensively. Much, much more formal evaluative work is needed. Even in the cases where much data has been generated, however, it is usually the case that such research is not placed in sources that are available to teachers. Research-translation journals like *The Reading Teacher, Educational Leadership,* and *The Elementary School Journal* are a start, but even more is required. One idea would be to create an encyclopedic source that summarizes available evaluations of strategic interventions in a fashion akin to the *Mental Measurements Handbook* (Mitchell, 1983). That more evaluation work is becoming available with every passing month and that there are some general summaries of strategies available that are well informed by research (e.g., Devine, 1987) makes it easy to conclude that more, better, and more available evaluations will be the rule in the not-too-distant future.

5. *There are individual differences in children such that some benefit from strategy instruction only given great commitment of resources.* Very young children have difficulty acquiring some strategies like interactive imagery (Pressley, 1982; Pressley, Borkowski, & Johnson, 1987). Mentally handicapped children can often learn strategies, but their continued use by these populations sometimes requires continuous prompting (e.g., Campione et al., 1982). Individual differences that are more subtle than age or global mental status have an influence on strategy generalization as well.

One of the most exciting directions in instructional research is the study of individual differences as predictors of strategy use and generalization. For instance, some strategies require content expertise in order to be executed in a content area at all. One such technique is activation of information that one knows about a topic as a method for facilitating learning of a passage on that topic (e.g., Hasselhorn & Körkel, 1986). Children who are impulsive may not take the time necessary to execute complicated strategies. Anxious children may be so caught up in their anxiety that there is little capacity left over for strategy execution. Girls seem to be competent with respect to some aspects of good strategy use before boys are. Girls use organizational strategies earlier (Cox & Waters, 1986), and grade-1 and -2 girls seem to be more aware of when they are doing well versus when they are doing poorly on cognitive tasks (Pressley, Levin, Ghatala, & Ahmad, 1987). Might there also be differences between the sexes in learning strategies given instruction?

A study by Kurtz and Borkowski (1984) illustrates the importance of individual differences research with respect to theories like the good strategy user model, but also highlights the important role that individual differences may play in classroom acquisition of strategies. The good strategy user model posits an important role in self-regulation for knowledge about when and where to use strategies. Such knowledge permits recognition of situations where strategies can be applied, which is one of the most critical steps in strategy transfer (Crisafi & Brown, 1986). Given the crucial role of this form of metacognition to generalization, Kurtz and Borkowski (1984) reasoned that children who possess more metamemory about strategies in general should be more likely to transfer strategic skills that they are taught. They specifically believed that children who possessed a great deal of prior understanding of cognitive functioning would be more likely to generalize new strategies that were taught with metacognitive embellishment.

Kurtz and Borkowski (1984) first assessed the metamemory competence of their grade-1 and grade-3 participants. The metamemory battery consisted of questions about knowledge of elaboration and other strategies for remembering, knowledge about planful behaviors for future events, knowledge of organized memory searches, knowledge about the relative difficulties of different tasks, and knowledge of memory monitoring. In addition, assessments were made of performance and strategy use during several tasks including learning of categorizable lists and learning of paired associates. Thus, this initial session established individual differences in general metamemory about strategy use and individual differences in competence on tasks for which the subjects would later be taught strategies.

Following these preliminary assessments, the children were divided into three training groups. Two of these groups received general metamemory training at this point. This consisted of group discussion sessions about how the mind works, emphasizing that memory can be enhanced by using strategies that are well matched to the requirements of particular memory tasks. Both strategic and nonstrategic behaviors were modeled. Some strategies (not ones that were later trained) were described and modeled as examples of deliberate strategic behavior—with both encoding and retrieval dynamics of these strategies emphasized. The following was a sample dialogue from the session:

Teacher 1: Did you ever hear anyone say, "Use your head"? What they meant was *stop* and *think* about what you're doing before you do it. Then after you've thought of the best possible way to learn or do something, do it that way.

Teacher 2: Our minds can work better and faster if we know how to use them. Today we're going to talk about some ways that we can use our minds better. There are two parts to remembering things. First, we have to fasten things in our minds, then we have to take out the things we put in. Today we're going to talk about things we can do to help us both put things in our mind and take them out.

Teacher 1: One of the things we can do to fasten things in our minds is to go over them many times. If we go over and over and over something, it will be easier to remember. Have you ever done that with anything? (Encourage dialogue.) How many of you know how to clean out

the sink at home? You know how to do that well because you've done it *many times*. How many of you know the roads from your house to school? I imagine that the first time you went to school you didn't know the way. But by the time you went over those roads *fifty* times, you hardly had to think about it anymore!
Teacher 2: We'll give you an example. Molly, I wish we didn't have to learn these spelling words today. . .they're *hard*.
Teacher 1: Yes, I'd rather go swimming. But I bet we can learn them pretty quickly. Let's see—(writes words slowly on the board).
Teacher 2: Hmmm—if I write these over and over, I bet I'll remember them better. (Writes words over and over. Makes mistakes at first and corrects, then gradually writes them all correctly.)
Teacher 1: (Writes words, stares at them awhile, writes a few, draws pictures on board, stares at words again.) Who learned the words faster? Why? (Encourage dialogue) Do you think that would work for other things too?" (pp. 341–342)

During the time corresponding to when the subjects in the two metamemory training conditions engaged in dialogue about metamemory, strategy-trained control subjects spent an equal amount of time in dialogue with the experimenters, except that cognitive awareness and increased efficiency of cognitive monitoring were not covered.

Following these sessions of dialogue, one of the two metamemory groups (hereafter the strategy-trained metamemory condition) and the strategy-trained control subjects were given task-specific strategy training. They were taught a categorization strategy for learning of categorizable lists and an elaboration strategy for paired associates. During this phase, the subjects in the third condition (metamemory control subjects) received no instruction about how to do the criteria tasks.

During the final session of the study, subjects first were required to perform tasks that could be accomplished using the strategies that were taught in the strategy-training conditions, but ones not experienced previously in the study. Then, the participants were given tasks identical to those used during training to assess whether strategy use was maintained.

As expected, strategy training had a dramatic effect on performance. Providing general metamemory training did not, except for one dramatically important result. Pre-experimental differences in metamemory correlated significantly (Pearson $r = 0.66$) with generalization performance in the metamemory-strategy training condition, but not so in the strategy-trained control ($r = 0.35$) or metamemory control ($r = -0.08$) conditions. Kurtz and Borkowski (1984) concluded that, "Apparently, an initially high level of metamemory enabled children to benefit more from instructions, and, specifically, to utilize additional metamemorial knowledge in generalizing a newly acquired strategy to other tasks (p. 348)."

There should be a lot of additional study of metamemorial differences between children as predictors of strategy generalization. In addition to Kurtz and Borkowski (1984), Borkowski and his associates have demonstrated the correlation between prior metacognition and strategy durability several times (e.g., Borkowski et al., 1983; Kendall, Borkowski, & Cavanaugh, 1980; see Pressley, Borkowski, & O'Sullivan, 1985, for a general overview). Other individual difference dimensions, however, probably play a role in determining whether a learner transfers strategies or not, and these should receive serious research attention as well. For instance, there are clearly differences between children of any given age in their functional short-term memory capacities (e.g., Case, 1985). Guttentag (1984) has argued and presented evidence that these differences are associated with differences in the likelihood that children will use short-term-capacity-demanding strategies. A hypothesis that follows is that children who have more short-term capacity will be more willing to transfer capacity-demanding strategies. A variation on this theme is that subjects who enjoy performing cognitively demanding tasks may be more willing than other children to try to use strategies in new situations (Cacioppo & Petty, 1982), a result that would be consistent with Salomon and Globerson's (1987) position that propensity toward mindfulness is an important determinant of intellectual competence.

SUMMARY

Despite the fact that strategy instruction is difficult, there are plenty of reasons to believe that progress is being made in determining how to increase the likelihood that classroom teachers can and will deliver such instruction. Progress will follow from additional research and research-informed dissemination efforts, especially if part of this dissemination includes revision of teacher education so that teachers are better prepared to deliver strategy instruction. One such program at Michigan State University is supervised by Gerald Duffy and Laura Roehler. Prospective teachers are taught a lot about strategies and information processing as part of course work that extends over a year. During this same time they participate in practicuum experience that is explicitly tied to the coursework, with some of the in-course coverage determined by problems that arise during the practicum. The participating student teachers also have opportunities to watch experienced instructors teach strategies to children. Thus, the teachers-in-training receive exposure to academic content and behavioral models; they learn by doing and reflecting on the difficulties that they encounter. The professor provides a lot of guidance along the way. The demands of direct explanation and reciprocal instruction probably require educational internships of this type. We hope that more such opportunities will become available as the process-oriented approaches to education gain in prominence (e.g., Gagné, 1985). Such changes in teacher education will almost certainly increase the amount of strategy instruction in schools. As cognitive-strategy instruction becomes more common, the frequency of good strategy use should be more evident.

Summary and Discussion

We opened this chapter by posing the question of whether there really are good strategy users. The best bet is that good strategy use is probably very domain specific. Thus, no viewer of the NCAA basketball tournament (U. S. collegiate championship) could doubt that the top coaches are consummately strategic. It seems unlikely that these same coaches display such a high degree of strategic savvy in all of the domains that humans operate in. In fact, the only globally strategic individuals that we have encountered are fictitious – the great detectives in the great detective novels. Sherlock Holmes, the Hardy Boys, and Fletch process all the right information in just the right ways at just the right times *all the time*. Anyone who does not believe that this is an impressive feat should try to write their own detective novel. One of us (M. P.) is doing so. It takes him months of research, writing, and rewriting in order to construct a half-dozen chapters of strategic detective activity. That captivating and convincing portraits of consistently excellent strategy use can be constructed by the likes of Sir Arthur Conan Doyle, Franklin W. Dixon, and Malcolm McDonald in no way guarantees that such globally capable performance is ever produced by real people operating in real time.

For the most part this chapter was about such real people, people who often fail to monitor their performances and who often fail to use strategies that they know and could deploy. Some of the failures described here might even be considered shocking – Many nonpsychologists would be surprised to find out that adults sometimes miss the types of errors that occur in the Markman stories or that even close transfer rarely follows automatically from learning a strategy.

More positively, it seems likely that people can be trained to be better strategy users, although we perceive that such training is not easy to accomplish. We also do not know if training could ever be complete enough so that most students would know a variety of strategies and deploy them appropriately across a host of domains – or whether such general use of strategies could be developed to the point that there was highly automatized use of many different procedures. The only way to find out how much training can improve functioning is to do intensive, extensive, and long-term strategy training. The development of compendia of strategies (e.g., Devine, 1987) is a first step; the development of training packages like those used at Kansas is also a move in the right direction; the training of teachers who are sensitive to the needs of process-oriented instruction is also desirable. The real challenge is to get all of these elements together and functioning for a long period of time with real students. Our point of view is that the many fine well-controlled laboratory studies aimed at specific aspects of memory (i.e., the studies that provided most of the data for this book) could and should be complemented by more ambitious field experiments aimed at improving memory and memory-strategy use as much as possible. It is time to start thinking big – to start thinking about realistic educational interventions that have the potential for broadly enhancing memory functioning in ways that directly improve ecologically valid intellectual performances of students.

8. Conclusions

Our focus in this book was the development of memory for verbal materials during childhood and adolescence. Most of the research can be interpreted within the general information processing framework. Our purpose in this chapter is to summarize briefly the most important conclusions that follow from what was reviewed here, as well as to comment on a few directions that might be profitably pursued in future research.

What Develops?

The earliest work on memory development was conducted at the end of the last century and early in this century. With a few exceptions (e.g., Brunswik et al., 1932), these early studies were limited to descriptions of developmental trends. That is, they neither tested theoretical models nor specific explanations of memory developments that were described. In contrast, modern researchers are more interested in determining the processes that mediate the developmental trends that have been observed. What has emerged from the research to date is a model that explains memory development in terms of changes in functional memory capacity, use of verbal memory strategies, nonstrategic knowledge, and metamemory.

FUNCTIONAL MEMORY CAPACITY

There was little agreement during the 1970s about the role of structural changes in memory development. There were arguments that memory capacity was invariant over the life span (at least after 3 to 5 years of age), a theoretical argument that seemed inconsistent with robust correlations between age and children's performance on memory-span tasks. Case's (1985; Case et al., 1982) developmental model became extremely popular because it reconciled the apparent contradictions between theory and data. Case argues that short-term memory consists of two subcomponents, a storage space and an operating space. Compared to younger children, older children can hold more information in short-term memory because they execute cognitive operations more efficiently than younger children. Older children have used these operations more – the more an operation has been used, the greater the automatic and efficient use of the operation. In addition, regardless of practice, it seems that there are developmental increases in the execution of cognitive operations (Dempster, 1981). Execution of cognitive operations consume less and less capacity with increasing age (i.e., the functional operating space decreases). Thus, there is increasing capacity available for storage of input, even though the total amount of structurally determined capacity does not change with development. Siegler (1986) provided the following analogy between developmental changes in functional capacity and apparent changes in the capacity of a trunk of an automobile:

> The capacity of a car's trunk does not change as the owner acquires experience in packing luggage into it. Nonetheless, the amount of material that can be packed into the trunk does change. Whereas the trunk at first might hold two or three suitcases, it might eventually come to hold four or five. As each packing operation is executed more efficiently, trunk space is freed for additional operations (p. 82).

We emphasize that the postulated developmental invariance in total memory capacity is an *intraindividual* characteristic. *Interindividual* differences in total memory capacity are important when trying to explain individual differences in memory performance. Measures of memory capacity are especially predictive of performance when memory tasks do not offer much opportunity for strategic mediation (Schneider, 1986). Whether people benefit from instructions to execute strategies that require a great deal of capacity to execute is also predictable from individual differences in capacity.

STRATEGIES

Developmental memory research certainly flourished following the adoption and developmental adaptation of the general information processing model (e.g., Atkinson & Shiffrin, 1968), including the differentiation made in these models between structural parameters and control or strategic processes. The study of strategies like rehearsal and organizational grouping (i.e., for list learning) quickly made it clear that a direct relationship existed between age-correlated changes in memory strategies and performance changes. Many developmental psychologists in the 1970s believed that much of memory development could be explained as the development of increasingly flexible and more general memory strategies (e.g., Hagen et al., 1975; Moely, 1977). Most of the research supporting this hypothesis was generated with grade-school children, since 5 to 11 years of age was considered to be an especially crucial period for strategy development. These conclusions were premature, however.

First, there is now a lot of evidence that strategy development begins before the grade-school years and continues into adulthood. For instance, intentional memory strategies are observable in preschool children when they are dealing with famliar tasks or contexts (e.g., hide-and-seek tasks). At the mature end of the developmental spectrum, however, Rohwer and Thomas and their colleagues (e.g., Christopoulos et al., 1987) have shown that even college students often fail to use sophisticated strategies when doing school learning. In addition, it has become clearer that studies focusing on input or output strategies alone, which was the case in most work on encoding and rehearsal strategies, failed to capture that the interaction of encoding and recall processes is often more important than encoding or retrieval activities alone (e.g., Ackerman, 1985a). Finally, it seems that some outcomes that were once believed to be due to use of intentionally deployed strategies are in fact due to automatically occurring processes that are not consciously controllable (and thus, not strategic following the definition presented in Chapter 3). Consider when young children learn lists of items, with the list members drawn from a few salient categories (e.g., five foods, five vehicles, and five furniture items). Recall is often organized categorically. Bjorklund's work (e.g., 1985, 1987) makes clear that such organization during recall often reflects associative processes during retrieval (i.e., recall of one member of a category cues recall of another member) rather than organization at input. In general, there has been increasing understanding during the last decade that knowledge factors can play a large role in developmental improvements in memory performance.

NONSTRATEGIC KNOWLEDGE BASE

The strong version of the knowledge-base hypothesis was that most developmental improvements in memory were not mediated by shifts in strategy use, but rather reflected changes in the extent and accessibility of the nonstrategic knowledge base. Especially supportive of this position were empirical demonstrations that children's learning does not vary with age when to-be-learned materials are equally familiar and meaningful to children at different developmental levels (e.g., Chechile & Richman, 1982). Comparisons of child experts and adults novices have also provided striking support for the hypothesis that nonstrategic knowledge is a powerful determinant of performance. Chi's (1978) demonstration that 10-year-old chess experts could learn meaningful chess positions better than adult chess novices is especially well known.

There has also been important work documenting that the use of strategies often depends on the nonstrategic knowledge base. For instance, Tarkin, Myers, and Ornstein (cited in Ornstein et al., in press) demonstrated that repetition strategies used by third graders vary as a function of the meaningfulness of the learning material. When grade-3 children learned especially meaningful materials, their rehearsal set sizes were as large as those typically produced by grade-6 students. On the other hand, grade-3 children's set sizes were much smaller when they processed relatively unfamiliar materials. Comparable results have been reported for use of categorical-organizational strategies (Frankel & Rollins, 1985; Schneider, 1986).

METAMEMORY

There was intensive study of metamemory during the last decade. Both knowledge of facts about memory and children's memory monitoring were analyzed.

Memory facts can be divided into knowledge about persons, tasks, strategies, and the interactions between persons, tasks, and strategies (Flavell, 1985; Wellman, 1983). The person category refers to whether children understand qualities of their own memories and those of other people. The task category consists of knowledge about what makes one task more difficult than another. The strategy category covers verbalizable knowledge about various encoding and retrieval strategies. Early research on children's knowledge of memory facts (e.g., Kreutzer et al., 1975) created the impression that knowledge about memory develops quite early and is reasonably complete by grade 3. More recent research has established that knowledge about persons, tasks, strategies, and the interactions of these variables continues to develop into adulthood.

Monitoring performance on a day-in, day-out basis increases understanding about the relative difficulties of memory tasks, thus, permitting predictions about future performance. That monitoring contributes to the knowledge of memory facts (e.g., that one memory task is more difficult than another) makes obvious that conceptual distinctions between various facets of metamemory (in this case, monitoring and knowledge of memory) are fuzzy indeed. Monitoring of performance in the present (which occurs in short-term memory) is distinctly different from knowledge about memory that is in long-term storage. For instance, monitoring yields on-line awareness of whether materials that are the current objects of study have been learned already or require additional study. Although children as young as 5 to 6 years of age have some rudimentary competence to monitor, monitoring develops slowly throughout childhood and adolescence. Striking monitoring failures are sometimes observed even in adults, however.

It has proven difficult to study and measure metamemory. There are always questions as to whether metamemory interviews yield complete and accurate information. When unambiguous information about monitoring is obtained, it is at great expense in that many potentially contaminating factors can only be controlled and evaluated using complex experiments that involve a number of conditions (e.g., Pressley, Levin, & Ghatala, 1984).

One of the most important research questions addressed by metamemory researchers was whether empirical support could be produced for theoretically specified connections between metamemory, strategic behaviors, and memory performances. The first wave of relevant studies failed to produce statistically significant connections between metamemory and strategic behaviors or memory performances, a conclusion emphasized in some prominent reviews (e.g., Cavanaugh &

Perlmutter, 1982). Close scrutiny of these studies revealed difficulties including measurement problems (e.g., ceiling effects). These problems were remedied in more recent studies that employed metamemory indicators that were directly relevant to the memory tasks used in the studies. This "second generation" of studies has produced significant relationships between knowledge, behaviors, and performances. The correlations found in the grade-school years were generally medium to high, increasing with increasing age of the children. The average correlation coefficient was .41.

SUMMARY

Most studies of memory development focused on one of the four factors in isolation. Thus, relatively little is known about how the four factors interact, although the situation is improving (e.g., recent interest in knowledge by strategy interactions). The lack of evidence pertaining to interactions makes it particularly difficult to draw definitive conclusions about the influence of the four memory development factors at different points in development. It is possible to provide a rough outline based on the evidence that is available.

The basic neurological architecture that supports memory development is established in the first five years. Only a few strategies are used during this preschool period, mostly ones that are deployed in familiar situations. Preschoolers have little knowledge of memory or variables affecting memory. In fact, they possess some knowledge that is wildly inconsistent with reality (e.g., that they can learn enormous amounts of material in a short period of time). There is little monitoring of performance. More positively, the nonstrategic knowledge base undergoes extensive development during this first five years.

During grade school (i.e., 5 to 11 years of age), speed of information processing increases. A number of memory strategies emerge and develop, with the development of rehearsal and organizational strategies for list learning documented in some detail. Factual knowledge about memory increases during this period, and monitoring improves. The knowledge base continues to develop and greatly facilitates learning of content that is related to knowledge already possessed by children (e.g., children who know a lot about soccer can learn new information about soccer more easily than children who lack knowledge of soccer). It must be emphasized, however, that development of memory is far from complete by the end of the grade-school years.

Processing speed continues to increase during adolescence. More strategies are acquired during this interval (e.g., elaboration). Old strategies (e.g., rehearsal, organization) continue to develop and are used more flexibly. Monitoring continues to improve. Eighteen-year-olds know more about memory and other things than do 12-year-olds. Nonetheless, good strategy use is a rare commodity even among adults. Although processing speed probably reaches a maximum in early adulthood (e.g., Salthouse, 1982), most adults possess only fraction of the strategies, metamemory, and nonstrategic knowledge base that they could possess.

What Next?

Despite the enormous amount of information that has been generated about memory development during this century, knowledge of children's memory is still incomplete. Most of the research to date was generated in a very few experimental paradigms, mostly laboratory tasks. Everyday memory has been ignored for the most part. Many researchers (ourselves included) accept a memory model in which contextual and motivational variables are presumed to be important determinants of memory. For the most part, however, these same researchers continue to study memory without regard to naturalistic situational or motivational states. See Perlmutter (in press) for more detailed criticisms.

We suspect that current theory will in fact stimulate a lot of additional research on memory development. Programmatic research on some real world memory problems is beginning to emerge and is being received enthusiastically (e.g., autobiographical memory, Rubin, 1986; eyewitness memory, Ceci, Toglia, & Ross 1986), and thus, there is reason to be optimistic that study of memory in natural contexts will be conducted in the next decade. Realistic and interesting models of motivational factors as determinants of memory (see Borkowski et al., in press) should fuel research directed at understanding how motivation affects memory. We have three particular recommendations for those undertaking this research.

1. *Complement traditional developmental and experimental methods with modern multivariate approaches like causal modeling.* Causal models permit the evaluation of models of memory functioning that are composed of a variety of factors in interaction (e.g., functional short-term memory capacity, strategies, metamemory, nonstrategic knowledge, contextual factors, motivational variables). In particular, the relative contributions of these variables and how they affect one another can be specified and evaluated. Researchers at the Max Planck Institute have had good success in using LISREL analyses, especially in predicting performance in sort-recall tasks (i.e., situations that can be mediated by use of semantic-organizational strategies). For instance, that group has determined that similar models predict sort-recall performance in grade-3, grade-5, and grade-7 children, as well as in adults. The model for the grade 5 level is displayed in Figure 8.1. It specifies that general intelligence affects memory performance directly, but also affects it through the "hope of success" and metamemory variables. Memory behavior affects memory performance directly; memory behavior is affected by both metamemory (knowledge of memory variables) and monitoring. Monitoring also has a direct effect on memory.

2. *Study potentially important individual differences more intensely.* Although there has been interest in potential sex differences in verbal memory since the beginning of the century (see Chapter 1), we still know almost nothing about whether there are sex differences in memory development. This is because sex differences were not even examined in most studies of children's memory. More positively, the recent studies by Waters and her colleagues (Cox & Waters, 1986) substantiated that sex differences (generally favoring females) are present. Why do we mention this finding? We want to emphasize that there has been neglect of many salient individual

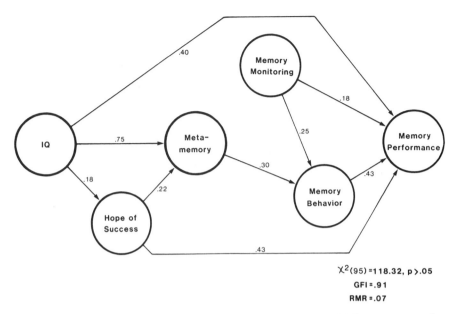

$$X^2(95) = 118.32, \, p > .05$$
$$GFI = .91$$
$$RMR = .07$$

FIGURE 8.1. Structural equation model (LISREL) describing and explaining memory performance in fifth graders (Schneider et al., 1987b).

differences variables. After all, there is no difference between children that is more obvious than sex.

Even those individual differences that have been considered have not been studied as analytically as they could be. For instance, consider the study of cultural differences in memory development. One finding is cited frequently based on this literature. Children in third-world and underdeveloped countries who experience western-type schooling are more likely to have the memory skills possessed by western children than children in those countries who are not western-schooled. More interesting are recent cross-cultural studies that report progress in identifying mechanisms that might mediate omnibus cross-cultural differences.

For example, Schneider et al. (1986) demonstrated differences in use of organizational strategies between German and American children performing a sort-recall task. The German children used organization more than the American children. Since the cause of this cross-cultural difference was not obvious, Kurtz et al. (1986) conducted a follow-up study with grade-2 German and American children. Once again, the German children used organization more than the Americans. In this study additional data were collected tapping the strategy teaching provided by parents and teachers. There was a clear cultural difference in that German children were much more likely to be taught memory strategies than American children. Complementary within-culture work (United States) has been produced by Moely and her colleagues (Moely, Hart, Santulli et al., 1986; Moely, Leal et al., 1986).

They concluded based on observation of actual classroom practice that individual differences in use of memory strategies correlate with differences in teaching emphasis. Children whose teachers introduce memory strategies were more likely to use strategies than children whose teachers failed to instruct strategies. Data such as these should stimulate additional research on the degree that differences in memory skills are related to differences in educational environments. (See Beuhring and Kee, 1987a, for fascinating reports by adolescents that their natural use of elaboration was prompted by memory strategy instruction that they had received in school.)

In addition to neglect of interindividual differences, there has also been neglect of intraindividual differences. Little is known about whether children's memory performances are consistent across situations. The few studies that have been conducted focused on whether there were consistent differences in use of strategies (i.e., Do children who use strategies in one situation use them in another one?). This problem was studied by Kail (1979) with third and sixth graders. Kail employed factor analytic methods and interpreted his results as being compatible with the assumption that there is a general strategy factor. Inspection of the simple correlations, however, makes it clear that there were great intraindividual inconsistencies. The intercorrelations between the various memory performances and strategy measures were generally low. Later studies have shown that the degree of intraindividual consistency over varying memory tasks depends on the similarities of the tasks and task demands (Cavanaugh & Borkowski, 1980; Knopf, Körkel, Schneider, & Weinert, in press). Nonetheless, a lot of work with a lot of different strategies must be done before there is any refined understanding of intraperson consistencies.

3. *Conduct longitudinal studies.* Perhaps the most frustrating aspect of the memory development literature is that very little is known about the mechanisms that account for the development of strategies (Ornstein et al., in press; Ornstein & Naus, 1985). More positively, there are hypotheses. Bjorklund (e.g., 1985). believes that strategies are sometimes abstracted from occasions when naturalistic mediation enhances performance; the Vygotskians believe that some strategies are passed from parent to child as the parent provides instruction that is compatible with the child's cognitive level (e.g., Rogoff & Mistry, 1985); we identify with the perspective that at least some strategies are taught explicitly to children in school (Beuhring & Kee, 1987a; Kurtz et al., 1986; Pressley, Goodchild, Fleet, Zajchowski, & Evans, in press). Nonetheless, there is only scanty support that any of these mechanisms mediates naturalistic acquisition of strategies.

An additional frustration is that there is little information about which memory activities can be viewed as precursors to later use of strategies. There has been no programmatic research to relate preschoolers' memory behaviors to the strategic activities of grade-school children. A similar situation holds true for the development of nonstrategic knowledge and metamemory. There are no clear data about how early nonstrategic knowledge and metamemory contribute to later development.

There is no doubt that the literature gaps bemoaned in the last two paragraphs cannot be filled by additional cross-sectional research. The cross-sectional paradigm (the approach used in the preponderance of memory research) can only provide information about developmental differences, not developmental changes. Mechanisms that might account for naturalistic changes can only be evaluated when there are opportunities to evaluate changes in memory performance following exposure to the mechanisms. Whether early person and environmental factors account for later memory characteristics can only be evaluated when it is possible to describe how particular individuals change and differ from one point in development to another.

It is obvious that these problems can only be studied longitudinally. The advantages of longitudinal studies are easy to enumerate (e.g., Ornstein et al., in press; Schneider & Weinert, in press). Most importantly, such research permits examination of relationships between early knowledge, characteristics, behaviors, and environments and later knowledge, characteristics, and behaviors. In-depth longitudinal studies of memory development could include long-term measurement of many factors believed to contribute to developmental improvements in memory performance. These factors could be examined alone and in interaction to determine which are more potent than others and whether there might be developmental changes in the mix of factors determining memory performance.

Such work would greatly enrich knowledge about memory development. Although the findings summarized in this book are valuable resources that should be considered in detail as part of the planning of longitudinal studies, it seems a good bet that the best memory development research is yet to come. Thus, we conclude confidently that this volume represents nothing more than a preliminary report. Much more will be discovered about memory between 2 and 20.

References and Bibliography

Ach, N. (1905). *Über die Willenstätigkeit und das Denken.* Göttingen: Vanderhoeck & Ruprecht.

Ackerman, B.P. (1982). Retrieval variability: The inefficient use of retrieval cues by young children. *Journal of Experimental Child Psychology, 33,* 413–428.

Ackerman, B.P. (1983). Encoding distinctiveness and the encoding shift penalty in children and adults. *Journal of Experimental Child Psychology, 36,* 257–283.

Ackerman, B.P. (1984). Item specific and relational encoding effects in children's recall and recognition memory for words. *Journal of Experimental Child Psychology, 37,* 426–450.

Ackerman, B.P. (1985a). Children's retrieval deficit. In C.J. Brainerd & M. Pressley (Eds.), *Basic processes in memory development* (pp. 1–46). New York: Springer.

Ackerman, B.P. (1985b). The effects of specific and categorical orienting on children's incidental and intentional memory for pictures and words. *Journal of Experimental Child Psychology, 39,* 300–325.

Ackerman, B.P. (1985c). Constraints on retrieval search for episodic information in children and adults. *Journal of Experimental Child Psychology, 40,* 152–180.

Ackerman, B.P. (1985d). Children's use of context and category cues to retrieve episodic information from memory. *Journal of Experimental Child Psychology, 40,* 420–438.

Ackerman, B.P. (1985e). Children's use of retrieval cues to "describe" episodic information in memory: Problems of constructability and discriminability. *Journal of Experimental Child Psychology, 40,* 193–217.

Ackerman, B.P. (1986a). The relation between attention to the incidental context and memory for words in children and adults. *Journal of Experimental Child Psychology, 41,* 149–183.

Ackerman, B.P. (1986b). Referential and causal coherence in the story comprehension of children and adults. *Journal of Experimental Child Psychology, 41,* 336–366.

Ackerman, B.P. (1987). Descriptions: A model of nonstrategic memory development. In H.W. Reese (Ed.), *Advances in child development and behavior* (Vol. 20). Orlando, FL: Academic Press.

Ackerman, B.P., & Hess, L. (1982). The effects of encoding distinctiveness on retrieval variability in children and adults. *Journal of Experimental Child Psychology, 33*, 465–474.

Ackerman, B.P., & Rathburn, J. (1984). Development differences in the use of retrieval cues to describe episodic information in memory. *Journal of Experimental Child Psychology, 38*, 147–173.

Ackerman, B.P., & Rust-Kahl, E. (1982). The effects of contrastive encoding of semantic information on children's memory for words. *Journal of Experimental Child Psychology, 34*, 414–434.

Adams, J.A. (1987). Historical review and appraisal of research on the learning, retention, and transfer of human motor skills. *Psychological Bulletin, 101*, 41–74.

Adams, L.T., & Worden, P.E. (1986). Script development and memory organization in preschool and elementary school children. *Discourse Processes, 9*, 149–166.

Allik, J.P., & Siegel, A.W. (1976). The use of the cumulative rehearsal strategy: A developmental study. *Journal of Experimental Child Psychology, 21*, 316–327.

Alvermann, D.E., Smith, L.C., & Readence, J.E. (1985). Prior knowledge activation and the comprehension of compatible and incompatible texts. *Reading Research Quarterly, 20*, 420–436.

Ammon, P. (1977). Cognitive development and early childhood education: Piagetian and neo-Piagetian theories. In L.H. Hom & P.A. Robinson (Eds.), *Psychological processes in early education* (pp. 157–202). New York: Academic Press.

Anderson, C.W. (1987). Strategic teaching in science. In B.F. Jones, A.S. Palincsar, D.S. Ogle, & E.G. Carr (Eds.), *Strategic teaching and learning: Cognitive instruction in the content areas*. Alexandria, VA: Association for Supervision and Curriculum Development.

Anderson, J.R. (1976). *Language, memory, and thought*. Hillsdale, NJ: Erlbaum & Associates.

Anderson, J.R. (1983). *The architecture of cognition*. Cambridge, MA: Harvard University Press.

Anderson, J.R. (1985). *Cognitive psychology and its implications*. San Francisco: W.H. Freeman & Co.

Anderson, R.C., & Pearson, P.D. (1984). A schema-theoretic view of basic processes in reading comprehension. In P.D. Pearson, M. Kamil, R. Barr, & P. Mosenthal (Eds.), *Handbook of reading research* (pp. 255–291). New York: Longman.

Anderson, R.C., & Pichert, J.W. (1978). Recall of previously unrecallable information following a shift in perspective. *Journal of Verbal Learning and Verbal Behavior, 17*, 1–12.

Andreassen, C., & Waters, H.S. (1984). *Organization during study: Relationships between meta-memory, strategy use, and performance*. Paper presented at the annual meeting of the American Research Association, New Orleans, LA.

Anglin, J.M. (1977). *Word, object, and conceptual development*. New York: Norton.

Appel, F.L., Cooper, R.G., McCarrell, N., Sims-Knight, J., Yussen, S.R., & Flavell, J.H. (1972). The development of the distinction between perceiving and memorizing. *Child Development, 43*, 1365–1381.

Appelbaum, M.I., & McCall, R.B. (1983). Design and analysis in developmental psychology. In P.H. Mussen (Ed.), *Handbook of child psychology* (Vol. 1, pp. 415–476). New York: Wiley.

Applebee, A.N. (1984). *Contexts for learning to write*. Norwood, NJ: Ablex.

Applebee, A.N. (1986). Problems in process approaches. Toward a reconceptualization of process instruction. In A.R. Petrosky, D. Bartholomae, & K.J. Rehage (Eds.), *The teaching of writing: Eighty-fifth yearbook of the National Society for the Study of Education* (pp. 95–113). Chicago, IL: University of Chicago Press.

Arnold, D.J., & Brooks, P.H. (1976). Influence of contextual organizing material on children's listening comprehension. *Journal of Educational Psychology, 68,* 711–716.

Asarnow, J.R., & Meichenbaum, D. (1979). Verbal rehearsal and serial recall. *Child Development, 50,* 1173–1177.

Ashcraft, M.A., & Kellas, G. (1974). Organization in normal and retarded children: Temporal aspects of storage and retrieval. *Journal of Experimental Psychology, 103,* 502–508.

Asher, S.R., Hymel, S., & Wigfield, A. (1978). Influence of topic interest on children's reading comprehension. *Journal of Reading Behavior, 10,* 35–47.

Ashmead, D.H., & Perlmutter, M. (1980). Infant memory in everyday life. In M. Perlmutter (Ed.), *New directions for child development: Children's memory* (pp. 1–16). San Francisco: Jossey-Bass.

Atkinson, R.C. (1975). Mnemotechnics in second-language learning. *American Psychologist, 30,* 821–828.

Atkinson, R.C., Hansen, D.N., & Bernbach, H.A. (1964). Short-term memory with young children. *Psychonomic Science, 1,* 255–256.

Atkinson, R.C., & Raugh, M.R. (1975). An application of the mnemonic keyword method to the acquisition of a Russian vocabulary. *Journal of Experimental Psychology: Human Learning and Memory, 104,* 126–133.

Atkinson, R.C., & Shiffrin, R.M. (1968). Human memory. A proposed system and its control processes. In K.W. Spence & J.T. Spence (Eds.), *The psychology of learning and motivation* (Vol. 2, pp. 90–197). New York: Academic Press.

Atkinson, R.C., & Shiffrin, R.M. (1971). The control of short-term memory. *Scientific American,* 82–90.

Baddeley, A. (1981). The concept of working memory: A view of its current state and probable future development. *Cognition, 10,* 17–23.

Baddeley, A. (1986). *Working memory.* New York: Oxford University Press.

Baker, L. (1985). How do we know when we don't understand? Standards for evaluating text comprehension. In D.L. Forrest-Pressley, G.E. MacKinnon, & T.G. Waller (Eds.), *Metacognition, cognition and human performance* (Vol. 1, pp. 155–205). Orlando, San Diego: Academic Press.

Baker, L., & Anderson, R.L. (1982). Effects of inconsistent information on text processing: Evidence for comprehension monitoring. *Reading Research Quarterly, 17,* 281–294.

Baker, L., & Brown, A.L. (1984). Metacognitive skills and reading. In P.D. Pearson, M. Kamil, R. Barr, & P. Mosenthal (Eds.), *Handbook of reading research (pp. 353–394).* New York: Longman.

Baker-Ward, L., Ornstein, P.A., & Holden, D.J. (1984). The expression of memorization in early childhood. *Journal of Experimental Child Psychology, 37,* 555–575.

Baldwin, R.S., Peleg-Bruckner, Z., & McClintock, A.H. (1985). Effects of topic interest and prior knowledge on reading comprehension. *Reading Research Quarterly, 20,* 497–504.

Ballstaedt, S.P., Mandl, H., Schnotz, N., & Tergan, S.O. (1981). *Texte verstehen—Texte gestalten.* München: Urban & Schwarzenberg.

Bandura, A. (1977). Self-efficacy: Toward a unifying theory of behavioral change. *Psychological Review, 84,* 191–215.

Bandura, A. (1982). Self-efficacy mechanism in human agency. *American Psychologist, 37,* 122–147.

Barclay, C.R. (1979). The executive control of mnemonic activity. *Journal of Experimental Child Psychology, 27,* 262–276.

Barclay, C.R. (1981). On the relation between memory and metamemory. *The Psychological Record, 31,* 153–156.

Baron, J. (1981). Reflective thinking as a goal of education. *Intelligence, 5,* 291–309.

Baron, J. (1985). *Rationality and intelligence.* Cambridge, England: Cambridge University Press.

Bartlett, F.C. (1932). *Remembering.* Cambridge, England: Cambridge University Press.

Battig, W.F., & Montague, W.E. (1969). Category norms for verbal items in 56 categories: A replication and extension of the Connecticut category norms. *Journal of Experimental Psychology Monographs, 80,* 3.

Beal, C.R. (1985). Development of knowledge about the use of cues to aid prospective retrieval. *Child Development, 56,* 631–642.

Beal, C.R., & Flavell, J.H. (1982). The effect of increasing the salience of message ambiguities on kindergartner's evaluations of communicative success and message adequacy. *Developmental Psychology, 18,* 43–48.

Beal, C.R., & Fleisig, W.E. (1987, April). *Preschooler's preparation for retrieval in object relocation tasks.* Paper presented at the biennial meeting of the Society for Research in Child Development, Baltimore, MD.

Bean, C.H. (1912). The curve of forgetting. *Archives of Psychology, 21,* 15–21.

Begg, I., & Anderson, M.C. (1976). Imagery and associative memory in children. *Journal of Experimental Child Psychology, 21,* 480–489.

Begg, I., & Young, B.J. (1977). An organizational analysis of the form class effect. *Journal of Experimental Child Psychology, 23,* 503–519.

Belloni, L.E., & Jongsma, E.A. (1978). The effects of interest on reading comprehension of low-achieving students. *Journal of Reading, 22,* 106–109.

Belmont, J.M., & Borkowski, J.G. (1988). A group test of children's metamemory. *Bulletin of the Psychonomic Society, 26,* 206–208.

Belmont, J.M., & Butterfield, E.C. (1969). The relations of short-term memory to development and intelligence. In L.P. Lipsitt & H.W. Reese (Eds.), *Advances in child development and behavior* (Vol. 4, pp. 30–83). New York: Academic Press.

Belmont, J.M., & Butterfield, E.C. (1971). What the development of short-term memory is. *Human Development, 14,* 236–248.

Belmont, J.M., & Butterfield, E.C. (1977). The instructional approach to developmental cognitive research. In R.V. Kail & J.W. Hagen (Eds.), *Perspectives on the development of memory and cognition* (pp. 437–481). Hillsdale, NJ: Erlbaum & Associates.

Belmont, J.M., Butterfield, E.C., & Borkowski, J.G. (1978). Training retarded people to generalize memorization methods across memory tasks. In M.M. Gruneberg, P.E. Morris, & R.M. Sykes (Eds.), *Practical aspects of memory* (pp. 418–425). London: Academic Press.

Belmont, J.M., Butterfield, E.C., & Ferretti, R.P. (1982). To secure transfer of training instruct self-management skills. In D.K. Detterman (Ed.), *How and how much can intelligence be increased* (pp. 147–154). Norwood, NJ: Ablex.

Bender, B.G., & Levin, J.R. (1976). Motor activity, anticipated motor activity, and young children's associative learning. *Child Development, 47,* 560–562.

Bentler, P.M. (1980). Multivariate analysis with latent variables: Causal modeling. *Annual Review of Psychology, 31,* 419–456.

Berch, D.B., & Evans, R.C. (1973). Decision processes in children's recognition memory. *Journal of Experimental Child Psychology, 16,* 148–164.

Bereiter, C., & Bird, M. (1985). Use of thinking aloud in identification and teaching of reading comprehension strategies. *Cognition and Instruction, 2,* 91–130.

Berliner, D.C. (1986). In pursuit of the expert pedagogue. *Educational Researcher, 15,* (7), 5–13.

Bernholtz, J.E., & Bjorklund, B.R. (1986). *The activation of semantic memory relations and its role in the development of strategic organization in children.* Paper presented at the conference on Human Development, Nashville, TN.

Bernstein, A., & Bogdanoff, T. (1905). Experimente über das Verhalten der Merkfähigkeit bei Schulkindern. In W. Stern (Ed.), *Beiträge zur Psychologie der Aussage, 2.Folge* (pp. 115–139). Leipzig: Barth.

Bernstein, M.R. (1955). Relationship between interest and reading comprehension. *Journal of Educational Research, 49,* 283–288.

Best, D.L., & Ornstein, P.A. (1986). Children's generation and communication of mnemonic organizational strategies. *Developmental Psychology, 22,* 845–853.

Beuhring, T., & Kee, D.W. (1987a). Developmental relationships among metamemory elaborative strategy use, and associative memory. *Journal of Experimental Child Psychology, 44,* 377–400.

Beuhring, T., & Kee, D.W. (1987b). Elaboration and associative memory development: The metamemory link. In M.A. McDaniel & M. Pressley (Eds.), *Imagery and related mnemonic processes: Theories and applications* (pp. 257–273). New York: Springer.

Bialystok, E., & Ryan, E.B. (1985). A metacognitive framework for the development of first and second language skills. In D.L. Forrest-Pressley, G.E. MacKinnon & T.G. Waller (Eds.), *Metacognition, cognition, and human performance* (Vol. 1, pp. 207–252). Orlando, San Diego: Academic Press.

Binet, H. (1904). *La fatigue intellectuelle.* Paris: Schleicher.

Binet, H. (1909). *Les idees modernes sur les enfants.* Paris: Schleicher.

Binet, H., & Henri, V. (1894a). La memoire des mots. *L'Annee Psychologique, 1,* 1–23.

Binet, H., & Henri, V. (1894b). La memoire des phrases. *L'Annee Psychologique, 1,* 24–59.

Bisanz, G.L., Vesonder, G.T., & Voss, J.F. (1978). Knowledge of one's own responding and the relation of such knowledge to learning. *Journal of Experimental Child Psychology, 25,* 116–128.

Bjorklund, D.F. (1976). *Children's identification and encoding of category information for recall.* Unpublished doctoral dissertation, University of North Carolina, Chapel Hill, NC.

Bjorklund, D.F. (1985). The role of conceptual knowledge in the development of organization in children's memory. In C.J. Brainerd & M. Pressley (Eds.), *Basic processes in memory development: Progress in cognitive development research* (pp. 103–142). New York: Springer.

Bjorklund, D.F. (1987). How age changes in knowledge base contribute to the development of children's memory: An interpretive review. *Developmental Review, 7,* 93–130.

Bjorklund, D.F., & Bernholtz, J.E. (1986). The role of knowledge base in the memory performance of good and poor readers. *Journal of Experimental Child Psychology, 41,* 362–393.

Bjorklund, D.F., & Bjorklund, B.R. (1985). Organization versus item effects of an elaborated knowledge base on children's memory. *Developmental Psychology, 21,* 1120–1131.

Bjorklund, D.F., & de Marchena, M.R. (1984). Developmental shifts in the basis of organization in memory: The role of associative versus categorical relatedness in children's free-recall. *Child Development, 55,* 952–962.

Bjorklund, D.F., & Harnishfeger, K.K. (1987). Developmental differences in the mental effort requirements for the use of an organizational strategy in free recall. *Journal of Experimental Child Psychology, 44*, 109–125.

Bjorklund, D.F., & Jacobs, J.W. (1984). A developmental examination of ratings of associative strengths. *Behavior Research Methods, Instruments & Computers, 16*, 568–569.

Bjorklund, D.F., & Jacobs, J.W. (1985). Associative and categorical processes in children's memory: The role of automaticity in the development of organization in free recall. *Journal of Experimental Child Psychology, 39*, 599–617.

Bjorklund, D.F., & Muir, J.E. (1988). Children's development of free recall memory: Remembering on their own. In R. Vasta (Ed.), *Annals of child development* (Vol. 5). Greenwich, CT: JAI Press.

Bjorklund, D.F., Ornstein, P.A., & Haig, J.R. (1977). Developmental differences in organization and recall: Training in the use of organizational techniques. *Developmental Psychology, 13*, 175–183.

Bjorklund, D.F., & Thompson, B.E. (1983). Category typicality effects in children's memory performance: Qualitative and quantitative differences in the processing of category information. *Journal of Experimental Child Psychology, 35*, 329–344.

Bjorklund, D.F., Thompson, B.E., & Ornstein, P.A. (1983). Developmental trends in children's typicality judgements. *Behavior Research Methods & Instruments, 15*, 350–356.

Bjorklund, D.F., & Weiss, S.C. (1985). Influence of socioeconomic status on children's classification and free recall. *Journal of Educational Psychology, 77*, 119–128.

Bjorklund, D.F., & Zeman, B.R. (1982). Children's organization and metamemory awareness in their recall of familiar information. *Child Development, 53*, 799–810.

Bjorklund, D.F., & Zeman, B.R. (1983). The development of organizational strategies in children's recall of familiar information: Using social organization to recall the names of classmates. *International Journal of Behavioral Development, 6*, 341–353.

Black, J.B., & Bower, G.H. (1980). Story understanding as a problem solving. *Poetics, 9*, 223–250.

Black, M.M., & Rollins, H.A. (1982). The effects of instructional variables on young children's organization and free recall. *Journal of Experimental Child Psychology, 33*, 1–19.

Blair, R., Perlmutter, M., & Myers, N.A. (1978). Effects of unlabeled and labeled picture cues on very young children's memory for location. *Bulletin of Psychonomic Society, 11*, 46–48.

Blonskii, P.P. (1935). *Memory and thinking.* Moscow: Prosveshchenie.

Bolton, T.L. (1892). The growth of memory in school children. *American Journal of Psychology, 4*, 362–382.

Borkowski, J.G. (1985). Signs of intelligence: Strategy, generalization and metacognition. In S.R. Yussen (Ed.), *The growth of reflection in children* (pp. 105–144). Orlando: Academic Press.

Borkowski, J.G., & Büchel, F.P. (1983). Learning and memory strategies in the mentally retarded. In M. Pressley & J.R. Levin (Eds.), *Cognitive strategy research: Psychological foundations* (pp. 103–128). New York: Springer.

Borkowski, J.G., Carr, M., & Pressley, M. (1987). "Spontaneous" strategy use: Perspectives from metacognitive theory. *Intelligence, 11*, 61–75.

Borkowski, J.G., Carr, M., Rellinger, E., & Pressley, M. (in press). Self-regulated cognition. Interdependence of metacognition, attributions, and self-esteem. In B.F. Jones & L. Idol (Eds.), *Dimensions of thinking and cognitive instruction.* Hillsdale, NJ: Erlbaum & Associates.

Borkowski, J.G., Johnston, N.B., & Reid, N.K. (1987). Metacognition, motivation, and the transfer of control processes. In S.J. Ceci (Ed.), *Handbook of cognitive, social, and neuro-psychological aspects of learning disabilities* (Vol. 2, pp. 147–173). Hillsdale, NJ: Erlbaum & Associates.

Borkowski, J.G., & Krause, A.J. (1985). Metacognition and attributional beliefs. *Proceedings of the 23rd International Congress of Psychology.* Amsterdam: Elsevier.

Borkowski, J.G., Levers, S., & Gruenenfelder, T.M. (1976). Transfer of mediational strategies in children: The role of activity and awareness during strategy acquisition. *Child Development, 47,* 779–786.

Borkowski, J.G., Peck, V.A., Reid, M.K., & Kurtz, B.E. (1983). Impulsivity and strategy transfer: Metamemory as mediator. *Child Development, 54,* 459–473.

Borkowski, J.G., Reid, M.K., & Kurtz, B.E. (1984). Metacognition and retardation: Paradigmatic, theoretical, and applied perspectives. In R. Sperber, C. McCauley, & P. Brooks (Eds.), *Learning and cognition in the mentally retarded* (pp. 55–75). Baltimore, MD: University Park Press.

Bourdon, B. (1894). Influence de l'age sur la memoire immediate. *Revue Philosophique, 38,* 25–39.

Bousfield, A.K., & Bousfield, W.A. (1966). Measurement of clustering and of sequential constancies in repeated free recall. *Psychological Reports, 19,* 935–942.

Bousfield, W.A. (1953). The occurrence of clustering in the recall of randomly arranged associates. *Journal of Genetic Psychology, 49,* 229–240.

Bousfield, W.A., Cohen, B.H., & Whitmarsh, G.A. (1958). Associative clustering in the recall of words of different taxonomic frequencies of occurrence. *Psychological Report, 4,* 39–44.

Bousfield, W.A., Esterson, J., & Whitmarsh, G.A. (1958). A study of the developmental changes in conceptual and perceptual associative clustering. *The Journal of Genetic Psychology, 98,* 95–102.

Bower, G.H. (1975). Cognitive psychology: An introduction. In W.K. Estes (Ed.), *Handbook of learning and cognitive processes* (Vol. 1, pp. 25–80). Hillsdale, NJ: Erlbaum & Associates.

Bower, G.H. (1978). Contacts of cognitive psychology with social learning theory. *Cognitive Therapy and Research, 2,* 123–146.

Bower, G.H., Black, J.B., & Turner, T.J. (1979). Scripts in memory for text. *Cognitive Psychology, 11,* 177–220.

Bower, G.H., & Hilgard, E.R. (1981). *Theories of learning.* Englewood Cliffs, NJ: Prentice-Hall.

Brainerd, C.J. (1982). Children's concept learning as rule-sampling systems with Markovian properties. In C.J. Brainerd (Ed.), *Children's logical and mathematical cognition: Progress in cognitive development research* (pp. 177–212). New York: Springer.

Brainerd, C.J. (1985a). Model-based approaches to storage and retrieval development. In C.J. Brainerd & M. Pressley (Eds.), *Basic processes in memory development* (pp. 143–208). New York: Springer.

Brainerd, C.J. (1985b). Three-state models of memory development: A review of advances in statistical methodology. *Journal of Experimental Child Psychology, 40,* 375–394.

Brainerd, C.J., Desrochers, A., & Howe, M.L. (1981). Stages-of-learning analysis of developmental interactions in memory. *Journal of Experimental Psychology: Human Learning and Memory, 7,* 1–14.

Brainerd, C.J., & Howe, M.L. (1982). Stages-of-learning analysis of developmental interactions in memory, with illustrations from developmental interactions in picture-word effects. *Developmental Review, 2,* 251–273.

Brainerd, C.J., Howe, M.L., & Desrochers, A. (1982). A general theory of two-stage learning: A mathematical review with illustrations from memory development. *Psychological Bulletin, 91*, 634–665.

Brainerd, C.J., Howe, M.L., Kingma, J., & Brainerd, S.H. (1984). On the measurement of storage and retrieval contributions to memory development. *Journal of Experimental Child Psychology, 37*, 478–499.

Brainerd, C.J., & Pressley, M. (1985a). Preface. In C.J. Brainerd & M. Pressley (Eds.), *Basic processes in memory development. Progress in cognitive development research* (pp. vii–x). New York: Springer.

Brainerd, C.J., & Pressley, M. (1985b). *Basic processes in memory development. Progress in cognitive development research.* New York: Springer.

Brainerd, C.J., Howe, M.L., & Kingma, J. (1982). An identifiable model of two stage learning. *Journal of Mathematical Psychology, 26*, 263–293.

Bransford, J.D., & Franks, J.J. (1972). The abstraction of linguistic ideas: A review. *Cognition, 2*, 211–249.

Bransford, J.D., & Johnson, M.K. (1972). Contextual prerequisites for understanding: Some investigations of comprehension and recall. *Journal of Verbal Learning and Verbal Behavior, 11*, 717–726.

Bransford, J.D., Stein, B.S., Shelton, T.S., & Owings, R.A. (1981). Cognition and adaptation: The importance of learning to learn. In J.H. Harvey (Ed.), *Cognition, social behavior, and the environment* (pp. 93–110). Hillsdale, NJ: Erlbaum & Associates.

Bransford, J.D., Stein, B.S., Vye, N.J., Franks, J.J., Auble, P.M., Mezynski, K.J., & Perfetto, G.A. (1982). Differences in approaches to learning: An overview. *Journal of Experimental Psychology: General, 111*, 390–398.

Braunshausen, N. (1914). *Die experimentelle Gedächtnisforschung—Ein Kapitel der experimentellen Pädagogik.* Langensalza: Beyer & Söhne.

Brophy, J. (1985). *Socializing students' motivation to learn.* Unpublished manuscript. East Lansing, MI: Institute for Research on Teaching, Michigan State University.

Brophy, J. (1986). *On motivating students* (Occasional Paper No. 101). East Lansing, MI: Institute for Research on Teaching, Michigan State University.

Brophy, J., & Kher, N. (1986). Teacher socialization as a mechanism for developing student motivation to learn. In R. Feldman (Ed.), *Social psychology applied to education* (pp. 257–288). Cambridge, England: Cambridge University Press.

Brown, A.L. (1975). The development of memory: Knowing, knowing about knowing, and knowing how to know. In H.W. Reese (Ed.), *Advances in child development and behavior* (Vol. 10, pp. 103–152). New York: Academic Press.

Brown, A.L. (1977). Development, schooling, and the acquisition of knowledge about knowledge: Comments on Chapter 7 by Nelson. In R.C. Anderson, R.F. Spiro, & W.E. Montague (Eds.), *Schooling and the acquisition of knowledge* (pp. 241–258). Hillsdale, NJ: Erlbaum & Associates.

Brown, A.L. (1978). Knowing when, where, and how to remember: A problem of metacognition. In R. Glaser (Ed.), *Advances in instrucional psychology* (pp. 77–165). Hillsdale, NJ: Erlbaum & Associates.

Brown, A.L. (1979). Theories of memory and the problems of development: Activity, growth and knowledge. In L.S. Cermak & F.I.M. Craik (Eds.), *Levels of processing in human memory* (pp. 225–258). Hillsdale, NJ: Erlbaum & Associates.

Brown, A.L. (1980). Metacognitive development and reading. In R.J. Spiro, B. Bruce, & W.F. Brewer (Eds.), *Theoretical issues in reading comprehension* (pp. 453–482). Hillsdale, NJ: Erlbaum & Associates.

Brown, A.L. (1982). Learning and development: The problems of compatibility, access and induction. *Human Development, 25,* 89–115.

Brown, A.L. (1984). Metakognition, Handlungskontrolle, Selbststeuerung und andere, noch geheimnisvollere Mechanismen. In F.E. Weinert & R.H. Kluwe (Eds.), *Metakognition, Motivation und Lernen* (pp. 60–109). Stuttgart: Kohlhammer.

Brown, A.L. (1985). Mental orthopedics, the training of cognitive skills: An interview with Alfred Binet. In S.F. Chipman, J.W. Segal, & R. Glaser (Eds.), *Thinking and learning skills* (Vol. 2, pp. 319–337). Hillsdale, NJ: Erlbaum & Associates.

Brown, A.L., & Barclay, C.R. (1976). The effects of training specific mnemonics on the metamnemonic efficiency of retarded children. *Child Development, 47,* 71–80.

Brown, A.L., Bransford, J.D., Ferrara, R.A., & Campione, J.C. (1983). Learning, remembering, and understanding. In J.H. Flavell & E.M. Markman (Eds.), *Handbook of child psychology, Vol. III, Cognitive development* (pp. 77–166). New York: Wiley.

Brown, A.L., Campione, J.C., & Barclay, C.R. (1979). Training self-checking routines for estimating test readiness: Generalization from list learning to prose recall. *Child Development, 50,* 501–512.

Brown, A.L., Campione, J.C., & Day, J.D. (1981). Learning to learn: On training students to learn from texts. *Educational Researcher, 10,* 14–21.

Brown, A.L., Campione, J.C., & Murphy, M.D. (1977). Maintenance and generalization of trained metamnemonic awareness by educable retarded children. *Journal of Experimental Child Psychology, 24,* 191–211.

Brown, A.L., & Day, J.D. (1983). Macrorules for summarizing texts: The development of expertise. *Journal of Verbal Learning and Verbal Behavior, 22,* 1–14.

Brown, A.L., & DeLoache, J.S. (1978). Skills, plans, and self-regulation. In R.S. Siegler (Ed.), *Children's thinking: What develops?* (pp. 3–36). Hillsdale, NJ: Erlbaum & Associates.

Brown, A.L., & Lawton, S.C. (1977). The feeling of knowing experience in educable retarded children. *Developmental Psychology, 13,* 364–370.

Brown, A.L., & Palincsar, A.S. (in press). Reciprocal teaching of comprehension strategies: A natural history of one program for enhancing learning. In J. Borkowski & J.D. Day (Eds.), *Intelligence and cognition in special children: Comparative studies of giftedness, mental retardation, and learning disabilities.* Norwood, NJ: Ablex.

Brown, A.L., & Smiley, S.S. (1977). Rating the importance of structural units of prose passages: A problem of metacognitive development. *Child Development, 48,* 1–8.

Brown, A.L., & Smiley, S.S. (1978). The development of strategies for studying texts. *Child Development, 49,* 1076–1088.

Brown, A.L., Smiley, S.S., Day, J.D., Townsend, M.A.R., & Lawton, S.C. (1977). Intrusion of a thematic idea in children's comprehension and retention of stories. *Child Development, 48,* 1454–1466.

Brown, A.L., Smiley, S.S., Lawton, S.C. (1978). The effects of experience on the selection of suitable retrieval cues for studying texts. *Child Development, 49,* 829–835.

Brown, R., & McNeill, D. (1966). The "tip of the tongue" phenomenon. *Journal of Verbal Learning and Verbal Behavior, 5,* 325–337.

Browning, M.M., & Cavanaugh, J. (1985). *Metamemory and cognitive tempo as predictors of strategy transfer.* Paper presented at the biennial meeting of the Society for Research in Child Development, Toronto, Canada.

Bruner, J.S. (1964). The course of cognitive growth. *American Psychologist, 19,* 1–15.

Bruner, J.S., Olver, R.R., & Greenfield, P.M. (1966). *Studies in cognitive growth.* New York: Wiley.

Brunswik, E., Goldscheider, L., & Pilek, E. (1932). Zur Systematik des Gedächtnisses. In E. Brunswik (Ed.), *Beihefte zur Zeitschrift für angewandte Psychologie* (Vol. 64, pp. 1–158).

Büchel, F.P., & Borkowski, J.G. (1983). *Predicting and explaining strategy generalization: Task analysis and strategy elements.* Berichte und Arbeiten aus dem Institut für Psychologie der Universität Basel.

Bühler, K. (1930). *Die geistige Entwicklung des Kindes.* Jena: Gustav Fischer.

Burtis, P.J. (1982). Capacity increase and chunking in the development of short-term memory. *Journal of Experimental Child Psychology, 34,* 387–413.

Buschke, H. (1974). Components of verbal learning in children: Analysis by selective reminding. *Journal of Experimental Child Psychology, 18,* 488–496.

Buss, R.R., Yussen, S.R., Mathews, S.R., Miller, G.E., & Rembold, K.L. (1983). Development of children's use of a story schema to retrieve information. *Developmental Psychology, 19,* 22–28.

Cacioppo, J.T., & Petty, R.E. (1982). The need for cognition. *Journal of Personality and Social Psychology, 42,* 116–131.

Campbell, D.T., & Fiske, D.W. (1959). Convergent and discriminant validation by the multitrait-multimethod matrix. *Psychological Bulletin, 56,* 81–105.

Campione, J.C., & Armbruster, B.B. (1985). Acquiring information from texts: An analysis of four approaches. In J.W. Segal, S.F. Chipman, & R. Glaser (Eds.), *Thinking and learning skills, Vol. 1, Relating instruction to research* (pp. 317–359). Hillsdale, NJ: Erlbaum & Associates.

Campione, J.C., & Brown, A.L. (1984). Learning ability and transfer propensity as sources of individual differences in intelligence. In P.H. Brooks, R. Sperber, & C. McCauley (Eds.), *Learning and cognition in the mentally retarded* (pp. 265–293). Hillsdale, NJ: Erlbaum & Associates.

Campione, J.C., Brown, A.L., Ferrara, R.A., Jones, R.S., & Steinberg, E. (1985). Breakdowns in flexible use of information: Intelligence-related differences in transfer following equivalent learning performance. *Intelligence, 9,* 297–316.

Campione, J.C., Nitsch, K., Bray, N., & Brown, A.L. (1982). Improving memory skills in mentally retarded children: Empirical research and strategies for intervention. In P. Karoly & J.J. Steffen (Eds.), *Improving children's competence: Advances in child behavioral analysis and therapy* (Vol. 1, pp. 207–235). Lexington, MA: Lexington Books, D.C. Heath & Co.

Cantor, D.S., Andreassen, C., & Waters, H.S. (1985). Organization in visual episodic memory: Relationships between verbalized knowledge, strategy use, and performance. *Journal of Experimental Child Psychology, 40,* 218–232.

Carey, S. (1985). Are children fundamentally different kind of thinkers and learners than adults? In S.F. Chipman, J.W. Segal, & R. Glaser (Eds.), *Thinking and learning skills* (Vol. 2, pp. 485–517). Hillsdale, NJ: Erlbaum & Associates.

Carey, S. (1985). *Conceptual change in childhood.* Cambridge, MA: MIT Press.

Carr, M., & Borkowski, J.G. (in press). Metamemory and giftedness. *Gifted Child Quarterly.*

Case, R. (1972). Validation of a neo-Piagetian mental capacity construct. *Journal of Experimental Child Psychology, 14,* 287–302.

Case, R. (1974). Mental strategies, mental capacity, and instruction: A neo-Piagetian investigation. *Journal of Experimental Child Psychology, 18,* 382–397.

Case, R. (1978). Intellectual development from birth to adulthood: A neo-Piagetian interpretation. In R.S. Siegler (Ed.), *Children's thinking: What develops?* (pp. 37–72). Hillsdale, NJ: Erlbaum & Associates.

Case, R. (1985). *Intellectual development: Birth to adulthood.* Orlando, FL: Academic Press.

Case, R., & Kurland, D.M. (1980). A new measure for determining children's subjective organization of speech. *Journal of Experimental Child Psychology, 30*, 206-222.

Case, R., Kurland, D.M., & Goldberg, J. (1982). Operational efficiency and the growth of short-term memory span. *Journal of Experimental Child Psychology, 33*, 386-404.

Case, R., & Serlin, R. (1979). A new processing model for predicting performance on Pascual-Leone's test of m-space. *Cognitive Psychology, 11*, 308-326.

Castaneda, A., Fahel, L., & Odom, R. (1961). Associative characteristics of sixty-three adjectives and their relation to verbal paired-associate learning in children. *Child Development, 32*, 297-304.

Catania, A.C. (1985). The two psychologies of learning. In S. Koch & D.E. Leary (Eds.), *A century of psychology as science* (pp. 322-335). New York: McGraw-Hill.

Cavanaugh, J.C., & Borkowski, J.G. (1979). The metamemory-memory "connection": Effects of strategy training and maintenance. *Journal of General Psychology, 101*, 161-174.

Cavanaugh, J.C., & Borkowski, J.G. (1980). Searching for metamemory-memory connections: A developmental study. *Developmental Psychology, 16*, 441-453.

Cavanaugh, J.C., & Perlmutter, M. (1982). Metamemory: A critical examination. *Child Development, 53*, 11-28.

Ceci, S.J. (1980). A developmental study of multiple encoding and its relationship to age-related changes in free recall. *Child Development, 51*, 892-895.

Ceci, S.J. (1983). Automatic and purposive semantic processing characteristics of normal and language/learning-disabled children. *Development Psychology, 19*, 427-439.

Ceci, S.J. (1984). A developmental study of learning disabilities and memory. *Journal of Experimental Child Psychology, 38*, 352-371.

Ceci, S.J. (1986). *Handbook of cognitive, social, and neuropsychological aspects of learning disabilities* (Vol. 1). Hillsdale, NJ: Erlbaum & Associates.

Ceci, S.J. (1987). *Handbook of cognitive, social, and neuropsychological aspects of learning disabilities* (Vol. 2). Hillsdale, NJ: Erlbaum & Associates.

Ceci, S.J., & Bronfenbrenner, U. (1985). Don't forget to take the cupcakes out of the oven: Prospective memory, strategic time-monitoring, and context. *Child Development, 56*, 152-164.

Ceci, S.J., Bronfenbrenner, U., & Baker, J. (in press). Memory development and ecological complexity: The case of prospective remembering. In F.E. Weinert & M. Perlmutter (Eds.), *Memory development: Universal changes and individual differences*. Hillsdale, NJ: Erlbaum & Associates.

Ceci, S.J., & Howe, M.J.A. (1978a). Age-related differences in free recall as a function of retrieval flexibility. *Journal of Experimental Child Psychology, 26*, 432-442.

Ceci, S.J., & Howe, M.J.A. (1978b). Semantic knowledge as a determinant of developmental differences in recall. *Journal of Experimental Child Psychology, 26*, 230-245.

Ceci, S.J., & Howe, M.J.A. (1982). Metamemory and the effects of attending, intending, and intending to attend. In G. Underwood (Ed.), *Aspects of consciousness* (Vol. 3, pp. 147-164). London: Academic Press.

Ceci, S.J., Lea, S.E.G., & Howe, M.J.A. (1980). Structural analysis of memory traces in children from 4 to 10 years of age. *Developmental Psychology, 16*, 203-212.

Ceci, S.J., Toglia, M.P., & Ross, D.F. (1986). *Children's eye witness testimony*. New York, Berlin: Springer.

Cecil, N.L. (1984). Impact of interest on the literal comprehension of beginning readers: A West Indian study. *The Reading Teacher, 37*, 750-753.

Chase, W.G., & Simon, H.A. (1973). Perception in chess. *Cognitive Psychology, 4*, 55-81.

Chechile, R.A., & Meyer, D.L. (1976). A Bayesian procedure for separately estimating storage and retrieval components of forgetting. *Journal of Mathematical Psychology, 13,* 269–295.

Chechile, R.A., Richman, C.L., Topinka, C., & Ehrensbeck, K. (1981). A developmental study of the storage and retrieval of information. *Child Development, 52,* 251–259.

Chechile, R.A., & Richman, C.L.V. (1982). The interaction of semantic memory with storage and retrieval processes. *Developmental Review, 2,* 237–250.

Chi, M.T.H. (1976). Short-term memory limitations in children: Capacity or processing deficits? *Memory & Cognition, 4,* 559–572.

Chi, M.T.H. (1977). Age differences in memory span. *Journal of Experimental Child Psychology, 23,* 266–281.

Chi, M.T.H. (1978). Knowledge structure and memory development. In R.S. Siegler (Ed.), *Children's thinking: What develops?* (pp. 73–96). Hillsdale, NJ: Erlbaum & Associates.

Chi, M.T.H. (1981). Knowledge development and memory performances. In M.P. Friedman, J.P. Das & N. O'Connor (Ed.), *Intelligence and learning* (pp. 221–229). New York: Plenum Press.

Chi, M.T.H. (1983). *Trends in memory development research.* Basel/München: Karger.

Chi, M.T.H. (1984). Bereichsspezifisches Wissen und Metakognition. In F.E. Weinert & R.H. Kluwe (Eds.), *Metakognition, Motivation und Lernen* (pp. 211–233). Stuttgart: Kohlhammer.

Chi, M.T.H. (1985a). Changing conception of sources of memory development. *Human Development, 28,* 50–56.

Chi, M.T.H. (1985b). Interactive roles of knowledge and strategies in the development of organized sorting and recall. In S.F. Chipman, J.W. Segal, & R. Glaser (Eds.), *Thinking and learning skills, Vol. 2, Research and open questions* (pp. 457–483). Hillsdale, NJ: Erlbaum & Associates.

Chi, M.T.H., Feltovich, P., & Glaser, R. (1981). Categorization and representation of physics problems by experts and novices. *Cognitive Science, 5,* 121–152.

Chi, M.T.H., & Gallagher, J.D. (1982). Speed and processing: A developmental source of limitation. *Topics in Learning and Learning Disabilities, 2,* 23–32.

Chi, M.T.H., & Koeske, R.D. (1983). Network representation of a child's dinosaur knowledge. *Developmental Psychology, 19,* 29–39.

Chi, M.T.H., & Rees, E.T. (1983). A learning framework for development. In M.T.H. Chi (Ed.), *Trends in memory development research* (pp. 71–107). Basel/München: Karger.

Chiesi, L., Spilich, G.J., & Voss, J.F. (1979). Acquisition of domain-related information in relation to high and low domain knowledge. *Journal of Verbal Learning and Verbal Behavior, 18,* 257–273.

Christie, D.J., & Schumacher, G.M. (1975). Developmental trends in the abstraction and recall of relevant versus irrelevant thematic information from connected verbal materials. *Child Development, 46,* 598–602.

Christopoulos, J.P., Rohwer, W.D., Jr., & Thomas, J.W. (1987). Grade level differences in students' study activities as a function of course characteristics. *Contemporary Educational Psychology, 12,* 303–323.

Clark, C.M., & Elmore, J.L. (1979). *Teacher planning in the first weeks of school* (Research Series No. 56). East Lansing, MI: Michigan State University, Institute for Research on Teaching.

Clark, E.V. (1978). Awareness of language: Some evidence from what children say and do. In A. Sinclair, R.J. Jarvella, & W.J.M. Levelt (Eds.), *The child's conception of language* (pp. 17–45). New York: Springer.

Clifford, M.M. (1984). Thoughts on a theory of constructive failure. *Educational Psychologist, 19,* 108–120.

Clifford, M.M. (1986a). The comparative effects of strategy and effort attributions. *British Journal of Educational Psychology, 56,* 75–83.

Clifford, M.M. (1986b). The effects of ability, strategy, and effort attributions for educational, business, and athletic failures. *British Journal of Educational Psychology, 56,* 169–179.

Cole, M., Frankel, F., & Sharp, D. (1971). Development of free recall in children. *Developmental Psychology, 4,* 109–123.

Cole, M., Gay, J., Glick, J., & Sharp, D. (1971). *The cultural context of learning and thinking.* New York: Basic Books.

Cole, M., & Scribner, S. (1977). Cross-cultural studies of memory and cognition. In R.V. Kail & J.W. Hagen (Eds.), *Perspectives on the development of memory and cognition.* Hillsdale, NJ: Erlbaum & Associates.

Collins, A.M., & Loftus, E.F. (1975). A spreading-activation theory of semantic processing. *Psychological Bulletin, 82,* 407–428.

Corsale, K. (1981). *Children's knowledge and strategic use of organizational structure in recall.* Paper presented at the biennial-annual meetings of the Society for Research in Child Development, Boston.

Corsale, K., & Ornstein, P.A. (1980). Developmental changes in children's use of semantic information in recall. *Journal of Experimental Child Psychology, 30,* 231–245.

Cox, D., & Waters, H.S. (1986). Sex differences in the use of organization strategies: A developmental analysis. *Journal of Experimental Child Psychology, 41,* 18–37.

Cox, G., & Paris, S.G. (1976). *Associative bases of encoding: An age-related dimension?* Paper presented at the 48th annual meeting of the Midwestern Psychological Association, Chicago.

Cox, G., & Paris, S.G. (1979). *Evaluation, selection, and use of mnemonic skills by children, young adults, and the elderly.* Paper presented at the annual meetings of the American Educational Research Association, San Francisco.

Craik, F.I.M., & Jacoby, L.L.A. (1975). A process view of short-term retention. In F. Restle, R.M. Shiffrin, N.J. Castellan, H.R., & Lindman & D. (Eds.), *Cognitive theory* (Vol. 1, pp. 173–192). Hillsdale, NJ: Erlbaum & Associates.

Craik, F.I.M., & Lockhart, R.S. (1972). Levels of processing: A framework for memory research. *Journal of Verbal Learning and Verbal Behavior, 11,* 671–684.

Craik, F.I.M., & Watkins, M.J. (1973). The role of rehearsal in short-term memory. *Journal of Verbal Learning and Verbal Behavior, 12,* 599–607.

Crano, W.D., & Mendoza, J.L. (1987). Maternal factors that influence children's positive behavior: Demonstration of a structural equation analysis of selected data from the Berkeley Growth Study. *Child Development, 58,* 38–48.

Craske, M.L. (1985). Improving persistence through observational learning and attribution retraining. *British Journal of Educational Psychology, 55,* 138–147.

Crisafi, M.A., & Brown, A.L. (1986). Analogical transfer in very young children: Combining two separately learned solutions to reach a goal. *Child Development, 57,* 953–968.

Cronbach, L.J., & Snow, R.E. (1977). *Aptitudes and instructional methods: A handbook for research on interactions.* New York, NY: Irvington.

Cultice, J.C., Somerville, S.C., & Wellman, H.M. (1983). Preschooler's memory monitoring: Feeling-of-knowing judgments. *Child Development, 54,* 1480–1486.

Cuvo, A.J. (1974). Incentive level influence on overt rehearsal and free recall as a function of age. *Journal of Experimental Child Psychology, 18,* 167–181.

Cuvo, A.J. (1975). Developmental differences in rehearsal and free recall. *Journal of Experimental Child Psychology, 19*, 265–278.

Daehler, M.W., & Greco, C. (1985). Memory in very young children. In M. Pressley & C.J. Brainerd (Eds.), *Cognitive learning and memory in children. Progress in cognitive development research* (pp. 49–79). New York: Springer.

Danner, F.W. (1976). Children's understanding of intersentence organization in the recall of short descriptive passages. *Journal of Educational Psychology, 68*, 174–183.

Danner, F.W., & Taylor, A.M. (1973). Integrated pictures and relational imagery training in children's learning. *Journal of Experimental Child Psychology, 16*, 47–54.

Davies, G., & Brown, L. (1978). Recall and organization in five-year-old children. *British Journal of Psychology, 69*, 343–349.

Davis, J.K. (1966). Mediated generalization and interference across five grade levels. *Psychonomic Science, 6*, 273–274.

Day, J.D. (1980). *Training summarization skills: A comparison of teaching methods.* Unpublished doctoral dissertation, University of Illinois, Champaign-Urbana, IL.

Day, J.D., & Hall, L.K. (1987). *Intelligence-related differences in learning and transfer and the enhancement of transfer in the retarded.* Manuscript submitted for publication.

DeLoache, J.S. (1980). Naturalistic studies of memory for object location in very young children. In M. Perlmutter (Ed.), *New directions for child development: Children's memory* (pp. 17–32). San Francisco: Jossey Bass.

DeLoache, J.S. (1984). "Oh where, oh where": Memory-based searching by very young children. In C. Sophian (Ed.), *Origins of cognitive skills* (pp. 57–80). Hillsdale, NJ: Erlbaum & Associates.

DeLoache, J.S., & Brown, A.L. (1983). Very young children's memory for the location of objects in a large-scale environment. *Child Development, 54*, 888–897.

DeLoache, J.S., & Brown, A.L. (1984). Where do I go next? Intelligent searching by very young children. *Developmental Psychology, 20*, 37–44.

DeLoache, J.S., Cassidy, D.J., & Brown, A.L. (1985). Precursors of mnemonic strategies in very young children's memory. *Child Development, 56*, 125–137.

Dempster, F.N. (1978). Memory span and short-term memory capacity: A developmental study. *Journal of Experimental Child Psychology, 26*, 419–431.

Dempster, F.N. (1981). Memory span: Sources of individual and developmental differences. *Psychological Bulletin, 89*, 63–100.

Dempster, F.N. (1985). Short-term memory development in childhood and adolescence. In C.J. Brainerd & M. Pressley (Eds.), *Basic processes in memory development. Progress in cognitive development research* (pp. 209–248). New York: Springer.

Denhiere, G. (1982). Do we really mean schemata? In J.F. Le Ny & W. Kintsch (Eds.), *Language and comprehension* (pp. 219–237). Amsterdam: Alphen.

Denhiere, G. (in press). Story comprehension and memorization by children: The role of input-, conservation-, and output processes. In F.E. Weinert & M. Perlmutter (Eds.), *Memory development: Universal changes and individual differences.* Hillsdale, NJ: Erlbaum & Associates.

Denhiere, G., Cession, A., & Deschenes, A.-J. (1986). *Learning from text: Effects of age and prior knowledge.* Paper presented at the annual meeting of the American Educational Research Association, San Francisco.

Denhiere, G., & Le Ny, J.F. (1980). Relative importance of meaningful units in comprehension and recall of narratives by children and adults. *Poetics, 9*, 147–161.

Denis, M. (1987). Individual imagery differences and prose processing. In M.A. McDaniel & M. Pressley (Eds.), *Imagery and related mnemonic processes* (pp. 204–217). New York, Berlin: Springer.

Denis, M., & Carfantan, M. (1985). People's knowledge about images. *Cognition*, *20*, 49–60.

Denney, N, & Ziobrowski, M. (1972). Developmental changes in clustering criteria. *Journal of Experimental Child Psychology*, *13*, 275–282.

Derry, S.J., & Murphy, D.A. (1986). Designing systems that train learning ability: From theory to practice. *Review of Educational Research*, *56*, 1–39.

Deshler, D.D., Alley, G.R., Warner, M.M., & Schumaker, J.B. (1981). Instructional practices for promoting skill acquisition and generalization in severely learning disabled adolescents. *Learning Disability Quarterly*, *4*, 415–421.

Deshler, D.D., Schumaker, J.B., & Lenz, B.K. (1984). Academic and cognitive interventions for LD adolescents: Part I. *Journal of Learning Disabilities*, *17*, 108–117.

Deshler, D.D., Schumaker, J.B., Lenz, B.K., & Ellis, E.S. (1984). Academic and cognitive interventions for LD adolescents: Part II. *Journal of Learning Disabilities*, *17*, 170–187.

Devine, T.G. (1987). *Teaching study skills: A guide for teachers*. New York: Allyn & Bacon.

Digdon, N., Pressley, M., & Levin, J.R. (1985). Preschoolers' learning when pictures do not tell the whole story. *Educational Communication and Technology Journal*, *33*, 139–145.

Dixon, R.A. (1985). *Metamemory and aging: Issues of structure and function*. Paper presented at the third G.A. Talland Memory Conference on Memory and Aging: Cape Cod, MA.

Dixon, R.A., & Hultsch, D.F. (1983a). Structure and development of metamemory in adulthood. *Journal of Gerontology*, *38*, 682–688.

Dixon, R.A., & Hultsch, D.F. (1983b). Metamemory and memory for text relationships in adulthood: A cross-validation study. *Journal of Gerontology*, *38*, 689–694.

Drinkwater, B.A. (1976). Visual memory skills of medium contact Aboriginal children. *Australian Journal of Psychology*, *28*, 37–43.

Dube, E.F. (1982). Literacy, cultural familiarity, and "intelligence" as determinants of story recall. In U. Neisser (Ed.), *Memory observed: Remembering in natural contexts* (pp. 274–292). San Francisco: Freeman.

Duffy, G.G., Roehler, L.R., & Putnam, J. (1987). Putting the teacher in control: Basal reading textbooks and instructional decision making. *The Elementary School Journal*, *87*, 357–366.

Duffy, G.G., Roehler, L.R., Sivan, E., Rackliffe, G., Book, C., Meloth, M., Vavrus, L., Wesselman, R., Putnam, J., & Bassiri, D. (1987). The effects of explaining the reasoning associated with using reading strategies. *Reading Research Quarterly*, *22*, 347–368.

Dufresne, A., & Kobasigawa, A. (1987, April). *Children's spontaneous allocation of study time in a paired-associate task*. Paper presented at the biennial meeting of the Society for Research in Child Development, Baltimore, MD.

Durkin, D. (1979). What classroom observations reveal about reading comprehension instruction. *Reading Research Quarterly*, *14*, 481–538.

Dweck, C.S. (1987). *Children's theories of intelligence: Implications for motivation and learning*. Paper presented at the annual meeting of the American Educational Research Association, Washington, DC.

Dweck, C.S., & Elliot, E.S. (1983). Achievement motivation. In P.H. Mussen (General Editor) & E.M. Hetherington (Volume Editor), *Handbook of child psychology, Vol. IV, Socialization, personality, and social development* (pp. 643–691). New York: Wiley.

Ebbinghaus, H. (1885). *Über das Gedächtnis*. Leipzig: Duncker.

Ebbinghaus, H. (1897). Über eine neue Methode zur Prüfung geistiger Fähigkeiten und ihre Anwendung bei Schulkindern. *Zeitschrift für Psychologie und Physiologie der Sinnesorgane*, *13*, 401–457.

Ebbinghaus, H. (1902). *Grundzüge der Psychologie* (Vol. 1). Leipzig: Veit & Comp.

Ebbinghaus, H. (1905). *Grundzüge der Psychologie I (2. Aufl.)*. Leipzig: Veit & Comp.

Elliott, S.N. (1980). *Sixth grade and college students' metacognitive knowledge of prose organization and study strategies.* Paper presented at the annual meeting of the American Educational Research Association, Boston.

Elliott-Faust, D.J. (1984). *The "delusion of comprehension" phenomenon in young children: An instructional approach to promoting listening comprehension monitoring capabilities in grade three children.* Unpublished doctoral dissertation. London, Ontario: University of Western Ontario, Department of Psychology.

Elliott-Faust, D.J., & Pressley, M. (1984). *The "delusion of comprehension" phenomena in young children: An instructional approach to promoting listening comprehension monitoring capabilities in grade 3 children.* Paper presented at the annual meeting of the American Educational Research Association, New Orleans.

Elliott-Faust, D.J., & Pressley, M. (1986). How to teach comparison processing to increase children's short- and long-term listening comprehension monitoring. *Journal of Educational Psychology, 78,* 27–33.

Ellis, E.S. (1986). The role of motivation and pedagogy on the generalization of cognitive strategy training. *Journal of Learning Disabilities, 19,* 66–70.

Ellis, E.S., & Lenz, B.K. (1987). *A component analysis of effective learning strategies for LD students.* Unpublished manuscript. Columbia, South Carolina: University of South Carolina, College of Education.

Ellis, N.R. (Ed.) (1979). *Handbook of mental deficiency: Psychological theory and research.* Hillsdale, NJ: Erlbaum & Associates.

Emmerich, H.J., & Ackerman, B.P. (1978). Developmental differences in recall: Encoding or retrieval? *Journal of Experimental Child Psychology, 25,* 514–525.

Engle, R.W., & Marshall, K. (1983). Do developmental changes in digit span result from acquisition strategies? *Journal of Experimental Child Psychology, 36,* 429–436.

Entwisle, N.J., & Ramsden, P. (1983). *Understanding student learning.* New York: Nichols Publishing Co.

Epstein, W., Glenberg, A.M., & Bradley, M. (1984). Coactivation and comprehension: Contributions of text variables to the illusion of knowing. *Memory & Cognition, 12,* 355–360.

Ericsson, K.A., & Simon, H.A. (1980). Verbal reports as data. *Psychological Review, 87,* 215–251.

Ericsson, K.A., & Simon, H.A. (1983). *Verbal protocol analysis.* Cambridge, MA: MIT Press.

Ericsson, K.A., & Simon, H.A. (1984). *Protocol analysis: Verbal reports as data.* Cambridge, MA: MIT Press.

Estes, T.H., & Vaughan, J.L. (1973). Reading interest and comprehension: Implications. *The Reading Teacher, 27,* 149–153.

Ewert, O.M., & Schumann, R. (1983). Entwicklungspsychologische Voraussetzungen von Benennungsflexibilität. *Zeitschrift für Entwicklungspsychologie und Pädagogische Psychologie, 15,* 121–138.

Eysenck, M.W. (1979). Anxiety, learning, and memory: A reconceptualization. *Journal of Research in Personality, 13,* 363–385.

Fabricius, W.V., & Hagen, J.W. (1984). The use of causal attributions about recall performance to assess metamemory and predict strategic memory behavior in young children. *Developmental Psychology, 20,* 975–987.

Fabricius, W.V., & Wellman, H.M. (1983). Children's understanding of retrieval cue utilization. *Developmental Psychology, 19,* 15–21.

Fagan, J.F. (1984). Infant memory: History, current trends, relations to cognitive psychology. In M. Moscovitch (Ed.), *Infant memory: Its relation to normal and pathological memory in humans and other animals* (pp. 1–27). New York: Plenum Press.

Fechner, B. (1965). Zur Psychologie des Gedächtnisses III: Zur Gruppenbildung sinnvoller sprachlicher Texte in Abhängigkeit vom Alter. *Zeitschrift für Psychologie, 80,* 2–21.

Ferrara, R.A., Brown, A.L., & Campione, J.C. (1986). Children's learning and transfer of inductive reasoning rules: Studies of proximal development. *Child Development, 57,* 1087–1099.

Feuerstein, R. (1980). *Instrumental enrichment: An intervention program for cognitive modifiability.* Baltimore, MD: University Park Press.

Finkenbinder, E.O. (1913). The curve of forgetting. *American Journal of Psychology, 24,* 8–32.

Fischer, K.W. (1980). A theory of cognitive development: The control and construction of hierarchies of skills. *Psychological Review, 87,* 477–531.

Fischer, P.M., & Mandl, H. (1981). Selbstdiagnostische und selbstregulative Aspekte der Verarbeitung von Studientexten: Eine kritische Übersicht über Ansätze zur Förderung und Beeinflussung von Lernstrategien. In H. Mandl (Ed.), *Zur Psychologie der Textverarbeitung* (pp. 389–477). München: Urban & Schwarzenberg.

Fischer, P.M., & Mandl, H. (1982). Metacognitive regulation of text processing: Aspects and problems concerning the relation between self-statements and actual performance. In A. Flammer & W. Kintsch (Eds.), *Discourse processing* (pp. 339–351). Amsterdam: North-Holland.

Fivush, R., Hudson, J., Nelson, K. (1984). Children's long-term memory for a novel event: An exploratory study. *Merrill-Palmer Quarterly, 30,* 303–316.

Fivush, R., & Mandler, J.M. (1985). Developmental changes in the understanding of temporal sequences. *Child Development, 56,* 1437–1446.

Flammer, A., & Lüthi, R. (in press). Strategies in selective recall. In F.E. Weinert & M. Perlmutter (Eds.), *Memory development: Universal changes and individual differences.* Hillsdale, NJ: Erlbaum & Associates.

Flavell, J.H. (1963). *The developmental psychology of Jean Piaget.* Princeton, NJ: Van Nostrand.

Flavell, J.H. (1970). Developmental studies of mediated memory. In H.W. Reese & L.P. Lipsitt (Eds.), *Advances in child development and behavior* (pp. 181–211). New York: Academic Press.

Flavell, J.H. (1971). First discussant's comments: What is memory development the development of? *Human Development, 14,* 272–278.

Flavell, J.H. (1976). Metacognitive aspects of problem solving. In L.B. Resnick (Ed.), *The nature of intelligence.* Hillsdale, NJ: Erlbaum & Associates.

Flavell, J.H. (1977). *Cognitive development.* Englewood Cliffs, NJ: Prentice-Hall.

Flavell, J.H. (1978). Metacognitive development. In J.M. Scandura & C.J. Brainerd (Eds.), *Structural/process theories of complex human behavior* (pp. 213–247). Alphen a. d. Rijn: Sijthoff & Noordhoff.

Flavell, J.H. (1979). Metacognition and cognitive monitoring. A new area of cognitive-developmental inquiry. *American Psychologist, 34,* 906–911.

Flavell, J.H. (1981). Cognitive monitoring. In P. Dickson (Ed.), *Children's oral communication skills* (pp. 35–60). New York: Academic Press.

Flavell, J.H. (1984). Annahmen zum Begriff Metakognition sowie zur Entwicklung von Metakognition. In F.E. Weinert & R.H. Kluwe (Eds.), *Metakognition, Motivation und Lernen* (pp. 223–231). Stuttgart: Kohlhammer.

Flavell, J.H. (1985). *Cognitive development (2nd edition).* Englewood Cliffs, NJ: Prentice-Hall.

Flavell, J.H., Beach, D.H., & Chinsky, J.M. (1966). Spontaneous verbal rehearsal in a memory task as a function of age. *Child Development, 37,* 283–299.

Flavell, J.H., Friedrichs, A.G., & Hoyt, J.D. (1970). Developmental changes in memorization processes. *Cognitive Psychology, 1*, 324–340.

Flavell, J.H., Speer, J.R., Green, F.L., & August, D.L. (1981). The development of comprehension monitoring and knowledge about communication. *Monographs of the Society for Research in Child Development, 46* (5, Ser. No. 192).

Flavell, J.H., & Wellman, H.M. (1977). Metamemory. In R.V. Kail & J.W. Hagen (Eds.), *Perspectives on the development of memory and cognition* (pp. 3–33). Hillsdale, NJ: Erlbaum & Associates.

Forrest-Pressley, D.L., & Waller, T. (1984). *Cognition, metacognition and reading.* New York: Springer.

Forrest-Pressley, D.L., MacKinnon, G.E., & Waller, T.G. (1985a). *Cognition, metacognition, and human performance* (Vol. 1). New York: Academic Press.

Forrest-Pressley, D.L., MacKinnon, G.E., & Waller, T.G. (1985b). *Cognition, metacognition, and human performance* (Vol. 2). New York: Academic Press.

Fowler, J.W., & Peterson, P.L. (1981). Increasing reading persistence and altering attributional style of learned helpless children. *Journal of Educational Psychology, 73*, 251–260.

Frank, H.S., & Rabinovitch, M.S. (1974). Auditory short-term memory: Developmental changes in rehearsal. *Child Development, 45*, 397–407.

Frankel, M.T., Hagan, B.J., & Rollins, H.A. (1984). *Training young children to organize free-recall: Associative and categorical approaches.* Paper presented at the Southeastern Conference on Human Development, Athens, GA.

Frankel, M.T., & Rollins, H.A. (1982). Age-related differences in clustering: A new approach. *Journal of Experimental Child Psychology, 34*, 113–122.

Frankel, M.T., & Rollins, H.A. (1985). Associative and categorical hypotheses of organization in the free recall of adults and children. *Journal of Experimental Child Psychology, 40*, 304–318.

Frederiksen, N. (1984). Implications of cognitive theory for instruction in problem solving. *Review of Educational Research, 54*, 363–408.

Fricke, R., & Treinies, G. (1985). *Einführung in die Metaanalyse.* Bern/Stuttgart: Huber.

Gagné, E.D. (1985). *The cognitive psychology of school learning.* Boston: Little, Brown, & Co.

Gagné, R.M. (1977). *The conditions of learning* (3rd edition). New York: Holt, Rinehart, and Winston.

Galbraith, R.C., Olsen, S.F., Duerden, D.S., & Harris, W.L. (1982). The differentiation hypothesis: Distinguishing between perceiving and memorizing. *American Journal of Psychology, 95*, 655–667.

Garner, R. (1987). *Metacognition and reading comprehension.* Norwood, NJ: Ablex.

Garner, R., & Anderson, J. (1982). Monitoring-of-understanding research: Inquiry directions, methodological dilemmas. *Journal of Experimental Education, 50*, 70–76.

Garrison, A. (1980). Categorical and spatial modes of representation in young children's recall. *Journal of Experimental Child Psychology, 30*, 383–388.

Gehringer, M., & Strube, G. (1985). *Organization and recall of life events: What's special in autobiographical memory?* Unpublished Paper, Max Planck Institute for Psychological Research, Munich.

Geis, M.F., & Hall, D.M. (1976). Encoding and incidental memory in children. *Journal of Experimental Child Psychology, 22*, 58–66.

Geis, M.F., & Hall, D.M. (1978). Encoding and congruity in children's incidental memory. *Child Development, 49*, 857–861.

Geis, M.F., & Lange, G. (1976). Children's cue utilization in a memory-for-location task. *Child Development, 47*, 759–766.

Geiselman, R.E., Woodward, J.A., & Beatty, J. (1982). Individual differences in verbal memory performance: A test of alternative information-processing models. *Journal of Experimental Psychology, 111*, 109–134.

Gelman, R. (1978). Cognitive development. *Annual Review of Psychology, 29*, 297–332.

Gelzheiser, L.M. (1984). Generalization from categorical memory tasks to prose by learning disabled adolescents. *Journal of Educational Psychology, 76*, 1128–1138.

Ghatala, E.S. (1984). Developmental changes in incidental memory as a function of meaningfulness and encoding condition. *Developmental Psychology, 20*, 208–211.

Ghatala, E.S., Blanks, P., Pressley, M., & Levin, J.R. (1987). *Children's regulation of reading time on a reading task.* Manuscript in preparation.

Ghatala, E.S., & Levin, J.R. (1981). Children's incidental memory for pictures: Item processing versus list organization. *Journal of Experimental Child Psychology, 31*, 231–244.

Ghatala, E.S., & Levin, J.R. (1982). Orienting versus learning instructions in children's free recall: New evidence. *Journal of Experimental Child Psychology, 33*, 504–513.

Ghatala, E.S., Levin, J.R., Foorman, B., & Pressley, M. (in press). Improving children's regulation of their reading PREP time. *Contemporary Educational Psychology.*

Ghatala, E.S., Levin, J.R., Pressley, M., & Goodwin, D. (1986). A componential analysis of the effects of derived and supplied strategy-utility information on children's strategy selection. *Journal of Experimental Child Psychology, 41*, 76–92.

Ghatala, E.S., Levin, J.R., Pressley, M., & Lodico, M.G. (1985). Training cognitive strategy monitoring in children. *American Educational Research Journal, 22*, 199–216.

Gibson, E.J. (1969). *Principles of perceptual learning and development.* New York: Appleton-Century-Crofts.

Gick, M.L., & Holyoak, K.J. (1980). Analogical problem solving. *Cognitive Psychology, 12*, 306–355.

Gick, M.L., & Holyoak, K.J. (1983). Schema induction and analogical transfer. *Cognitive Psychology, 15*, 1–38.

Glaser, R. (1985). Learning and instruction: A letter for a time capsule. In S.F. Chipman, J.W. Segal, & R. Glaser (Eds.), *Thinking and learning skills, Vol. 2, Research and open questions* (pp. 609–618). Hillsdale, NJ: Erlbaum & Associates.

Glass, G.V. (1978). Integrating findings: The meta-analysis of research. In L.V. Hedges & I. Olkin (Eds.), *Review of research in education* (Vol. 5, pp. 351–379). Ithasca, IL: Plecock.

Glass, G.V., McGaw, B., & Smith, M.L. (1981). *Meta-analysis in social research.* Beverly Hills, CA: Sage.

Glenberg, A.M., & Epstein, W. (1985). Calibration of comprehension. *Journal of Experimental Psychology: Learning, Memory, and Cognition, 11*, 702–718.

Glenberg, A.M., & Epstein, W. (1987). Inexpert calibration of comprehension. *Memory & Cognition, 15*, 84–93.

Glenberg, A.M., Sanocki, T., Epstein, W., & Morris, C. (1986). *Enhancing calibration.* Program Report 86-14. Madison, WI: University of Wisconsin, Wisconsin Center for Education Research.

Glenberg, A.M., Wilkinson, A.C., & Epstein, W. (1982). The illusion of knowing: Failure in the self-assessment of comprehension. *Memory & Cognition, 10*, 597–602.

Globerson, T. (1983). Mental capacity and cognitive functioning: Developmental and social class differences. *Developmental Psychology, 2*, 225–230.

Goodman, C., & Gardiner, J.M. (1981). How well do children remember what they have recalled? *British Journal of Educational Psychology, 51,* 97–101.

Gordon, F.R., & Flavell, J.H. (1977). The development of intuitions about cognitive cueing. *Child Development, 48,* 1027–1033.

Goulet, L.R. (1968). Verbal learning in children: Implications for developmental research. *Psychological Bulletin, 5,* 359–376.

Graesser, A.C., & Nakamura, G.V. (1982). The impact of a schema on comprehension and memory. In G.H. Bower (Ed.), *The psychology of learning and motivation: Advances in research and theory* (Vol. 16). New York: Academic Press.

Greenfield, D.B., & Scott, M.S. (1985). A cognitive approach to preschool screening. *Learning Disabilities Research, 1,* 42–49.

Greeno, J.G. (1968). Identifiability and statistical properties of two-stage learning with no successes in the initial stage. *Psychometrika, 33,* 173–216.

Greeno, J.G. (1970). How associations are memorized. In D.A. Norman (Ed.), *Models of human memory* (pp. 261–284). New York: Academic Press.

Greeno, J.G., James, C.T., Da Polito, F.J., & Polson, P.G. (1978). *Associative learning: A cognitive analysis.* Englewood Cliffs, NJ: Prentice-Hall.

Groeben, N. (1982). *Leserpsychologie: Textverständnis—Textverständlichkeit.* Münster: Aschendorff.

Gruenenfelder, T.M., & Borkowski, J.G. (1975). Transfer of cumulative-rehearsal strategies in children's short-term memory. *Child Development, 46,* 1019–1024.

Guttentag, R.E. (1984). The mental effort requirement of cumulative rehearsal: A developmental study. *Journal of Experimental Child Psychology, 37,* 92–106.

Guttentag, R.E. (1985). Memory and aging: Implications for theories of memory development during childhood. *Developmental Review, 5,* 56–82.

Guttentag, R.E., Ornstein, P.A., Siemens, L. (1987). Children's spontaneous rehearsal: Transitions in strategy acquisition. *Cognitive Development, 2,* 307–326.

Guttmann, J., Levin, J.R., & Pressley, M. (1977). Pictures, partial pictures, and young children's oral prose learning. *Journal of Educational Psychology, 69,* 473–480.

Haake, R.J., Somerville, S.C., & Wellman, H.M. (1980). Logical ability of young children in searching a large-scale environment. *Child Development, 51,* 1299–1302.

Hagen, J.W. (1971). Some thoughts on how children learn to remember. *Human Development, 14,* 262–271.

Hagen, J.W. (1975). Commentary. *Monographs of the Society for Research in Child Development, 40* (Serial No. 159).

Hagen, J.W., Hargrave, S., & Ross, W. (1973). Prompting and rehearsal in short-term memory. *Child Development, 44,* 201–204.

Hagen, J.W., Jongeward, R.H., & Kail, R.V. (1975). Cognitive perspectives on the development of memory. In H.W. Reese (Ed.), *Advances in child development and behavior* (Vol. 10, pp. 57–101). New York, San Francisco, London: Academic Press.

Hagen, J.W., & Kail, R.V. (1973). Facilitation and distraction in short-term memory. *Child Development, 44,* 831–836.

Hagen, J.W., & Kingsley, P.R. (1968). Labeling effects in short-term memory. *Child Development, 39,* 113–121.

Hagen, J.W., & Stanovich, K.G. (1977). Memory: Strategies of acquisition. In R.V. Kail & J.W. Hagen (Eds.), *Perspectives on the development of memory and cognition.* Hillsdale, NJ: Erlbaum & Associates.

Hall, J.W., Murphy, J., Humphreys, M.S., & Wilson, K.P. (1979). Children's cued recall: Developmental differences in retrieval operations. *Journal of Experimental Child Psychology, 27,* 501–511.

Halperin, M.S. (1974). Developmental changes in the recall and recognition of categorized word lists. *Child Development, 45,* 144–151.

Hansen, J., & Pearson, P.D. (1983). An instructional study: Improving the inferential comprehension of good and poor fourth-grade readers. *Journal of Educational Psychology, 75,* 821–829.

Harris, G.J., & Burke, D. (1972). The effects of grouping on short-term serial recall of digits by children: Developmental trends. *Child Development, 43,* 710–716.

Harris, P.L. (1984). Commentary: Landmarks and movement. In C. Sophian (Ed.), *Origins of cognitive skills* (pp. 113–128). Hillsdale, NJ: Erlbaum & Associates.

Hart, J.T. (1965). Memory and the feeling of knowing experience. *Journal of Educational Psychology, 56,* 208–216.

Hasher, L., & Clifton, D. (1974). A developmental study of attribute encoding in free recall. *Journal of Experimental Child Psychology, 17,* 332–346.

Hasher, L., & Zacks, R.T. (1979). Automatic and effortful processes in memory. *Journal of Experimental Psychology: General, 108,* 356–388.

Hasselhorn, M. (1986). *Differentielle Bedingungsanalyse verbaler Gedächtnisleistungen bei Schulkindern.* Frankfurt a. Main: Peter Lang.

Hasselhorn, M. (1987). Lern- und Gedächtnisförderung bei Kindern: Ein systematischer Überblick über die experimentelle Trainingsforschung. *Zeitschrift für Entwicklungspsychologie und Pägdagogische Psychologie, 19,* 116–142.

Hasselhorn, M., Hager, W., & Möller, H. (1986). *Metacognitive and motivational components in the prediction of one's own memory performance: A closer look at an often used paradigm.* Unpublished Paper, University of Göttingen, Göttingen, FRG.

Hasselhorn, M., & Körkel, J. (1986). Metacognitive versus traditional reading instructions: The mediating role of domain-specific knowledge on children's text-processing. *Human Learning, 5,* 75–90.

Hatano, G. (1982). Cognitive consequences of practice in cultural specific procedural skills. *Newsletter of the Laboratory of Comparative Human Cognition, 4,* 15–18.

Hayes, J.R., & Simon, H.A. (1977). Psychological differences among problem isomorphs. In N.J. Castellan, Jr., D.P. Pisoni, & G.R. Potts (Eds.), *Cognitive theory* (Vol. 2). Hillsdale, NJ: Erlbaum & Associates.

Haynes, C.R., & Kulhavy, R.W. (1976). Conservation level and category clustering. *Developmental Psychology, 12,* 179–184.

Heckhausen, H. (1977). Achievement motivation and its constructs: A cognitive model. *Motivation and Emotion, 1,* 283–329.

Heckhausen, H. (1982). The development of achievement motivation. In W.W. Hartup (Ed.), *Review of child development research* (Vol. 6, pp. 600–668). Chicago: University of Chicago Press.

Hedges, L.V., & Olkin, I. (1985). *Statistical methods for meta-analysis.* Orlando, FL: Academic Press.

Heller, M.S., Gädike, A.K., & Weinläder, H. (1976). *Kognitiver Fähigkeitstest für 4. bis 13. Klassen (KFT 4-13).* Weinheim: Beltz.

Helmke, A., Schneider, W., & Weinert, F.E. (1986). Quality of instruction and classroom learning outcomes: The German contribution to the IEA classroom environment study. *Teaching and Teacher Education, 2,* 1–18.

Herrmann, D.J. (1982). Know thy memory: The use of questionnaires to assess and study memory. *Psychological Bulletin, 92,* 434–452.

Herrmann, D.J. (1984). Questionnaires about memory. In J.E. Harris & P.E. Morris (Eds.), *Everyday memory, actions and absent-mindedness* (pp. 133–151). London: Academic Press.

Herrmann, D.J., Grubs, L., Sigmundi, R.A., & Grueneich, R. (1986). Awareness of memory ability before and after relevant memory experience. *Human Learning*, *5*, 91–108.

Herrmann, T. (1982). Über begriffliche Schwächen kognitivistischer Kognitionstheorien: Begriffsinflation und Akteur-System-Kontamination. *Sprache und Kognition*, *1*, 3–14.

Higbee, K.L. (1977). *Your memory: How it works and how to improve it.* Englewood Cliffs, NJ: Prentice-Hall.

Higbee, K.L. (1987). Process mnemonics: Principles, prospects, and problems. In M.A. McDaniel & M. Pressley (Eds.), *Imagery and related mnemonic processes: Theories, individual differences, and applications* (pp. 407–427). New York: Springer.

Hilgard, E.R. (1951). Methods and procedures in the study of learning. In S.S. Stevens (Ed.), *Handbook of experimental psychology* (pp. 517–567). New York: Wiley.

Hinde, R.A., Perret-Clermont, A.-N., & Stevenson-Hinde, J. (1985). *Social relationships and cognitive development.* Oxford, England: Oxford University Press.

Holt, J.H. (1964). *How children fail.* New York: Dell.

Hoppe-Graff, S. (1984). Verstehen als kognitiver Prozeß. Psychologische Ansätze und Beiträge zum Textverstehen. *Zeitschrift für Literaturwissenschaft und Linguistik*, *55*, 10–37.

Hoppe-Graff, S., & Schöler, H. (1980). *Wie gut verstehen und behalten Kinder einfache Geschichten?* In Arbeiten der Forschungsgruppe Sprache und Kognition, Ber. Nr. 17 (Ed.), Mannheim: Universität Mannheim.

Hoppe-Graff, S., Schöler, H. (1981). Was sollen und was können Geschichtengrammatiken leisten? In H. Mandl (Ed.), *Zur Psychologie der Textverarbeitung* (pp. 307–333). München: Urban & Schwarzenberg.

Horn, H., & Myers, N.A. (1978). Memory for location and picture cues at ages two and three. *Child Development*, *49*, 845–856.

Howe, M.L. (1985). Storage and retrieval of associative clusters: A stage-of-learning analysis of associative memory traces. *Canadian Journal of Psychology*, *39*, 34–53.

Howe, M.L., Brainerd, C.J., & Kingma, J. (1985a). Development of organization in recall: A stages-of-learning analysis. *Journal of Experimental Child Psychology*, *39*, 230–251.

Howe, M.L., Brainerd, C.J., & Kingma, J. (1985b). Storage-retrieval processes of normal and learning-disabled children. A stage-of-learning analysis of picture-word effects. *Child Development*, *56*, 1120–1133.

Hudson, J., & Fivush, R. (1983). Categorical and schematic organization and the development of retrieval strategies. *Journal of Experimental Child Psychology*, *36*, 32–42.

Hudson, J., & Nelson, K. (1983). Effects of script structure on children's story recall. *Developmental Psychology*, *19*, 625–635.

Hunter, J.E., Schmidt, F.L., & Jackson, G.B. (1982). *Meta-analysis: Cumulating research findings across studies.* Beverly Hills, CA: Sage.

Hunter, W.S. (1917). The delayed reaction in a child. *Psychological Review*, *24*, 75–87.

Hunter-Blanks, P., Ghatala, E.S., Pressley, M., & Levin, J.R. (in press). A comparison of monitoring during study and during testing on a sentence-learning task. *Journal of Educational Psychology*.

Hurlock, E.B., & Schwartz, R. (1932). Biographical records of memory in preschool children. *Child Development*, *3*, 230–239.

Huttenlocher, J., & Burke, D. (1976). Why does memory span increase with age? *Cognitive Psychology*, *8*, 1–31.

Inhelder, B. (1969). Memory and intelligence in the child. In D. Elkind & J. Flavell (Eds.), *Studies in cognitive development* (pp. 335–364). New York: Oxford University Press.

Istomina, Z.M. (1977). The development of voluntary memory in preschool-age children. *Soviet Psychology*, *13*, 5–64.

Jablonski, E.M. (1974). Free recall in children. *Psychological Bulletin, 81*, 522–539.

Jacobs, J. (1887). Experiments on "Prehension." *Mind, 12*, 75–79.

Jacobs, J.E., & Paris, S.G. (1987). Children's metacognition about reading: Issues in definition measurement, and instruction. *Educational Psychologist, 22*, 255–278.

Jacoby, L.L., & Craik, F.I.M. (1979). Effects of elaboration of processing at encoding and retrieval: Trace distinctiveness and recovery of initial context. In L. Cermak & F.I.M. Craik (Eds.), *Levels of processing and human memory* (pp. 1–21). Hillsdale, NJ: Erlbaum & Associates.

James, W. (1890). *The principles of psychology* (Vol. 1). New York: Holt.

Jenkins, J.J. (1971). Second discussant's comments: What's left to say? *Human Development, 14*, 279–286.

Jenkins, J.J. (1974). Remember that old theory of memory? Well, forget it! *American Psychologist, 29*, 785–795.

Jenkins, J.J. (1979). Four points to remember: A tetrahedral model of memory experiments. In L.S. Cermak & F.I.M. Craik (Eds.), *Levels of processing in human memory* (pp. 429–446). Hillsdale, NJ: Erlbaum & Associates.

Jensen, A.R., & Rohwer, W.D. (1965). Syntactical mediation of serial and paired-associate learning as a function of age. *Child Development, 36*, 601–608.

Johnson, C.N., & Wellman, H.M. (1980). Children's developing understanding of mental verbs: "Remember," "know," and "guess." *Child Development, 51*, 1095–1102.

Johnson, N.S., & Mandler, J.M. (1980). A tale of two structures: Underlying surface forms in stories. *Poetics, 9*, 51–86.

Johnson, R.E. (1970). Recall of prose as a function of the structural importance of the linguistic units. *Journal of Verbal Learning and Verbal Behavior, 9*, 12–20.

Jöreskog, K.G., & Sörbom, D. (1984). *LISREL VI – Analysis of linear structural relationships by maximum likelihood instrumental variables, and least squares methods. (Users Guide).* Mooresville: Scientific Software.

Justice, E.M. (1985). Categorization as a preferred memory strategy: Developmental changes during elementary school. *Developmental Psychology, 21*, 1105–1110.

Justice, E.M. (1986). Developmental changes in judgments of relative strategy effectiveness. *British Journal of Developmental Psychology, 4*, 75–81.

Justice, E.M., & Bray, N.W. (1979). *The effects of context and feedback on metamemory in young children.* Unpublished manuscript, Old Dominion University, Norfolk, VA.

Kagan, J., & Klein, R.E. (1973). Cross-cultural perspectives on early development. *American Psychologist, 28*, 947–961.

Kagan, J., Klein, R.E., Finley, G.E., Rogoff, B., & Nolan, E. (1979). A cross-cultural study of cognitive development. *Monographs of the Society for Research in Child Development, 44*.

Kahnemann, D. (1973). *Attention and effort.* Englewood Cliffs, NJ: Prentice-Hall.

Kail, R.V. (1979). Use of strategies and individual differences in children's memory. *Developmental Psychology, 15*, 251–255.

Kail, R.V. (1984). *The development of memory in children (2nd ed.).* New York: Freeman.

Kail, R.V., & Hagen, J.W. (1977a). Preface. In R.V. Kail & J.W. Hagen (Eds.), *Perspectives on the development and cognition* (pp. xi–xiii). Hillsdale, NJ: Erlbaum & Associates.

Kail, R.V., & Hagen, J.W. (1977b). *Perspectives on the development of memory and cognition.* Hillsdale, NJ: Erlbaum & Associates.

Kail, R.V., & Hagen, J.W. (1982). Memory in childhood. In B.B. Wolman (Ed.), *Handbook of developmental psychology* (pp. 350–366). Englewood Cliffs, NJ: Prentice-Hall.

Kail, R.V., & Strauss, M.S. (1984). The development of human memory: An historical overview. In R. Kail & N.E. Spear (Eds.), *Comparative perspectives on the development of memory* (pp. 3–22). Hillsdale, NJ: Erlbaum & Associates.

Katz, A.N. (1987). Individual differences in the control of imagery processing: Knowing how, knowing when, and knowing self. In M. Pressley & J.R. Levin (Eds.), *Cognitive strategy research: Educational applications* (pp. 177–203). New York: Springer.

Kearins, J.M. (1981). Visual spatial memory in Australian aboriginal children of desert regions. *Cognitive Psychology, 13,* 434–460.

Kearins, J.M. (1983). A quotient of awareness. *Education News, 18,* 18–22.

Keating, D.P., & Bobbitt, B.L. (1978). Individual and developmental differences in cognitive-processing components of mental ability. *Child Development, 49,* 155–167.

Kee, D.W., & Bell, T.S. (1981). The development of organizational strategies in the storage and retrieval of categorical items in free-recall learning. *Child Development, 52,* 1163–1171.

Kee, D.W., & Davies, L. (in press). Mental effort and elaboration. A developmental analysis. *Contemporary Educational Psychology.*

Keeney, F.J., Cannizzo, S.R., & Flavell, J.H. (1967). Spontaneous and induced verbal rehearsal in a recall task. *Child Development, 38,* 953–966.

Keil, F.C. (1981). Constraints on knowledge and cognitive development. *Psychological Review, 88,* 197–227.

Kellas, G., Ashcraft, M.H., & Johnson, N.S. (1973). Rehearsal processes in the short-term memory performance of mildly retarded adolescents. *American Journal of Mental Deficiency, 77,* 670–679.

Kelly, M., Scholnick, E.K., Travers, S.H., & Johnson, J.W. (1974). *The representation of meaning in memory.* Hillsdale, NJ: Erlbaum & Associates.

Kelly, M., Scholnick, E.K., Travers, S.H., & Johnson, J.W. (1976). Relations among memory, memory appraisal, and memory strategies. *Child Development, 47,* 648–659.

Kemler, D.G., & Jusczyk, P.W. (1975). A developmental study of facilitation by mnemonic instruction. *Journal of Experimental Child Psychology, 20,* 400–410.

Kemsies, F. (1900). Gedächtnisuntersuchungen an Schülern. *Zeitschrift für Pädagogische Psychologie und Pathologie, 2,* 84–95.

Kemsies, F. (1901). Gedächtnisuntersuchungen an Schülern. *Zeitschrift für pädagogische Psychologie und Pathologie, 3.*

Kendall, C.R., Borkowski, J.G., & Cavanaugh, J.C. (1980). Metamemory and the transfer of an interrogative strategy by EMR children. *Intelligence, 4,* 255–270.

Kendall, P.C., & Braswell, L. (1985). *Cognitive-behavioral therapy for impulsive children.* New York: The Guilford Press.

Keniston, A.H., & Flavell, J.H. (1979). A developmental study of intelligent retrieval. *Child Development, 50,* 1144–1152.

Kennedy, B.A., & Miller, D.J. (1976). Persistent use of verbal rehearsal as a function of information about its value. *Child Development, 47,* 566–569.

Kennedy, F. (1898). On the experimental investigation of memory. *Psychological Review, 5,* 477–499.

Kennedy, S.P., & Suzuki, N.S. (1977). Spontaneous elaboration in Mexican-American and Anglo-American high school seniors. *American Educational Research Journal, 14,* 383–388.

Keppel, G. (1964). Verbal learning in children. *Psychological Bulletin, 61,* 63–80.

Kesselring, M. (1911). Experimentelle Untersuchungen zur Theorie des Stundenplans. *Zeitschrift für Pädagogische Psychologie und Experimentelle Pädagogik, 12,* 314–324.

Kestner, J., & Borkowski, J.G. (1979). Children's maintenance and generalization of an inter-rogative learning strategy. *Child Development, 50*, 485–494.

King, J.F., Zechmeister, E.B., & Shaughnessy, J.J. (1980). Judgments of knowing: The influence of retrieval practice. *American Journal of Psychology, 93*, 329–343.

Kingsley, P.R., & Hagen, J.W. (1969). Induced versus spontaneous rehearsal in short-term memory in nursery school children. *Developmental Psychology, 1*, 40–46.

Kintsch, W. (1975). Memory representations of text. In R.L. Solso (Ed.), *Information processing and cognition* (pp. 269–294). Hillsdale, NJ: Erlbaum & Associates.

Kintsch, W. (1977). *Memory and cognition*. New York: Wiley.

Kintsch, W. (1982). *Gedächtnis und Kognition*. Berlin/Heidelberg/New York: Springer.

Kintsch, W., & Greene, E. (1978). The role of culture-specific schemata in the comprehension and recall of stories. *Discourse Processes, 1*, 1–13.

Kintsch, W., & van Dijk, T.A. (1978). Toward a model of text comprehension and production. *Psychological Review, 85*, 363–394.

Kirkpatrick, E.A. (1894). An experimental study of memory. *Psychological Review, 1*, 602–609.

Kleinfeld, J. (1971). Visual memory in village Eskimo and urban Caucasian children. *Arctic, 24*, 132–137.

Klix, F. (1984). *Gedächtnis, Wissen, Wissensnutzung*. Berlin: Verlag Deutscher Wissenschaften.

Kluwe, R.H. (1979). *Wissen und Denken*. Stuttgart: Kohlhammer.

Kluwe, R.H. (1980). *Metakognition: Komponenten einer Theorie zur Kontrolle und Steuerung eigenen Denkens*. Unveröffentliches Manuskript, Universität München.

Kluwe, R.H. (1981). Metakognition. In W. Michaelis (Ed.), *Bericht über den 32. Kongreß der Deutschen Gesellschaft für Psychologie* (pp. 246–258). Göttingen: Hogrefe.

Kluwe, R.H. (1982). Cognitive knowledge and executive control: Metacognition. In D. Griffin (Ed.), *Animal mind – human mind* (pp. 201–224). New York: Springer.

Kluwe, R.H., & Friedrichsen, G. (1984). Mechanisms of control and regulation in problem solving. In J. Kuhl & J. Beckmann (Eds.), *Action-control: From cognition to behavior* (pp. 183–218). New York: Springer.

Kluwe, R.H., & Schiebler, K. (1984). Entwicklung exekutiver Prozesse und kognitiver Leistungen. In F.E. Weinert & R.H. Kluwe (Eds.), *Metakognition, Motivation und Lernen* (pp. 31–60). Stuttgart: Kohlhammer.

Kluwe, R.H., & Spada, H. (1981). *Studien zur Denkentwicklung*. Bern/Stuttgart: Huber.

Knopf, M. (1986). *Metagedächtnis und Gedächtnis*. Unveröffentlichte Dissertation, Universität Heidelberg.

Knopf, M., Körkel, J., Schneider, W., & Weinert, F.E. (in press). Human memory as a faculty versus human memory as a set of specific abilities: Evidence from a life-span approach. In F.E. Weinert & M. Perlmutter (Eds.), *Memory development: Universal changes and individual differences*. Hillsdale, NJ: Erlbaum & Associates.

Knopf, M., & Waldmann, M.R. (1985). *Repräsentation von Alltagsereignissen und Gedächtnisentwicklung bei 4- und 6-jährigen*. Vortrag auf der 7. Tagung Entwicklungspsychologie, Trier.

Kobasigawa, A. (1974). Utilization of retrieval cues by children in recall. *Child Development, 45*, 127–134.

Kobasigawa, A. (1977). Retrieval strategies in the development of memory. In R.V. Kail & J.W. Hagen (Eds.), *Perspectives on the development of memory and cognition* (pp. 177–201). Hillsdale, NJ: Erlbaum & Associates.

Kobasigawa, A. (1983). Monitoring retrieval processes by children. *The Journal of Genetic Psychology, 142*, 259–269.

Kobasigawa, A., & Dufresne, A. (in press). Children's utilization of study time: Differential and sufficient aspects. In M. Pressley, G.E. Miller, & C.B. McCormick (Eds.), *Cognitive strategy research: Theoretical analyses and educational applications*. Berlin, New York: Springer.

Kobasigawa, A., & Middleton, D.B. (1972). Free recall of categorized items by children at three grade levels. *Child Development, 43*, 1067–1072.

Kobasigawa, A., & Orr, R. (1973). Free recall and retrieval speed of categorized items by kindergarten children. *Journal of Experimental Child Psychology, 15*, 187–192.

Koppenaal, R.J., Krull, A., & Katz, H. (1964). Age, interference and forgetting. *Journal of Experimental Child Psychology, 1*, 360–375.

Körkel, J., Schneider, W., Vogel, K., & Weinert, F.E. (1983). *Developmental changes in the metamemory-memory behavior relationship*. Poster presented at the 7th biennial meeting of the ISSBD, Munich.

Körkel, J. (1987). *Die Entwicklung von Gedächtnis- und Metagedächtnisleistungen in Abhängigkeit von bereichsspezifischen Vorkenntnissen*. Frankfurt a. Main: Lang.

Kosslyn, S.M. (1980). *Image and mind*. Cambridge, MA: Harvard University Press.

Kramer, J.J., & Engle, R. (1981). Teaching awareness of strategic behavior in combination with strategy training: Effects of children's memory. *Journal of Experimental Child Psychology, 32*, 513–530.

Kreutzer, M.A., Leonard, C., & Flavell, J.H. (1975). An interview study of children's knowledge about memory. *Monographs of the Society for Research in Child Development, 40* (1, Serial No. 159).

Kuhl, J. (1984). Volitional aspects of achievement motivation and learned helplessness. Toward a comprehensive theory of action control. In B.A. Maher (Ed.), *Progress in experimental personality research* (Vol. 13, pp. 100–171). Orlando, FL: Academic Press.

Kuhl, J. (1985). Volitional mediators of cognition-behavior consistency: Self-regulatory processes and action control versus state orientation. In J. Kuhl & J. Beckmann (Eds.), *Action control: From cognition to behavior* (pp. 101–128). New York: Springer.

Kuhl, J., & Schneider, W. (1987). *Emotional control in school children*. Unpublished manuscript, Max-Planck-Institute for Psychological Research, Munich, FRG.

Kun, A. (1977). Development of the magnitude-covariation and compensation schemata in ability and effort attributions of performance. *Child Development, 48*, 862–873.

Kunzinger, E.L. (1985). A short-term longitudinal study of memorial development during early grade school. *Developmental Psychology, 21*, 642–646.

Kunzinger, E.L., & Witryol, S.L. (1984). The effects of differential incentives on second-grade rehearsal and free recall. *The Journal of Genetic Psychology, 144*, 19–30.

Kurtz, B.E., & Borkowski, J.G. (1984). Children's metacognition: Exploring relations among knowledge, process, and motivational variables. *Journal of Experimental Child Psychology, 37*, 335–354.

Kurtz, B.E., & Borkowski, J.G. (1987). Developmental of strategic skills in impulsive and reflective children: A developmental study of metacognition. *Journal of Experimental Child Psychology, 43*, 129–148.

Kurtz, B.E., Reid, M.K., Borkowski, J.G., & Cavanaugh, J.C. (1982). On the reliability and validity of children's metamemory. *Bulletin of the Psychonomic Society, 19*, 137–140.

Kurtz, B.E., & Schneider, W. (in press). The effects of age, study time, and importance of text units on strategy use and memory for texts. *European Journal of the Psychology of Education*.

Kurtz, B.E., Schneider, W., Turner, L., & Carr, M. (1986). *Memory performance in German and American children: Differing roles of metacognitive and motivational variables.* Paper presented at the annual meeting of the American Educational Reearch Association, San Francisco.

Laboratory of Comparative Human Cognition (1979). Cross-cultural psychology's challenges to our ideas of children and development. *American Psychologist, 34,* 827–833.

Laboratory of Comparative Human Cognition (1983). Culture and cognitive development. In P.H. Mussen (Ed.), *Handbook of child psychology* (Vol. 1, pp. 295–356). New York: Wiley.

Lachman, J.L., & Lachman, R. (1979). Comprehension and cognition: A state of the art inquiry. In L.S. Cermak & F.I.M. Craik (Eds.), *Levels of processing in human memory* (pp. 183–209). Hillsdale, NJ: Erlbaum. & Associates.

Lachman, J.L., & Lachman, R. (1980). New directions in memory and aging. In L.W. Poon, J.L. Fozard, L.S., Cermak, D. Ahrenberg & L.W. Thompson (Eds.), *New directions in memory and aging* (pp. 545–550). Hillsdale, NJ: Erlbaum & Associates.

Lachman, J.L., Lachman, R., & Thronesbery, C. (1979). Metamemory through the adult life span. *Developmental Psychology, 15,* 543–551.

Lange, G. (1973). The development of conceptual and rote recall skills among school age children. *Journal of Experimental Child Psychology, 15,* 394–406.

Lange, G. (1978). Organization-related processes in children's recall. In P.A. Ornstein (Ed.), *Memory development in children* (pp. 101–128). Hillsdale, NJ: Erlbaum & Associates.

Lange, G., & Griffith, S.B. (1977). The locus of organization failures in children's recall. *Child Development, 48,* 1498–1502.

Lange, G., & Jackson, P. (1974). Personal organization in children's free recall. *Child Development, 45,* 1060–1067.

Laurence, M.W. (1966). Age differences in performance and subjective organization in the free-recall learning of pictorial material. *Canadian Journal of Psychology, 20,* 388–399.

Lawson, M.J., & Fuelop, S. (1980). Understanding the purpose of strategy training. *British Journal of Educational Psychology, 50,* 175–180.

Leal, L., Crays, N., & Moely, B.E. (1985). Training children to use a self-monitoring study strategy in preparation for recall: Maintenance and generalization effects. *Child Development, 56,* 643–653.

Ledger, G.W., & Ryan, E.B. (1985). Semantic integration: Effects of imagery, enaction, and sentence repetition training on prereaders' recall for pictograph sentences. *Journal of Experimental Child Psychology, 39,* 531–545.

Leontjev, A.N. (1931). *Development of memory.* Moscow: Uchpedgiz.

Leontjev, A.N. (1977). *Probleme der Entwicklung des Psychischen.* Kronberg, Ts.: Athenäum.

Levelt, W.J.M. (1974). *Formal grammars in linguistics and psycholinguistics* (Vol. 3). Den Haag: Mouton.

Levin, J.R. (1976). What have we learned about maximizing what children can learn? In J.R. Levin & V.L. Allen (Eds.), *Cognitive learning in children.* New York: Academic Press.

Levin, J.R. (1981a). The mnemonic '80s: Keywords in the classroom. *Educational Psychologist, 16,* 65–82.

Levin, J.R. (1981b). On functions of pictures in prose. In F.J. Pirozzolo & M.C. Wittrock (Eds.), *Neuropsychological and cognitive processes in reading* (pp. 203–228). New York: Academic Press.

Levin, J.R. (1982). Pictures as prose-learning devices. In A. Flammer & W. Kintsch (Eds.), *Discourse processing* (pp. 412–444). Amsterdam: North-Holland.

Levin, J.R. (1983). Pictorial strategies for school learning: Practical illustrations. In M. Pressley & J.R. Levin (Eds.), *Cognitive strategy research: Educational applications* (pp. 213–237). New York: Springer.

Levin, J.R. (1985a). Educational applications of mnemonic pictures: Possibilities beyond your wildest imagination. In A.A. Sheikh (Ed.), *Imagery in educational: Imagery in the educational process* (pp. 63–87). Farmingdale, NY: Baywood.

Levin, J.R. (1985b). Yodai features = mnemonic procedures: A commentary on Higbee and Kunihira. *Educational Psychologist, 20,* 73–76.

Levin, J.R., Bender, B.G., & Pressley, M. (1979). Pictures, imagery, and children's recall of central versus peripheral sentence information. *Educational Communication and Technology Journal, 27,* 89–95.

Levin, J.R., & Ghatala, E. (1982). Orienting versus learning instructions in children's free recall: New evidence. *Journal of Experimental Child Psychology, 33,* 504–513.

Levin, J.R., Johnson, D.D., Pittelman, S.D., Hayes, B.L., Levin, K.M., Shriberg, L.K., & Toms-Bronowski, S. (1984). A comparison of semantic- and mnemonic-based vocabulary-learning strategies. *Reading Psychology, 5,* 1–15.

Levin, J.R., McCabe, A.E., & Bender, B.G. (1975). A note on imagery-inducing motor activity in young children. *Child Development, 46,* 263–266.

Levin, J.R., McCormick, C.B., Miller, G.E., Berry, J.K., & Pressley, M. (1982). Mnemonic versus nonmnemonic vocabulary-learning strategies for children. *American Educational Research Journal, 19,* 121–136.

Levin, J.R., & Pressley, M. (1978). A test of the developmental imagery hypothesis in children's associative learning. *Journal of Educational Psychology, 70,* 691–694.

Levin, J.R., & Pressley, M. (1981). Improving children's prose comprehension: Selected strategies that seem to succeed. In C. Santa & E. Bittayes (Eds.), *Children's prose comprehension: Research and practice* (pp. 44–71). Newark, DE: International Reading Association.

Levin, J.R., Shriberg, L.K., Miller, G.E., McCormick, G.B., & Levin, B.B. (1980). The keyword method in the classroom: How to remember the states and their capitals. *Elementary School Journal, 80,* 185–191.

Levin, J.R., Yussen, S.R., De Rose, T.M., & Pressley, M. (1977). Developmental changes in assessing recall and recognition memory capacity. *Developmental Psychology, 13,* 608–615.

Liben, L.S. (1977). Memory in the context of cognitive development: The Piagetian approach. In R.V. Kail & J.W. Hagen (Eds.), *Perspectives on the development of memory and cognition* (pp. 297–331). Hillsdale, NJ: Erlbaum & Associates.

Liben, L.S. (1982). The developmental study of children's memory. In T.M. Field, A. Huston, H.C. Quay, L. Troll, & G.E. Finley (Eds.), *Review of human development* (pp. 269–284). New York: Wiley.

Liberty, C., & Ornstein, P.A. (1973). Age differences in organization and recall: The effects of training in categorization. *Journal of Experimental Child Psychology, 15,* 169–186.

Licht, B.G., & Kistner, J.A. (1986). Motivational problems of learning-disabled children: Individual differences and their implications for treatment. In J.K. Torgeson & B.Y.L. Wong (Eds.), *Psychological and educational perspectives on learning disabilities* (pp. 225–255). Orlando, FL: Academic Press.

Lindberg, M.A. (1980). Is knowledge base development a necessary and sufficient condition for memory development? *Journal of Experimental Child Psychology, 30,* 401–410.

Lipson, M.Y. (1982). Learning new information from text: The role of prior knowledge and reading ability. *Journal of Reading Behavior, 14,* 243–261.

List, J.A., Keating, D.P., Merriman, W.E. (1985). Differences in memory retrieval: A construct validity investigation. *Child Development, 56,* 138–151.

Lobsien, M. (1902a). Experimentelle Untersuchungen über die Gedächtnisentwicklung bei Schulkindern. *Zeitschrift für Psychologie und Physiologie der Sinnesorgane, 27,* 34–76.

Lobsien, M. (1902b). Memorieren. *Zeitschrift für Pädagogische Psychologie, Pathologie und Hygiene, 4*, 293–306.

Lobsien, M. (1911a). Zur Entwicklung des akustischen Wortgedächtnisses der Schüler. *Zeitschrift für Pädagogische Psychologie und Experimentelle Pädagogik, 12*, 238–245.

Lobsien, M. (1911b). Korrelationen zwischen Zahlengedächtnis und Rechenleistung. *Zeitschrift für Pädagogische Psychologie und Experimentelle Pädagogik, 12*, 54–60.

Lockhart, R.S. (1984). What do infants remember? In M. Moscovitch (Ed.), *Infant memory: Its relation to normal and pathological memory in humans and other animals* (pp. 131–143). New York: Plenum Press.

Lockhart, R.S., Craik, F.I.M., & Jacoby, L.L. (1976). Depth of processing, recognition and recall. In J. Brown (Ed.), *Recall and recognition*. New York: Wiley.

Lodico, M.G., & Ghatala, E.S., Levin, J.R., Pressley, M., & Bell, J.A. (1983). The effects of strategy-monitoring on children's selection of effective memory strategies. *Journal of Experimental Child Psychology, 35*, 263–277.

Logan, G.D. (1985). Skill and automaticity: Relations, implications, and future directions. *Canadian Journal of Psychology, 39*, 367–386.

Lohmöller, J.-B. (1984). *LVPLS program manual*. Köln: Zentralarchiv für Empirische Sozialforschung.

Loughlin, K.A., & Daehler, M.A. (1973). The effects of distraction and added perceptual cues on the delayed reaction of very young children. *Child Development, 44*, 384–388.

Lovelace, E.A. (1984). Metamemory: Monitoring future recallability. *Journal of Experimental Psychology: Learning, Memory, & Cognition, 10*, 756–766.

Lovelace, E.A., & Marsh, G.R. (1984). Metacomprehension of text material. *Journal of Gerontology, 40*, 192–197.

Lucariello, J., & Nelson, K. (1982). *Context of categories in young children's memory.* Paper presented at the Southeastern Conference on Development, Baltimore, MD.

Lucariello, J., & Nelson, K. (1985). Slot-filler categories as memory organizers for young children. *Developmental Psychology, 21*, 272–282.

Lyon, D.R. (1977). Individual differences in immediate serial recall: A matter of mnemonics? *Cognitive Psychology, 9*, 403–411.

Lyons, W. (1986). *The disappearance of introspection*. Cambridge, MA: MIT Press.

Maccoby, E.E. (1964). Developmental psychology. *Annual Review of Psychology, 15*, 203–250.

Maccoby, E.E., & Hagen, J.W. (1965). Effects of distraction upon central versus incidental recall: Developmental trends. *Journal of Experimental Child Psychology, 2*, 280–289.

Maki, R.H., & Berry, S.L. (1984). Metacomprehension of text material. *Journal of Experimental Psychology: Learning, Memory, & Cognition, 10*, 663–679.

Mandler, J.M. (1978). A code in the node: The use of a story scheme in retrieval. *Discourse Processes, 1*, 14–35.

Mandler, J.M. (1979). Categorical and schematic organization in memory. In C.R. Puff (Ed.), *Memory, organization, and structure* (pp. 259–299). New York: Academic Press.

Mandler, J.M. (1982). Recent research on story grammars. In J.-F. Le Ny & W. Kintsch (Eds.), *Language and comprehension* (pp. 207–218). Amsterdam: Alphen.

Mandler, J.M. (1983). Representation. In J.H. Flavell & E.M. Markman (Eds.), *Handbook of child psychology* (Vol. 3, pp. 420–493). New York: Wiley.

Mandler, J.M. (1984). *Stories, scripts and scenes: Aspects of schema theory.* Hillsdale, NJ: Lawrence Erlbaum & Associates.

Mandler, J.M. (1986). The development of event memory. In F. Klix & H. Hagendorf (Eds.), *Human memory and cognitive capabilities* (Vol. A, pp. 459–467). Amsterdam: Elsevier (North-Holland).

Mandler, J.M., & DeForest, M. (1979). Is there more than one way to recall a story? *Child Development*, *50*, 886–889.

Mandler, J.M., & Johnson, N.S. (1977). Remembrance of things passed: Story structure and recall. *Cognitive Psychology*, *9*, 111–151.

Mandler, J.M., Scribner, S., Cole, M., & De Forest, M. (1980). Cross-cultural invariance in story recall. *Child Development*, *51*, 19–26.

Markman, E.M. (1973). *Factors affecting the young child's ability to monitor his memory.* Unpublished doctoral dissertation, University of Pennsylvania, Philadelphia, PA.

Markman, E.M. (1977). Realizing that you don't understand: A preliminary investigation. *Child Development*, *48*, 986–992.

Markman, E.M. (1979). Realizing that you don't understand: Elementary school children's awareness of inconsistencies. *Child Development*, *50*, 643–655.

Markman, E.M. (1981). Comprehension monitoring. In W.P. Dickson (Ed.), *Children's oral communication skills* (pp. 61–84). New York: Academic Press.

Markman, E.M. (1984). An analysis of hierarchical classification. In R. Sternberg (Ed.), *Advances in the psychology of human intelligence* (pp. 325–366). Hillsdale, NJ: Erlbaum & Associates.

Markman, E.M. (1985). Comprehension monitoring: Developmental and educational issues. In S.F. Chipman, J.W. Segal, & R. Glaser (Eds.), *Thinking and learning skills, Vol. 2, Research and open questions* (pp. 275–292). Hillsdale, NJ: Erlbaum & Associates.

Markman, E.M., & Callahan, M. (1984). An analysis of hierarchical classification. In R. Sternberg (Ed.), *Advances in the psychology of human intelligence* (pp. 325–366). Hillsdale, NJ: Erlbaum & Associates.

Markman, E.M., Cox, B., & Machida, S. (1981). The standard object-sorting task as a measure of conceptual organization. *Developmental Psychology*, *17*, 115–117.

Markman, E.M., & Gorin, L. (1981). Children's ability to adjust their standards for evaluating comprehension. *Journal of Educational Psychology*, *73*, 320–325.

Markus, H., & Nurius, P. (1986). Possible selves. *American Psychologist*, *41*, 954–969.

Marshall, G.R., & Cofer, C.N. (1970). Single-word free-association norms for 328 responses from the Connecticut cultural norms for verbal items in categories. In L. Postman & G. Keppel (Eds.), *Norms of word association* (pp. 321–360). New York: Academic Press.

Mastropieri, M.A., Scruggs, T.E., & Levin, J.R. (1987). Mnemonic instruction in special education. In M.A. McDaniel & M. Pressley (Eds.), *Imagery and related mnemonic processes: Theories, individual differences, and applications* (pp. 358–376). New York: Springer.

Masur, E.F., McIntyre, C.W., & Flavell, J.H. (1973). Developmental changes in apportionment of study time among items in a multitrial free recall task. *Journal of Experimental Child Psychology*, *15*, 237–246.

McCarver, R.B. (1972). A developmental study of the effects of organizational cues on short-term memory. *Child Development*, *43*, 1317–1325.

McClure, E., Mason, J., & Barnitz, J. (1979). An exploratory study of story structure and age effects on children's ability to sequence stories. *Discourse Processes*, *2*, 213–249.

McCombs, B.L. (1986). *The role of the self-system in self-regulated learning.* Paper presented at the annual meeting of the American Educational Research Association, San Francisco.

McCombs, B.L. (1987). *The role of affective variables in autonomous learning.* Paper presented at the annual meeting of the American Educational Research Association, Washington, DC.

McCormick, C.B., & Levin, J.R. (1986). Manuscript in preparation (cited in McCormick & Levin, 1987).

McCormick, C.B., & Levin, J.R. (1987). Mneomonic prose-learning strategies. In M.A. McDaniel & M. Pressley (Eds.), *Imagery and related mnemonic processes: Theories, individual differences, and applications* (pp. 392–406). New York: Springer.

McGeoch, J.A., & Irion, A.L. (1952). *The psychology of human learning.* New York: Longmans, Green & Co.

McGivern, J., Levin, J.R., Pressley, M., & Ghatala, E.S. (1985). *A developmental study of memory monitoring and strategy use.* Paper presented at the annual meeting of the American Educational Research Association, Chicago.

Meacham, J.A. (1975). Patterns of memory abilities in two cultures. *Developmental Psychology, 11,* 50–63.

Meacham, J.A. (1977). Soviet investigations of memory development. In R.V. Kail & J.W. Hagen (Eds.), *Perspectives on the development of memory and cognition* (pp. 273–295). Hillsdale, NJ: Erlbaum & Associates.

Medway, F.M., & Venino, G.R. (1982). The effects of effort feedback and performance patterns on children's attribution and task persistence. *Contemporary Educational Psychology, 7,* 26–34.

Meichenbaum, D.M. (1977). *Cognitive behavior modification. An integrative approach.* New York: Plenum Press.

Meichenbaum, D., Burland, S., Gruson, L., & Cameron, R. (1985). Metacognitive assessment. In S. Yussen (Ed.), *The growth of reflection in children* (pp. 3–30). New York: Academic Press.

Melkman, R., & Deutsch, C. (1977). Memory functioning as related to developmental changes in bases of organization. *Journal of Experimental Child Psychology, 23,* 84–97.

Melkman, R., Tversky, B., & Baratz, D. (1981). Developmental trends in the use of perceptual and conceptual attributes in grouping, clustering, and retrieval. *Journal of Experimental Child Psychology, 31,* 470–486.

Merkel, S.P., & Hall, V.C. (1982). The relationship between memory for order and other cognitive tasks. *Intelligence, 6,* 437–441.

Mervis, C.B., & Rosch, E.M. (1981). The internal structure of basic and non-basic color categories. *Language, 57,* 384–405.

Messer, S.B. (1976). Reflection-impulsivity: A review. *Psychological Bulletin, 83,* 1026–1052.

Meumann, E. (1907a). Sechste Vorlesung: Entwicklung der einzelnen geistigen Fähigkeiten beim Kinde (Fortsetz.). *Vorlesungen zur Einführung in die Experimentelle Pädagogik (Bd. 1).* Leipzig: Wilhelm Engelmann.

Meumann, E. (1907b). Elfte Vorlesung: Die geistige Arbeit des Kindes. *Vorlesungen zur Einführung in die Experimentelle Pädagogik (Bd. 1 u.2).* Leipzig: Wilhelm Engelmann.

Meumann, E. (1912). Beobachtungen über differenzierte Einstellung bei Gedächtnisversuchen. *Zeitschrift für Pädagogische Psychologie, 13,* 456–463.

Milgram, N.A. (1967). Verbal context versus visual compound in paired-associate learning in children. *Journal of Experimental Child Psychology, 5,* 597–603.

Milgram, N.A. (1968). The effects of MA and IQ on verbal mediation in paired associate learning. *Journal of Genetic Psychology, 113,* 129–143.

Miller, C.A. (1956). The magical number seven, plus or minus two: Some limits on our capacity for processing information. *Psychological Review, 63,* 81–97.

Miller, G.E., & Pressley, M. (1987). Partial picture effects on children's memory for sentences containing implicit information. *Journal of Experimental Child Psychology, 43,* 300–310.

Mischel, W. (1981). Metacognition and the rules of delay. In J. Flavell & L. Ross (Eds.), *Cognitive social development: Frontiers and possible futures* (pp. 240–271). New York: Cambridge University Press.

Misciones, J.L., Marvin, R.S., O'Brien, R.G., & Greenburg, M.T. (1978). A developmenetal study of preschool children's understanding of the words "know" and "guess." *Child Development*, *48*, 1107–1113.

Mistry, J.J., & Lange, G.W. (1985). Children's organization and recall of information in scripted narratives. *Child Development*, *56*, 953–961.

Mitchell, J.V., Jr. (1983). *Tests in print III: An index to tests, test reviews, and the literature on specific tests.* Lincoln, Nebraska: University of Nebraska-Lincoln, The Buros Institute of Mental Measurements.

Möbus, C., & Schneider, W. (Eds.) (1986). *Strukturmodelle für Längsschnittdaten und Zeitreihen.* Bonn/Stuttgart: Hans Huber.

Moely, B.E. (1977). Organizational factors in the development of memory. In R.V. Kail & J.W. Hagen (Eds.), *Perspectives on the development of memory and cognition* (pp. 203–236). Hillsdale, NJ: Erlbaum & Associates.

Moely, B.E., Hart, S.S., Leal, L., Johnson-Baron, T., Santulli, K.A., & Rao, N. (1986). *An investigation of how teachers establish stable use and generalization of memory strategies through the use of effective training techniques.* Paper presented at the annual meetings of the American Educational Research Association, San Francisco.

Moely, B.E., Hart, S.S., Santulli, K., Leal, L., Johnson, T., Rao, N., & Burney, L. (1986). How do teachers teach memory skills? *Educational Psychologist*, *21*, 55–72.

Moely, B.E., & Jeffrey, W.E. (1974). The effects of organization training on children's free recall of category items. *Child Development*, *45*, 135–143.

Moely, B.E., Leal, L., Pechman, E., Johnson, T., Santulli, K., Rao, N., Hart, S., & Burney, L. (1986). *Relationships between teachers' cognitive instruction and children's memory skills.* Paper presented at the biennial meeting of the Southwestern Society for Research in Child Development, San Antonio, TX.

Moely, B.E., Olson, F.A., Halwes, T.G., & Flavell, J.H. (1969). Production deficiency in young children's clustered recall. *Developmental Psychology*, *1*, 26–34.

Monroe, E.K., & Lange, G. (1977). The accuracy with which children judge the composition of their free recall. *Child Development*, *48*, 381–387.

Moore, J.M., & Haith, M. (1979). *Executive processes during memory retrieval.* Paper presented at the biennial meeting of the Society for Research in Child Development, San Francisco.

Morrison, F.J., & Lord, C. (1982). Age differences in recall of categorized material: Organization or retrieval? *The Journal of Genetic Psychology*, *141*, 233–241.

Moscovitch, M. (Ed.) (1984). *Infant memory: Its relation to normal and pathological memory in humans and other animals.* New York: Plenum.

Moynahan, E.D. (1973). The development of knowledge concerning the effect of categorization upon free recall. *Child Development*, *44*, 238–246.

Moynahan, E.D. (1976). The development of the ability to assess recall performance. *Journal of Experimental Child Psychology*, *21*, 94–97.

Moynahan, E.D. (1978). Assessment and selection of paired associate strategies: A developmental study. *Journal of Experimental Child Psychology*, *26*, 257–266.

Müller, G.E., & Pilzecker, A. (1900). Experimentelle Beiträge zur Lehre vom Gedächtnis. *Ergänzungsband der Zeitschrift für Psychologie.*

Müller, G.E., & Schuhmann, F. (1894). Experimentalle Beiträge zur Untersuchung des Gedächtnisses. *Zeitschrift für Psychologie*, *6*, 89–121.

Munn, N.L. (1954). Learning in children. In P. Mussen (Ed.), *Carmichael's manual of child psychology (3rd edition)* (pp. 374–458). New York: Wiley.

Murphy, M.D. (1979). Measurement of category clustering in free recall. In C.R. Puff (Ed.), *Memory, organization, and structure* (pp. 51–83). New York: Academic Press.

Murphy, M.D., & Brown, A.L. (1975). Incidental learning in preschool children as a function of level of cognitive analysis. *Journal of Experimental Child Psychology, 19,* 509–523.

Murphy, M.D., & Puff, C.R. (1982). Free recall: Basic methodology and analyses. In C.R. Puff (Ed.), *Handbook of research methods in human memory and cognition* (pp. 99–128). New York: Academic Press.

Myers, M., & Paris, S.G. (1978). Children's metacognitive knowledge about reading. *Journal of Educational Psychology, 70,* 680–690.

Myers, N.A., & Perlmutter, M. (1978). Memory in the years from two to five. In P.A. Ornstein (Ed.), *Memory development in children* (pp. 191–218). Hillsdale, NJ: Erlbaum & Associates.

Nagy, L. (1930). Experimentelle Untersuchungen über die Entwicklung der Gedächtnis- und Denkformen der Knaben und Mädchen zwischen 7 - 19 Jahren. In H. Volkelt (Ed.), *Bericht über den 11. Kongreß für Experimentelle Psychologie in Wien vom 9.-13. April 1929* (pp. 113–122). Jena; Gustav Fischer.

Nakayama, S.Y., & Kee, D.W. (1980). Automatic encoding of superordinate and subordinate taxonomic categories in different populations. *Journal of Educational Psychology, 72,* 386–393.

Naus, M.J., & Halasz, F.G. (1979). Developmental perspectives on cognitive processing and semantic memory structure. In L.S. Cermak & F.I.M. Craik (Eds.), *Levels of processing in human memory* (pp. 259–288). Hillsdale, NJ: Erlbaum & Associates.

Naus, M.J., & Ornstein, P.A. (1983). Development of memory strategies: Analysis, questions, and issues. In M.T.H. Chi (Ed.), *Trends in memory development research* (Vol. 9, pp. 1–30). Basel: Karger.

Naus, M.J., Ornstein, P.A., & Aivano, S. (1977). Developmental changes in memory: The effects of processing time and rehearsal instructions. *Journal of Experimental Child Psychology, 23,* 237–251.

Naus, M.J., Ornstein, P.A., & Kreshtool, K. (1977). Developmental differences in recall and recognition: The relationship between rehearsal and memory as test expectation changes. *Journal of Experimental Child Psychology, 23,* 252–265.

Neimark, E.D. (1976). The natural history of spontaneous mnemonic activities under conditions of minimal experimental constraint. In A.D. Pick (Ed.), *Minnesota Symposia on Child Psychology* (pp. 84–118). Hillsdale, NJ: Erlbaum & Associates.

Neimark, E., Slotnick, N.S., & Ulrich, T. (1971). Development of memorization strategies. *Developmental Psychology, 5,* 427–432.

Nelson, K. (1978). How young children represent knowledge of their world in and out of language. In R. Siegler (Ed.), *Children's thinking: What develops?* (pp. 255–273). Hillsdale, NJ: Erlbaum & Associates.

Nelson, K., & Brown, A.L. (1978). The semantic-episodic distinction in memory development. In P.A. Ornstein (Ed.), *Memory development in children* (pp. 233–242). Hillsdale, NJ: Erlbaum & Associates.

Nelson, K., Fivush, R., Hudson, J., & Lucariello, J. (1983). Scripts and the development of memory. In M.T.H. Chi (Ed.), *Trends in memory development research* (pp. 52–70). Basel: Karger.

Nelson, K., & Gründel, J. (1981). Generalized event representations. Basic building blocks of cognitive development. In M.E. Lamb & A.L. Brown (Eds.), *Advances in developmental psychology* (Vol. 1, pp. 131–158). Hillsdale, NJ: Erlbaum & Associates.

Nelson, K., & Hudson, J. (in press). Scripts and memory: Functional relationship in development. In F.E. Weinert & M. Perlmutter (Eds.), *Memory development: Universal changes and individual differences.* Hillsdale, NJ: Erlbaum & Associates.

Nelson, K., & Ross, G. (1980). The generalities and specifics of long-term memory in infants and young children. In M. Perlmutter (Ed.), *New directions for child development: Children's memory* (pp. 87–101). San Francisco, Jossey-Bass.

Nelson, T.O. (1984). A comparison of current measures of the accuracy of feeling-of-knowing predictions. *Psychological Bulletin, 95,* 109–133.

Nelson, T.O., & Narens, L. (1980). Norms of 300 general-information questions: Accuracy of recall, latency of recall, and feeling-of-knowing ratings. *Journal of Verbal Learning and Behavior, 19,* 338–368.

Netschajeff, A. (1900). Experimentelle Untersuchungen über die Gedächtnisentwicklung bei Schulkindern. *Zeitschrift für Psychologie und Physiologie der Sinnesorgane, 24,* 322–351.

Netschajeff, A. (1902). Über Memorieren. *Sammlung von Abhandlungen aus dem Gebiete der Pädagogischen Psychologie und Physiologie, 5,* 293–329.

Neuringer, A. (1981). Self-experimentation: A cell for change. *Behaviorism, 9,* 79–94.

Newcombe, N., Rogoff, B., & Kagan, J. (1977). Developmental changes in recognition memory for pictures of objects and scenes. *Developmental Psychology, 13,* 337–341.

Nezworski, T. (1982). Story structure versus content in children's recall. *Journal of Verbal Learning and Verbal Behavior, 21,* 196–206.

Nicholls, J.G. (1978). The development of the concepts of effort and ability of academic attainment, and the understanding that difficult tasks require more ability. *Child Development, 49,* 800–814.

Nicholls, J.G. (in press). What is ability and why are we mindful of it? A developmental perspective. In J. Kolligian & R.J. Sternberg (Eds.), *Perspectives of competence across the lifespan.* New Haven, CT: Yale University Press.

Nicolson, R. (1981). The relationship between memory span and processing speed. In M.J. Friedman, J.P. Das, & N. O'Connor (Eds.), *Intelligence and learning* (pp. 179–183). New York: Plenum Press.

Nisbett, R.E., & Wilson, T.D. (1977). Telling more than we can know: Verbal reports on mental processes. *Psychological Review, 84,* 231–259.

Norman, D.A., & Bobrow, D.G. (1979). Descriptions: An intermediate stage in memory retrieval. *Cognitive Psychology, 11,* 107–123.

Norman, D.A., & Rumelhart, D.E. (1975). *Explorations in cognition.* San Francisco: Freeman.

O'Brien, E.J., & Myers, J.L. (1985). When comprehension difficulty improves memory for text. *Journal of Experimental Psychology: Learning, Memory, and Cognition, 11,* 12–21.

Oerter, R. (1985). Die Formung von Kognition und Motivation durch Schule: Wie Schule auf das Leben vorbereitet. *Unterrichtswissenschaft, 13,* 203–219.

Oerter, R., & Schuster-Oeltzschner, M. (1987). Gedächtnis und Wissen. In R. Oerter & L. Montada (Eds.), *Entwicklungspsychologie (2. Auflage)* (pp. 537–571). München: Urban & Schwarzenberg.

Offner, M. (1924). *Das Gedächtnis.* Berlin: Reuther & Reichard.

Oka, E.R., & Paris, S.G. (1987). Patterns of motivation and reading skills in underachieving children. In S.J. Ceci (Ed.), *Handbook of cognitive, social, and neuropsychological aspects of learning disabilities* (Vol. 2, pp. 115–146). Hillsdale, NJ: Erlbaum & Associates.

Olson, G.M., & Sherman, T. (1984). Learning and memory in infants. In J.R. Anderson & S.M. Kosslyn (Eds.), *Tutorials in learning and memory* (pp. 1–29). San Francisco: Freeman.

Olson, G.M., & Sherman, T. (1983). Attention, learning and memory in infants. In P.H. Mussen (Ed.), *Handbook of child psychology* (Vol. 2, pp. 1001–1080). New York: Wiley.

Olson, G.M., & Strauss, M.S. (1984). The development of infant memory. In M. Moscovitch (Ed.), *Infant memory* (pp. 29–48). New York: Plenum Press.

Omanson, R.C., Warren, W.H., & Trabasso, T. (1978). Goals, inferential comprehension, and recall of stories by children. *Discourse Processes, 1*, 337–354.

Ornstein, P.A. (1978a). Introduction: The study of children's memory. In P.A. Ornstein (Ed.), *Memory development in children* (pp. 1–20). Hillsdale, NJ: Erlbaum & Associates.

Ornstein, P.A. (1978b). *Memory development in children.* Hillsdale, NJ: Erlbaum & Associates.

Ornstein, P.A., Baker-Ward, L., & Naus, M.J. (in press). The development of mnemonic skill. In F.E. Weinert & M. Perlmutter (Eds.), *Memory development: Universal changes and individual differences.* Hillsdale, NJ: Erlbaum & Associates.

Ornstein, P.A., & Corsale, K. (1979). Organizational factors in children's memory. In C.R. Puff (Ed.), *Memory, organization, and structure* (pp. 219–257). New York: Academic Press.

Ornstein, P.A., Medlin, R.G., Stone, B.P., & Naus, M.J. (1985). Retrieving for rehearsal: An analysis of active rehearsal in children's memory. *Developmental Psychology, 21*, 633–641.

Ornstein, P.A., & Naus, M.J. (1978). Rehearsal processes in children's memory. In P.A. Ornstein (Ed.), *Memory development in children* (pp. 69–99). Hillsdale, NJ: Erlbaum & Associates.

Ornstein, P.A., & Naus, M.J. (1985). Effects of the knowledge base on children's memory strategies. In H.W. Reese (Ed.), *Advances in child development and behavior* (Vol. 19, pp. 113–148). New York: Academic Press.

Ornstein, P.A., Naus, M.J., & Liberty, C. (1975). Rehearsal and organizational processes in children's memory. *Child Development, 46*, 818–830.

Ornstein, P.A., Naus, M.J., & Miller, T.D. (1977). The effects of list organization and rehearsal activity in memory. *Child Development, 48*, 292–295.

Ornstein, P.A., Naus, M.J., & Stone, B.P. (1977). Rehearsal training and developmental differences in memory. *Developmental Psychology, 13*, 15–24.

O'Sullivan, J.T., & Pressley, M. (1984). Completeness of instruction and strategy transfer. *Journal of Experimental Child Psychology, 38*, 275–288.

Owings, R.A., & Baumeister, A.A. (1979). Levels of processing, encoding strategies, and memory development. *Journal of Experimental Child Psychology, 28*, 100–118.

Owings, R.A., Petersen, G.A., Bransford, J.D., Morris, C.D., & Stein, B.S. (1980). Spontaneous monitoring and regulation of learning: A comparison of successful and less successful fifth graders. *Journal of Educational Psychology, 72*, 250–256.

Paivio, A.U. (1963). Learning of adjective-noun paired-associates as a function of adjective-noun word order and noun abstractness. *Canadian Journal of Psychology, 17*, 370–379.

Paivio, A.U. (1965). Abstractness, imagery, and meaningfulness in paired-associate learning. *Journal of Verbal Learning and Verbal Behavior, 4*, 32–38.

Paivio, A.U. (1971). *Imagery and verbal processes.* New York: Holt, Rinehart, & Winston.

Paivio, A.U. (1986). *Mental representation: A dual-coding approach.* New York: Oxford University Press.

Paivio, A.U., & Harshman, R.A. (1983). Factor analysis of a questionnaire on imagery and verbal habits and skills. *Canadian Journal of Psychology, 37,* 461–483.

Paivio, A.U., & Yuille, J.C. (1966). Word abstractness, meaningfulness, and paired-associate learning in children. *Journal of Experimental Child Psychology, 4,* 81–89.

Palermo, D.S. (1961). Backward associations in the paired-associate learning of fourth and sixth grade children. *Psychological Reports, 9,* 227–233.

Palermo, D.S. (1962). Mediated association in a paired-associate transfer task. *Journal of Experimental Psychology, 64,* 234–238.

Palermo, D.S., Flamer, G.B., & Jenkins, J.J. (1964). Association value of responses in the paired-associate learning of children and adults. *Journal of Verbal Learning and Verbal Behavior, 3,* 171–175.

Palincsar, A.S. (1986). The role of dialogue in providing scaffolded instruction. *Educational Psychologist, 21,* 73–98.

Palincsar, A.S., & Brown, A.L. (1984). Reciprocal teaching of comprehension-fostering and comprehension-monitoring activities. *Cognition and Instruction, 1,* 117–175.

Palincsar, A.S., & Brown, A.L. (in press). Advances in the cognitive instruction of handicapped students. In M.C. Wang, H.J. Walberg, & M. Reynolds (Eds.), *The handbook of special education: Research and practice.* New York: Pergamon Press.

Paris, S.G. (1975). Integration and inference in children's comprehension and memory. In F. Restle, R.M. Shiffrin, J. Castellan, H. Lindman, & D. Pisoni (Eds.), *Cognitive theory* (Vol. 1, pp. 223–246). Hillsdale, NJ: Erlbaum & Associates.

Paris, S.G. (1978a). Coordination of means and goals in the development of mnemonic skills. In P. Ornstein (Ed.), *Memory development in children* (pp. 259–273). Hillsdale, NJ: Erlbaum & Associates.

Paris, S.G. (1978b). The development of inference and transformation as memory operations. In P. Ornstein (Ed.), *Memory development in children* (pp. 129–156). Hillsdale, NJ: Erlbaum & Associates.

Paris, S.G. (in press). Memory development across the life-span. In F.E. Weinert & M. Perlmutter (Eds.), *Memory development: Universal changes and individual differences.* Hillsdale, NJ: Erlbaum & Associates.

Paris, S.G., & Carter, A.Y. (1973). Semantic and constructive aspects of sentence memory in children. *Developmental Psychology, 9,* 109–113.

Paris, S.G., Cross, D.R., & Lipson, M.Y. (1984). Informed strategies for learning: A program to improve children's reading awareness and comprehension. *Journal of Educational Psychology, 76,* 1239–1252.

Paris, S.G., & Jacobs, J.E. (1984). The benefits of informed instruction for children's reading awareness and comprehension skills. *Child Development, 55,* 2083–2093.

Paris, S.G., & Lindauer, B.K. (1976). The role of inference in children's comprehension and memory for sentences. *Cognitive Psychology, 8,* 217–227.

Paris, S.G., & Lindauer, B.K. (1977). Constructive aspects of children's comprehension and memory. In R.V. Kail & J.W. Hagen (Eds.), *Perspectives on the development of memory and cognition* (pp. 35–60). Hillsdale, NJ: Erlbaum & Associates.

Paris, S.G., & Lindauer, B.K. (1982). The development of cognitive skills during childhood. In B. Wolman (Ed.), *Handbook of Developmental Psychology* (pp. 33–349). Englewood Cliffs, NJ: Prentice-Hall.

Paris, S.G., Lipson, M.Y., & Wixson, K.K. (1983). Becoming a strategic reader. *Contemporary Educational Psychology, 8,* 293–316.

Paris, S.G., & Myers, N.A. (1981). Comprehension monitoring memory and study strategies of good and poor readers. *Journal of Reading Behavior, 13,* 5–22.

Paris, S.G., Newman, R.S., & Jacobs, J.E. (1985). Social contexts and functions of children's remembering. In M. Pressley & C.J. Brainerd (Eds.), *Cognitive learning and memory in children* (pp. 81–115). New York: Springer.

Paris, S.G., Newman, R.S., & McVey, K.A. (1982). Learning the functional significance of mnemonic actions: A microgenetic study of strategy acquisition. *Journal of Experimental Child Psychology, 34,* 490–509.

Paris, S.G., & Oka, E.R. (1986). Children's reading strategies, metacognition, and motivation. *Developmental Review, 6,* 25–56.

Paris, S.G., & Upton, L.R. (1976). Children's memory inferential relationships in prose. *Child Development, 47,* 660–668.

Paris, S.G., Wixson, K.K., & Palinscar, A.S. (in press). Instructional approaches to reading comprehension. *Review of Research in Education.* Washington, DC: American Educational Research Association.

Pascual-Leone, J. (1970). A mathematical model for the transition rule in Piaget's developmental stages. *Acta Psychologia, 63,* 301–345.

Pascual-Leone, J. (1978). Compounds, confounds, and models in developmental information processing: A reply to Trabasso and Foellinger. *Journal of Experimental Child Psychology, 26,* 18–40.

Pascual-Leone, J. (1980). Constructive problems for constructive theories: The current relevance of Piaget's work and a critique of information-processing stimulation. In R.H. Kluwe & H. Spada (Eds.), *Developmental models of thinking* (pp. 263–296). New York: Academic Press.

Pascual-Leone, J., & Sparkman, E. (1980). The dialectics of empiricism and rationalism: A last methodological reply to Trabasso. *Journal of Experimental Child Psychology, 28,* 88–101.

Patterson, C.J., Cosgrove, J.M., & O'Brien, R.G. (1980). Nonverbal indicants of comprehension and noncomprehension in children. *Developmental Psychology, 16,* 38–48.

Pearson, P.D., Hansen, J., & Gordon, C. (1979). The effect of background knowledge on young children's comprehension of explicit and implicit information. *Journal of Reading Behavior, 11,* 201–209.

Pedersen, R.H. (1905). Experimentelle Untersuchung der visuellen und akustischen Erinnerungsbilder, angestellt an Schulkindern. *Archiv für Gesamte Psychologie, 4,* 520–534.

Peeck, J., van den Bosch, A.B., & Kreupeling, W.J. (1982). Effect of mobilizing prior knowledge in learning from text. *Journal of Educational Psychology, 74,* 771–777.

Pellegrino, J.W., & Hubert, J.L. (1982). The analysis of organization and structure in free recall. In C.R. Puff (Ed.), *Handbook of research methods in human memory and cognition* (pp. 129–172). New York: Academic Press.

Pellegrino, J.W., & Ingram, A.L. (1979). Processes, products, and measures of memory organization. In C.R. Puff (Ed.), *Memory, organization, and structure* (pp. 21–49). New York: Academic Press.

Perlmutter, M. (1978). What is memory aging the aging of? *Developmental Psychology, 14,* 330–345.

Perlmutter, M. (1980). *New directions for child development. Children's memory.* San Francisco, Jossey-Bass.

Perlmutter, M. (1982). Experimental and observational studies of preschool children's memory. In N. Nir-Janiv & B. Spodek (Eds.), *Early childhood education—An international perspective* (pp. 65–78). New York: Plenum Press.

Perlmutter, M. (1984). Continuities and discontinuities in early human memory paradigms, processes, and performance. In R. Kail & N.E. Spear (Eds.), *Comparative perspectives on the development of memory* (pp. 253–284). Hillsdale, NJ: Erlbaum & Associates.

Perlmutter, M. (in press). Research on memory and its development: Past, present, and future. In F.E. Weinert & M. Perlmutter (Eds.), *Memory development: Universal changes and individual differences*. Hillsdale, NJ: Erlbaum & Associates.

Perlmutter, M., Hazen, N., Mitchell, D.B., Grady, J.G., Cavanaugh, J.C., & Flook, J.P. (1981). Picture cues and exhaustive search facilitate very young children's memory for location. *Developmental Psychology, 17*, 104–110.

Perlmutter, M., & Lange, G. (1978). A developmental analysis of recall-recognition distinctions. In P.A. Ornstein (Ed.), *Memory development in children* (pp. 243–258). Hillsdale, NJ: Erlbaum & Associates.

Perlmutter, M., & Myers, N.A. (1979). Development of recall in 2- to 4-year-old children. *Developmental Psychology, 15*, 78–83.

Perlmutter, M., & Ricks, M. (1979). Recall in preschool children. *Journal of Experimental Child Psychology, 27*, 423–436.

Perlmutter, M., Schork, E.J., & Lewis, D. (1982). Effects of semantic and perceptual orienting tasks on preschool children's memory. *Bulletin of Psychonomic Society, 19*, 65–68.

Piaget, J. (1952). *The origin of intelligence in children*. New York: International Universities Press.

Piaget, J. (1968). *On the development of memory and identity*. Barre, MA: Clark University Press.

Piaget, J. (1970). Piaget's theory. In P.H. Mussen (Ed.), *Carmichael's manual of child psychology (3rd edition)* (Vol. 1, pp. 703–732). New York: Wiley.

Piaget, J., & Inhelder, B. (1971). *Mental imagery in the child*. New York: Basic Books.

Piaget, J., & Inhelder, B. (1973). *Memory and intelligence*. New York: Basic Books.

Pichert, J.W., & Anderson, R.C. (1977). Taking different perspectives on a story. *Journal of Educational Psychology, 69*, 309–315.

Pohlmann, A. (1906). *Einfluß der Lokalisation auf das Behalten. Experimentelle Beiträge zur Lehre vom Gedächtnis*. Berlin: Gerdes & Hödel.

Pollnac, R.B., & Jahn, G. (1976). Culture and memory revisited. An example from Buganda. *Journal of Cross-Cultural Psychology, 7*, 73–86.

Posnansky, C.J. (1978a). Age- and task-related differences in the use of category-size information for the retrieval of categorized items. *Journal of Experimental Child Psychology, 26*, 373–382.

Posnansky, C.J. (1978b). Category norms for verbal items in 25 categories for children in grades 2–6. *Behavior Research Methods & Instruments, 10*, 819–832.

Postman, L. (1961). The present status of interference theory. In C.N. Cofer (Ed.), *Verbal learning and verbal behavior* (pp. 152–179). New York: McGraw-Hill.

Poulsen, D., Kintsch, E., Kintsch, W., & Premack, D. (1979). Children's comprehension and memory for stories. *Journal of Experimental Child Psychology, 28*, 379–403.

Pressley, M. (1977). Imagery and children's learning: Putting the picture in developmental perspective. *Review of Educational Research, 47*, 586–622.

Pressley, M. (1982). Elaboration and memory development. *Child Development, 53*, 296–309.

Pressley, M. (1985). Review of Borkowski's insights. In S.R. Yussen (Ed.), *The growth of reflection in children* (pp. 145–148). Orlando, FL: Academic Press.

Pressley, M. (1986). The relevance of the good strategy user model to the teaching of mathematics. *Educational Psychologist, 21*, 139–161.

Pressley, M. (1987). Are keyword methods limited to slow presentation rates? An empirically-based reply to Hall and Fuson (1986). *Journal of Educational Psychology, 79*, 333–335.

Pressley, M., & Ahmad, M. (1986). Transfer of imagery-based mnemonics by adult learners. *Contemporary Educational Psychology, 11*, 150–160.

Pressley, M., Borkowski, J.G., & Johnson, C.J. (1987). The development of good strategy use: Imagery and related mnemonic strategies. In M.A. McDaniel & M. Pressley (Eds.), *Imagery and related mnemonic processes: Theories, individual differences, and applications* (pp. 274–301). New York: Springer.

Pressley, M., Borkowski, J.G., & O'Sullivan, J.T. (1984). Memory strategy instruction is made of this: Metamemory and durable strategy use. *Educational Psychology, 19*, 94–107.

Pressley, M., Borkowski, J.G., & O'Sullivan, J.T. (1985). Children's metamemory and the teaching of memory strategies. In D.L. Forrest-Pressley, G.E. MacKinnon, & T.G. Waller (Eds.), *Metacognition, cognition, and human performance* (pp. 111–153). Orlando, FL: Academic Press.

Pressley, M., Borkowski, J.G., & Schneider, W. (1987). Cognitive strategies: Good strategy users coordinate metacognition and knowledge. In R. Vasta & G. Whitehurst (Eds.), *Annals of Child Development* (Vol. 5, pp. 89–129). New York: JAI-Press.

Pressley, M., & Brainerd, C.J. (Eds.) (1985). *Cognitive learning and memory in children.* New York: Springer.

Pressley, M., Cariglia-Bull, T., Deane, S., & Schneider, W. (1987). Short-term memory, verbal competence, and age as predictors of imagery instructional effectiveness. *Journal of Experimental Child Psychology, 43*, 194–211.

Pressley, M., Cariglia-Bull, T., & Snyder, B.L. (1987). Are there programs that can really teach thinking and learning skills?: A review of Segal, Chipman, & Glaser's *Thinking and learning skills, Vol. 1, Relating instruction to research. Contemporary Education Research* (pp. 81–120). Orlando, FL: Academic Press.

Pressley, M., & Dennis-Rounds, J. (1980). Transfer of a mnemonic keyword strategy at two age levels. *Journal of Educational Psychology, 72*, 575–582.

Pressley, M., Forrest-Pressley, D.J., Elliott-Faust, D.J., & Miller, G.E. (1985). Children's use of cognitive strategies, how to teach strategies, and what to do if they can't be taught. In M. Pressley & C.J. Brainerd (Eds.), *Cognitive learning and memory in children* (pp. 1–47). New York: Springer.

Pressley, M., Forrest-Pressley, D.J., & Elliott-Faust, D.J. (in press). What is strategy instructional enrichment and how to study it: Illustrations from research on children's prose memory and comprehension. In F.E. Weinert & M. Perlmutter (Eds.), *Memory development: Universal changes and individual differences.* Hillsdale, NJ: Erlbaum & Associates.

Pressley, M., & Ghatala, E.S. (in press). Metacognitive benefits of taking a test. *Journal of Experimental Child Psychology.*

Pressley, M., & Ghatala, E.S. (in press). Delusions about performance on a multiple-choice comprehension test. *Reading Research Quarterly.*

Pressley, M., Goodchild, F., Fleet, J., Zajchowski, R., & Evans, E.D. (in press). The challenges of classroom strategy instruction. *Elementary School Journal.*

Pressley, M., Heisel, B.E., McCormick, C.G., & Nakamura, G.V. (1982). Memory strategy instruction with children. In C.J. Brainerd & M. Pressley (Eds.), *Progress in cognitive development research, Vol. 2, Verbal processes in children* (pp. 125–159). New York: Springer.

Pressley, M., Johnson, C.J., & Symons, S. (1987). Elaborating to learn and learning to elaborate. *Journal of Learning Disabilities, 20*, 76–91.

Pressley, M., & Levin, J.R. (1977a). Developmental differences in subjects' associative learning strategies and performance: Assessing a hypothesis. *Journal of Experimental Child Psychology, 24*, 431–439.

Pressley, M., & Levin, J.R. (1977b). Task parameters affecting the efficacy of a visual imagery learning strategy in younger and older children. *Journal of Experimental Child Psychology, 24*, 53–59.

Pressley, M., & Levin, J.R. (1978). Developmental constraints associated with children's use of the keyword method for foreign language vocabulary learning. *Journal of Experimental Child Psychology, 26*, 359–372.

Pressley, M., & Levin, J.R. (1980). The development of mental imagery retrieval. *Child Development, 51*, 558–560.

Pressley, M., & Levin, J.R. (1981). The keyword method and recall of vocabulary words from definitions. *Journal of Experimental Psychology: Human Learning and Memory, 7*, 72–76.

Pressley, M., & Levin, J.R. (1983a). *Cognitive strategy research: Educational applications.* New York: Springer.

Pressley, M., & Levin, J.R. (1983b). *Cognitive strategy research: Psychological foundations.* New York: Springer.

Pressley, M., & Levin, J.R. (1987). Elaborative learning strategies for the inefficient learner. In S.J. Ceci (Ed.), *Handbook of cognitive, social, and neuropsychological aspects of learning disabilities* (Vol. 2, pp. 175–212). Hillsdale, NJ: Erlbaum & Associates.

Pressley, M., Levin, J.R., & Bryant, S.L. (1983). Memory strategy instruction during adolescence: When is explicit instruction needed? In M. Pressley & J.R. Levin (Eds.), *Cognitive strategy research: Psychological foundations* (pp. 25–49). New York: Springer.

Pressley, M., Levin, J.R., & Delaney, H.D. (1982). The mnemonic keyword method. *Review of Educational Research, 56*, 61–92.

Pressley, M., Levin, J.R., Digdon, N., Bryant, S.L., & Ray, K. (1983). Does method of item presentation affect keyword method effectiveness? *Journal of Educational Psychology, 75*, 686–691.

Pressley, M., Levin, J.R., & Ghatala, E.S. (1984). Memory strategy monitoring in adults and children. *Journal of Verbal Learning and Verbal Behavior, 23*, 270–288.

Pressley, M., Levin, J.R., & Ghatala, E.S. (1988). Strategy-comparison opportunities promote long-term strategy use. *Contemporary Educational Psychology, 13*, 157–168.

Pressley, M., Levin, J.R., Ghatala, E.S., & Ahmad, M. (1987). Test monitoring in young grade school children. *Journal of Experimental Child Psychology, 43*, 96–111.

Pressley, M., Levin, J.R., Kuiper, N.A., Bryant, S.L., & Michener, S. (1982). Mnemonic versus nonmnemonic vocabulary-learning strategies: Additional comparisons. *Journal of Educational Psychology, 74*, 693–707.

Pressley, M., Levin, J.R., & McCormick, C.B. (1980). Young children's learning of foreign language vocabulary: A sentence variation of the keyword method. *Contemporary Educational Psychology, 5*, 22–29.

Pressley, M., Levin, J.R., & McDaniel, M.A. (1987). Remembering versus inferring what a word means: Mnemonic and contextual approaches. In M.G. McGeown & M.E. Curtis (Eds.), *The nature of vocabulary acquisition* (Vol. 5, pp. 107–127). Hillsdale, NJ: Erlbaum & Associates.

Pressley, M., & MacFadyen, J. (1983). Mnemonic mediator retrieval at testing by preschool and kindergarten children. *Child Development, 54*, 474–479.

Pressley, M., McDaniel, M.A., Tannenbaum, R., & Wood, E. (1988). *What happens when adult readers try to answer prequestions that accompany textbook material?* Unpublished manuscript, London, Canada, University of Western Ontario.

Pressley, M., McDaniel, M.A., Turnure, J.E., Wood, E., & Ahmad, M. (1987). Generation and precision of elaboration: Effects on intentional and incidental learning. *Journal of Experimental Psychology: Learning memory, and cognition, 13*, 291–300.

Pressley, M., & Miller, G.E. (1987). The effects of illustrations on children's listening comprehension and oral prose memory. In D.M. Willows & H.A. Houghton (Eds.), *Illustrations, graphs, and diagrams: Psychological theory and educational practice* (pp. 87–114). New York: Springer.

Pressley, M., Ross, K.A., Levin, J.R., & Ghatala, E.S. (1984). The role of strategy utility knowledge in children's strategy decision making. *Journal of Experimental Child Psychology, 38*, 491–504.

Pressley, M., Samuel, J., Hershey, M.M., Bishop, S.L., & Dickinson, D. (1981). Use of a mnemonic technique to teach young children foreign language vocabulary. *Contemporary Educational Psychology, 6*, 110–116.

Pressley, M., Snyder, B.L., & Cariglia-Bull, T. (1987). How can good strategy use be taught to children? Evaluation of six alternative approaches. In S. Cormier & J. Hagman (Eds.), *Transfer of learning: Contemporary research and applications* (pp. 81–120). Orlando, FL: San Diego: Academic Press.

Pressley, M., Snyder, B.L., Levin, J.R., Murray, H.G., & Ghatala, E.S. (1987). Perceived readiness for examination performance (PREP) produced by initial reading of text and text containing adjunct questions. *Reading Research Quarterly, 22*, 219–236.

Price, L.E. (1963). Learning and performance in verbal paired-associate tasks with preschool children. *Psychological Reports, 12*, 847–850.

Prytulak, L.S. (1971). Natural language mediation. *Cognitive Psychology, 2*, 1–56.

Pylyshen, Z.W. (1984). *Computation and cognition: Toward a foundation for cognitive science.* Cambridge, MA: MIT Press.

Raaijmakers, J.G.W., & Shiffrin, R.M. (1980). SAM: A theory of probabilistic search of associative memory. In G.H Bower (Ed.), *The psychology of learning and motivation* (Vol. 14, pp. 208–262). New York: Academic Press.

Raaijmakers, J.G.W., & Shiffrin, R.M. (1981). Search of associative memory. *Psychological Review, 88*, 92–134.

Rabinowitz, J.C., Ackerman, B.P., Craik, F.I.M., & Hinchley, J.L. (1982). Aging and metamemory: The roles of relatedness and imagery. *Journal of Gerontology, 37*, 688–695.

Rabinowitz, M. (1984). The use of categorical organization: Not an all-or-none situation. *Journal of Experimental Child Psychology, 38*, 338–351.

Rabinowitz, M., & Chi, M.T.H. (1987). An interactive model of strategic processing. In S.J. Ceci (Ed.), *Handbook of the cognitive, social, and physiological characteristics of learning disabilities* (Vol. 2, pp. 83–102). Hillsdale, NJ: Erlbaum & Associates.

Rabinowitz, M., & Mandler, J.M. (in press). Organization and information retrieval. *Journal of Experimental Psychology: Learning, Memory, and Cognition.*

Radossawljewitsch, P.R. (1907). Das Behalten und Vergessen bei Kindern und Erwachsenen nach experimentellen Untersuchungen. In E. Meumann (Ed.), *Pädagogische Monographien (Band 1)* (pp. 128–181). Leipzig: Otto Nemnich.

Rahmani, L. (1973). *Soviet psychology: Philosophical, theoretical, and experimental issues.* New York: International Universities Press.

Ranschburg, P. (1901). Apparat und Methode zur Untersuchung des optischen Gedächtnisses für medizinische und pädagogisch - psychologische Zwecke. *Monatsschrift für Psychiatrie und Neurologie, 10*, 17–51.

Ratner, H. (1980). The role of social context in memory development. In M. Perlmutter (Ed.), *New directions for child development: Children's memory* (pp. 49–67). San Francisco: Jossey-Bass.

Ratner, H.H., & Myers, N.A. (1980). Related picture cues and memory for hidden-object location at age two. *Child Development, 51*, 561–564.

Redfield, D.L., & Rousseau, E.W. (1981). Meta-analysis of experimental research in teacher questioning behavior. *Review of Educational Research, 51*, 237–245.

Reed, S.K., Ernst, G.W., & Banjeri, R. (1974). The role of analogy in transfer between similar problem states. *Cognitive Psychology, 6*, 436–450.

Reese, H.W. (1962). Verbal mediation as a function of age level. *Psychological Bulletin, 59*, 502–509.

Reese, H.W. (1976). The development of memory: Life-span perspectives. In H.W. Reese (Ed.), *Advances in child development and behavior* (Vol. 11, pp. 190–212). New York: Academic Press.

Reese, H.W. (1977). Imagery and associative memory. In R.V. Kail & J.W. Hagen (Eds.), *Perspectives on the development of memory and cognition* (pp. 113–175). Hillsdale, NJ: Erlbaum & Associates.

Reese, H.W. (1979). Gedächtnisentwicklung im Verlauf des Lebens - empirische Befunde und theoretische Modelle. In L. Montada (Ed.), *Brennpunkte der Entwicklungspsychologie* (pp. 90–102). Stuttgart: Kohlhammer.

Reid, M.K., & Borkowski, J.G. (1985). *The influence of attribution training on strategic behaviors, self-management, and beliefs about control in hyperactive children.* Paper presented at the biennial meeting of the Society for Research in Child Development, Toronto, Canada.

Renninger, K.A., & Wozniak, R.H. (1985). Effect of interest on attentional shift, recognition, and recall in young children. *Developmental Psychology, 21*, 624–632.

Revelle, G.L., Wellman, H.M., & Karabenick, J.D. (1985). Comprehension monitoring in preschool children. *Child Development, 56*, 654–663.

Richman, C.L., Nida, S., & Pittman, L. (1976). Effects of meaningfulness on children's free-recall learning. *Developmental Psychology, 12*, 460–465.

Rickards, J.P. (1976). Interaction of position and conceptual level of adjunct questions on immediate and delayed retention of text. *Journal of Educational Psychology, 68*, 210–217.

Rickards, J.P., & DiVesta, F.J. (1974). Type and frequency of questions in processing text material. *Journal of Educational Psychology, 66*, 354–362.

Riegel, K.F. (1974). The structure of the structuralists. *Contemporary Psychology, 19*, 811–813.

Riegel, K.F. (1975). Structure and transformation in modern intellectual history. In K.F. Riegel & G.C. Rosenwald (Eds.), *Structure and transformation: Developmental and historical aspects.* New York: Wiley.

Rigney, J.W. (1980). Cognitive learning strategies and dualities in information processing. In R.E. Snow, P. Federico, & W.E. Montague (Eds.), *Aptitude, learning, and instruction* (Vol. 1, pp. 315–343). Hillsdale, NJ: Erlbaum & Associates.

Ringel, B.A., & Springer, C.J. (1980). On knowing how well one is remembering: The persistence of strategy use during transfer. *Journal of Experimental Child Psychology, 29*, 322–333.

Ritter, K. (1978). The development of knowledge of an external retrieval cue strategy. *Child Development, 49*, 1227–1230.

Ritter, K., Kaprove, B.H., Fitch, J.P., & Flavell, J.H. (1973). The development of retrieval strategies in young children. *Cognitive Psychology, 5*, 310–321.

Roehler, L.R., & Duffy, G.G. (1984). Direct explanation of comprehension processes. In G.G. Duffy, L.R. Roehler, & J. Mason (Eds.), *Comprehension instruction: Perspectives and suggestions* (pp. 265–280). New York: Longman.

Roenker, D.L., Thompson, C.P., & Brown, S.C. (1971). Comparison of measures for the estimation of clustering in free recall. *Psychological Bulletin, 76*, 45–48.

Rogoff, B. (1981). Schooling and development of cognitive skills. In H.C. Triandis & A. Heron (Eds.), *Handbook of cross-cultural psychology* (Vol. 4, pp. 233–294). Boston: Allyn & Bacon.

Rogoff, B., & Mistry, J. (1985). Memory development in cultural context. In M. Pressley & C.J. Brainerd (Eds.), *Cognitive learning and memory in children* (pp. 117–142). New York: Springer.

Rogoff, B., Newcombe, N., & Kagan, J. (1974). Planfulness and recongition memory. *Child Development, 45,* 972–977.

Rogoff, B., & Waddell, K.J. (1982). Memory of information organized in a scene by children from two cultures. *Child Development, 53,* 1224–1228.

Rohwer, W.D., Jr. (1973). Elaboration and learning in childhood and adolescence. In H.W. Reese (Ed.), *Advances in child development and behavior* (Vol. 8, pp. 1–57). New York: Academic Press.

Rohwer, W.D. (1980). An elaborative conception of learner differences. In R.E. Snow, P.A. Federico, & W.E. Montague (Eds.), *Aptitude, learning, and instruction, Vol. 2: Cognitive process analyses of learning and problem* (pp. 23–46). Hillsdale, NJ: Erlbaum & Associates.

Rohwer, W.D., Jr., & Bean, J.P. (1973). Sentence effects and noun-pair learning: A developmental interaction during adolescence. *Journal of Experimental Child Psychology, 15,* 521–533.

Rohwer, W.D., & Dempster, F.N. (1977). Memory development and educational processes. In R.V. Kail & J.W. Hagen (Eds.), *Perspectives on the development of memory and cognition* (pp. 407–435). Hillsdale, NJ: Erlbaum & Associates.

Rohwer, W.D., & Litrownik, J. (1983). Age and individual differences in the learning of a memorization procedure. *Journal of Educational Psychology, 75,* 799–810.

Rohwer, W.D., Jr., Rabinowitz, M., & Dronkers, N.F. (1982). Event knowledge, elaborative propensity, and the development of learning proficiency. *Journal of Experimental Child Psychology, 33,* 492–503.

Rohwer, W.D., Raines, J.M., Eoff, J., & Wagner, M. (1977). The development of elaborative propensity during adolescence. *Journal of Experimental Child Psychology, 23,* 472–492.

Rosch, E.H. (1973). On the internal structure of perceptual and semantic categories. In T.E. Moore (Ed.), *Cognitive development and the acquisition of language* (pp. 111–144). New York: Academic Press.

Rosch, E.H. (1975). Cognitive representations of semantic categories. *Journal of Experimental Psychology: General, 7,* 192–233.

Ross, B.H. (1984). Remindings and their effects in learning a cognitive skill. *Cognitive Psychology, 16,* 371–416.

Ross, B.M., & Millsom, C. (1970). Repeated memory of oral prose in Ghana and New York. *International Journal of Psychology, 5,* 173–181.

Rossi, S., & Wittrock, M.C. (1971). Developmental shifts in verbal recall between mental ages two and five. *Child Developmen, 42,* 333–338.

Roth, C. (1983). Factors affecting developmental changes in the speed of processing. *Journal of Experimental Child Psychology, 35,* 509–528.

Rubin, D.C. (Ed.) (1986). *Autobiographical memory.* Cambridge, England: Cambridge University Press.

Ruff, H. (1984). Infant memory from a Gibsonian point of view. In M. Moscovitch (Ed.), *Infant memory* (pp. 49–73). New York: Plenum Press.

Rumelhart, D.E. (1980). Schemata: The building blocks of cognition. In R. Spiro, B. Bruce, & W. Brewer (Eds.), *Theoretical issues in reading comprehension* (pp. 35–58). Hillsdale, NJ: Erlbaum & Associates.

Rumelhart, D.E. (1980). On evaluating story grammars. *Cognitive Science, 4*, 313–316.

Rundus, D. (1971). Analysis of rehearsal processes in free recall. *Journal of Experimental Child Psychology, 89*, 63–77.

Ryan, E.B., Weed, K.A., & Short, E.J. (1986). Cognitive behavior modification: Promoting active, self-regulatory learning styles. In J.K. Torgeson & B.Y.L. Wong (Eds.), *Psychological and educational perspectives on learning disabilities* (pp. 367–397). Orlando, FL: Academic Press.

Saarnio, D.A., & Bjorklund, D.F. (1984). Children's memory for objects in self-generated scenes. *Merrill-Palmer Quarterly, 30*, 287–301.

Salatas, H., & Flavell, J.H. (1976a). Retrieval of recently learned information: Development of strategies and control skills. *Child Development, 47*, 941–948.

Salatas, H., & Flavell, J.H. (1976b). Behavioral and metamnemonic indicators of strategic behaviors under remember instructions in first grade. *Child Development, 47*, 81–89.

Salomon, G., & Globerson, T. (1987). *Skill is not enough: The role of mindfulness in learning and transfer.* Technical Report No. 11, Tel Aviv, Israel: Tel Aviv University, School of Education.

Salthouse, T.A. (1982). *Adult cognition.* New York: Springer.

Samuel, A.G. (1978). Organizational vs retrieval factors in the development of digit span. *Journal of Experimental Child Psychology, 26*, 308–319.

Sarason, I.G. (1972). Experimental approaches to test anxiety: Attention and the uses of information. In C.D. Spielberger (Ed.), *Anxiety: Current trends in theory and research* (Vol. 2, pp. 303–408). New York: Academic Press.

Schank, R.C. (1975). *Conceptual information processing.* New York: Elsevier.

Schank, R.C. (1982). *Dynamic memory: A theory of reminding and learning in computers and people.* New York: Cambridge University Press.

Schank, R.C., & Abelson, R. (1977). *Scripts, plans, goals, and understanding.* Hillsdale, NJ: Erlbaum & Associates.

Schmidt, C.R., Paris, S.G., & Stober, S. (1979). Inferential distance and children's memory for pictorial sequences. *Developmental Psychology, 15*, 395–405.

Schneider, W., & Shiffrin, R.M. (1977). Controlled and automatic human information processing: I. Direction, search, and attention. *Psychological Review, 84*, 1–66.

Schneider, W., Dumais, S.T., & Shiffrin, R.M. (1984). Automatic and control processing and attention. In R. Parasuraman & D.R. Davies (Eds.), *Varieties of attention* (pp. 1–27). Orlando, FL: Academic Press.

Schneider, W. (1984). Die Entwicklung des Metagedächtnisses—Wie Kinder mit ihrem Gedächtnis umzugehen lernen. *Umschau, 84*, 378–380.

Schneider, W. (1985a). *Critique: Memory strategy and metamemory development.* Paper presented at the annual meeting of the American Educational Research Association, Chicago.

Schneider, W. (1985b). Metagedächtnis, gedächtnisbezogenes Verhalten und Gedächtnisleistung - Eine Analyse der empirischen Zusammenhänge bei Grundschülern der dritten Klassenstufe. *Zeitschrift für Entwicklungspsychologie und Pädagogische Psychologie, 17*, 1–16.

Schneider, W. (1985c). Developmental trends in the metamemory-memory behavior relationship: An integrative review. In D.L. Forrest-Pressley, G.E. MacKinnon, & T.G. Waller (Eds.), *Cognition, metacognition, and human performance* (Vol. 1, pp. 57–109). New York: Academic Press.

Schneider, W. (1986). The role of conceptual knowledge and metamemory in the development of organizational processes in memory. *Journal of Experimental Child Psychology, 42*, 318–336.

Schneider, W., Borkowski, J.G., Kurtz, B.E., & Kerwin, K. (1986). Metamemory and motivation: A comparison of strategy use and performance in German and American children. *Journal of Cross-Cultural Psychology, 17*, 315–336.

Schneider, W., & Brun, H. (1987). The role of context in young children's memory performance: Istomina revisited. *British Journal of Developmental Psychology, 5*, 333–341.

Schneider, W., Körkel, J., & Vogel, K. (1987). Zusammenhänge zwischen Metagedächtnis, srategischem Verhalten und Gedächtnisleistungen im Grundschulalter: Eine entwicklungspsychologische Studie. *Zeitschrift für Entwicklungspsychologie und Pädagogische Psychologie, 19*, 99–115.

Schneider, W., Körkel, J., & Weinert, F.E. (1987a). The knowledge base and memory performance: A comparison of academically successful and unsuccessful learners. Paper presented at the annual meetings of the American Educational Research Association, Washington, DC.

Schneider, W., Körkel, J., & Weinert, F.E. (1987b). The effects of intelligence, self-concept, and attributional style on metamemory and memory behavior. *International Journal of Behavioral Development, 10*, 281–299.

Schneider, W., & Sodian, B. (1988). Metamemory-memory relationships in preschool children: Evidence from a memory-for-location task. *Journal of Experimental Child Psychology, 45*, 209–233.

Schneider, W., & Treiber, B. (1984). Classroom differences in the determination of achievement changes. *American Educational Research Journal, 21*, 195–211.

Schneider, W., & Weinert, F.E. (in press). Memory development: Universal changes and individual differences. In A. de Ribaupierre (Ed.), *Transitional mechanisms in cognitive-emotional child development*. New York: Cambridge University Press.

Schoenfeld, A.H. (1985). *Mathematical problem solving*. Orlando, FL: Academic Press.

Schumaker, J.B., Deshler, D.D., & Ellis, E.S. (1986). Intervention issues related to the education of LD adolescents. In J.K. Torgeson & B.Y.L. Wong (Eds.), *Psychological and educational perspectives on learning disabilities* (pp. 329–365). Orlando, FL: Academic Press.

Scott, M.S., Greenfield, D.B., & Urbano, R.C. (1985). A comparison of complementary and taxonomic utilizations: Significance of the dependent measure. *International Journal of Behavioral Development, 8*, 241–256.

Scribner, S. (1974). Developmental aspects of categorized recall in a West African society. *Cognitive Psychology, 6*, 475–494.

Scribner, S., & Cole, M. (1972). Effects of constrained recall training on children's performance in a verbal memory task. *Child Development, 43*, 845–857.

Selz, O. (1913). Über die Gesetze des geordneten Denkverlaufs. Stuttgart: Spemann.

Shallice, T. (1979). Neuropsychological research and the fractionation of memory systems. In L.-G. Nilsson (Ed.), *Perspectives on memory research: Essays in honor of Uppsala University's 500th anniversary* (pp. 257–277). Hillsdale, NJ: Erlbaum & Associates.

Shapiro, S.S. (1965). Paired-associate learning in children. *Journal of Verbal Learning and Verbal Behavior, 4*, 170–174.

Sharp, D., Cole, M., & Lave, C. (1979). Education and cognitive development: The evidence from experimental research. *Monographs of the Society for Research in Child Development, 44* (Serial No. 178).

Shatz, M., & Gelman, R. (1973). The development of communication skills: Modifications in the speech of young children as a function of listener. *Monographs of the Society for Research on Child Development 38* (5, Serial No. 152).

Shaughnessy, J. (1981). Memory monitoring accuracy and modification of rehearsal strategies. *Journal of Verbal Learning and Verbal Behavior, 20*, 216–230.

Shaw, R., & Bransford, J.D. (1977). Introduction: Psychological approaches to the problem of knowledge. In R. Shaw & J.D. Bransford (Eds.), *Perceiving, acting, and knowing* (pp. 1–39). Hillsdale, NJ: Erlbaum & Associates.

Shiffrin, R.M., & Schneider, W. (1977). Controlled and automatic human information processing: II. Perceptual learning, automatic attending, and a general theory. *Psychological Review, 84,* 127–190.

Short, E.J., & Miller, D.J. (1981). Metamemory in preschoolers: The 4- and 5-year-old's sensitivity to memory instructions in a game-like context. *Genetic Psychology Monographs, 103,* 221–241.

Short, E.J., & Ryan, E.B. (1984). Metacognitive differences between skilled and less skilled readers: Remediating deficits through story grammar and attribution training. *Journal of Educational Psychology, 76,* 225–235.

Shriberg, L.K., Levin, J.R., McCormick, C.B., & Pressley, M. (1982). Learning about "famous" people via the keyword method. *Journal of Educational Psychology, 74,* 238–247.

Shure, M.B., & Spivack, G. (1978). *Problem-solving techniques in childrearing.* San Francisco: Jossey-Bass.

Siaw, S.N. (1984). Developmental and population comparisons of taxonomic and thematic organization in free recall. *Journal of Educational Psychology, 76,* 755–765.

Siegler, R.S. (1983). Information processing approaches to development. In P.H. Mussen (Ed.), *Handbook of child psychology, Vol. 1, History, theory, and methods* (pp. 129–211). New York: Wiley.

Siegler, R.S. (1986). Children's thinking. Englewood Cliffs, NJ: Prentice-Hall.

Simon, H.A. (1974). How big is a chunk? *Science, 183,* 482–488.

Slackman, E., & Nelson, K. (1984). Acquisition of an unfamiliar script in story form by young children. *Child Development, 55,* 329–340.

Slung, M. (1985). *The absent-minded professor's memory book.* New York: Ballantine Books.

Smirnov, A.A. (1973). *Problems of the psychology of memory.* New York: Plenum Press.

Smirnov, A.A., & Zinchenko, P.I. (1969). Problems in the psychology of memory. In M. Cole & J. Maltzman (Eds.), *A handbook of contemporary Soviet psychology* (pp. 452–502). New York: Basic Books.

Smith, L.C., Readence, J.E., & Alvermann, D.E. (1984). Effects of activating background knowledge on comprehension of expository prose. *33rd Yearbook of the National Reading Conference* (pp. 188–192). Rochester, NY: National Reading Conference.

Sodian, B. (1986). *Wissen durch Denken? Über den naiven Empirismus im Denken von Vorschulkindern.* Münster: Aschendorff.

Sodian, B., Schneider, W., & Perlmutter, M. (1986). Recall, clustering, and metamemory in young children. *Journal of Experimental Child Psychology, 41,* 395–410.

Somerville, S.C., Wellman, H.M., & Cultice, J.C. (1983). Young children's deliberate reminding. *The Journal of Genetic Psychology, 143,* 87–96.

Sophian, C. (1984). Developing search skills in infancy and early childhood. In C. Sophian (Ed.), *Origins of cognitive skills* (pp. 27–56). Hillsdale, NJ: Erlbaum & Associates.

Sophian, C., & Hagen, J.W. (1978). Involuntary memory and the development of retrieval skills in young children. *Journal of Experimental Child Psychology, 26,* 458–471.

Sophian, C., Larkin, J.H., & Kadane, J.B. (1985). A developmental model of search: Stochastic estimation of children's rule use. In H.M. Wellman (Ed.), *Children's searching: The development of search skill and spatial representation* (pp. 185–214). Hillsdale, NJ: Erlbaum & Associates.

Sophian, C., & Wellman, H.M. (1980). Selective information use in the development of search behavior. *Developmental Psychology, 16,* 323–336.

Sophian, C., & Wellman, H.M. (1983). Selective information use and perseveration in the search behavior of infants and young children. *Journal of Experimental Child Psychology*, *35*, 369–390.

Speer, J.R., & Flavell, J.H. (1979). Young children's knowledge of the relative difficulty of recognition and recall memory tasks. *Developmental Psychology*, *15*, 214–217.

Spiker, C.C. (1960). Associative transfer in verbal paired-associate learning. *Child Development*, *31*, 73–87.

Spring, C., & Capps, C. (1974). Encoding speed, rehearsal, and probed recall of dyslexic boys. *Journal of Educational Psychology*, *66*, 780–786.

Springer, C.J. (1979). Children's use of category-size information for the retrieval of information. *Bulletin of the Psychonomic Society*, *14*, 471–474.

Stein, B.S., & Bransford, J.D. (1979). Constraints on effective elaboration: Effects of precision and subject generation. *Journal of Verbal Learning and Verbal Behavior*, *18*, 769–777.

Stein, B.S., Littlefield, J., Bransford, J.D., & Persampieri, M. (1984). Elaboration and knowledge acquisition. *Memory & Cognition*, *12*, 522–529.

Stein, N.L., & Glenn, C.G. (1975). *A developmental study of children's recall of story material*. Paper presented at the Society for Research in Child Development, Denver, CO.

Stein, N.L., & Glenn, C.G. (1979). An analysis of story comprehension in elementary school children. In R. Freedle (Ed.), *New directions in discourse processing* (pp. 53–120). Norwood, NJ: Ablex.

Stein, N.L., & Nezworski, T. (1978). The effects of organization and instructional set on story memory. *Discourse Processes*, *1*, 177–193.

Stein, N.L., & Trabasso, T. (1981). What's in a story: Critical issues in story comprehension. In R. Glaser (Ed.), *Advances in the psychology of instruction* (pp. 213–267). Hillsdale, NJ: Erlbaum & Associates.

Stern, C., & Stern, W. (1909). *Erinnerung, Aussage und Lüge*. Leipzig: Barth.

Sternberg, R.J. (1979). The nature of mental abilities. *American Psychologist*, *34*, 214–230.

Sternberg, R.J. (1980). Sketch of a componential subtheory of human intelligence. *The Behavioral and Brain Sciences*, *3*, 573–584.

Sternberg, R.J. (1984). Mechanisms of cognitive development: A componential approach. In R.J. Sternberg (Ed.), *Mechanisms of cognitive development* (pp. 163–186). New York: Freeman.

Sternberg, R.J., & Powell, J.S. (1983). The development of intelligence. In P.H. Mussen (Ed.), *Handbook of child psychology (4th edition)* (Vol. 3, pp. 341–419). New York: Wiley.

Steuck, K.W. (1984). *The effects of task demands on children's metamemorial decisions*. Paper presented at the annual meeting of the American Educational Research Association, New Orleans.

Stevens, K. (1980). The effect of topic interest on the reading comprehension of higher ability students. *Journal of Educational Research*, *73*, 365–368.

Stevenson, H.W., Parker, T., Wilkinson, A., Bonnevaux, B., & Gonzalez, M. (1978). Schooling, environment, and cognitive development: A cross-cultural study. *Monographs of the Society for Research in Child Development*, *43* (Serial No. 175).

Stipek, D.J., Roberts, T.A., & Sanborn, M.E. (1984). Preschool-age children's performance expectations for themselves and another child as a function of the incentive value of success and the salience of past performance. *Child Development*, *55*, 1983–1989.

Strage, A., Tyler, A.B., Rohwer, W.D., Jr., & Thomas, J.W. (1987). An analytic framework for assessing distinctive course features with and across grade levels. *Contemporary Educational Psychology*, *12*, 280–302.

Strube, G. (1984). *Assoziation - Der Prozeß des Erinnerns und die Struktur des Gedächtnisses*. Berlin/Heidelberg: Springer.

Sydow, H. (1979). Probleme und Ergebnisse der kinderpsychologischen Gedächtnisforschung. *Probleme und Ergebnisse der Psychologie, 69*, 81–95.

Taylor, A.M., & Turnure, J.E. (1979). Imagery and verbal elaboration with retarded children: Effects on learning and memory. In N.R. Ellis (Ed.), *Handbook of mental deficiency, psychological theory and research* (pp. 659–697). Hillsdale, NJ: Erlbaum & Associates.

Tenney, Y.J. (1975). The child's conception of organization and recall. *Journal of Experimental Child Psychology, 19*, 100–114.

Tergan, S.-O. (1986). *Modelle der Wissensrepräsentation als Grundlage qualitativer Wissensdiagnostik.* Opladen: Westdeutscher Verlag.

Thompson, A.G. (1985). Teachers' conceptions of mathematics and the teaching of problem solving. In E.A. Silver (Ed.), *Teaching and learning mathematical problem solving* (pp. 281–294). Hillsdale, NJ: Erlbaum & Associates.

Thompson, C.P., & Barnett, C. (1985). Review, recitation, and memory monitoring. *Journal of Educational Psychology, 77*, 533–538.

Thorndike, E.L., & Woodworth, R.S. (1901). The influence of improvement in one mental function upon the efficiency of other functions. *Psychological Review, 8*, 247–261, 384–395, 553–564.

Tierney, R.J., & Cunningham, J.W. (1984). Research on teaching reading comprehension. In P.D. Pearson (Ed.), *Handbook of reading research* (pp. 609–655). New York: Longman.

Tobias, S. (1977). A model of research on the effect of anxiety on instruction. In J.E. Sieber, H.F. O'Neil, Jr., & S. Tobias (Eds.), *Anxiety, learning, and instruction* (pp. 223–240). Hillsdale, NJ: Erlbaum & Associates.

Tobias, S. (1979). Anxiety research in educational psychology. *Journal of Educational Psychology, 71*, 573–582.

Todd, C.M., & Perlmutter, M. (1980). Reality recalled by preschool children. In M. Perlmutter (Ed.), *New directions for child development: Children's memory (No. 10)* (pp. 69–86). San Francisco: Jossey-Bass.

Trabasso, T. (1978). On the estimation of parameters and the evaluation of a mathematical model: A reply to Pascual-Leone. *Journal of Experimental Child Psychology, 26*, 41–45.

Trabasso, T., & Foellinger, D.B. (1978). Information processing capacity in children: A test of Pascual-Leone's model. *Journal of Experimental Child Psychology, 26*, 1–17.

Trabasso, T., & Nicholas, D.W. (1980). Memory and inferences in the comprehension of narratives. In F. Wilkening, J. Becker, & T. Trabasso (Eds.), *Information integration by children* (pp. 215–242). Hillsdale, NJ: Erlbaum & Associates.

Tulving, E. (1962a). Subjective organization in free recall of unrelated words. *Psychological Review, 69*, 344–354.

Tulving, E. (1962b). The effect of alphabetical subjective organization on memorizing unrelated words. *Canadian Journal of Psychology, 16*, 185–191.

Tulving, E. (1972). *Episodic and semantic memory.* New York: Academic Press.

Tulving, E. (1979). Relation between encoding specificity and levels of processing. In L.S. Cermak & F.M. Craik (Eds.), *Levels of processing in human memory* (pp. 405–418). Hillsdale, NJ: Erlbaum & Associates.

Tulving, E., & Madigan, S. (1970). Memory and verbal learning. *Annual Review of Psychology, 21*, 437–484.

Tulving, E., & Thomson, D.M. (1973). Encoding specificity and retrieval processes in episodic memory. *Psychological Review, 80*, 352–373.

Turner, L.A., Kurtz, B.E., Schneider, W., Carr, M., & Borkowski, J.G. (1987). *Strategy acquisition and transfer: Cultural and environmental influences.* Unpublished manuscript, Vanderbilt University, Nashville, TN.

Turnure, J.E. (1985). Communication and cues in the functional cognition of the mentally retarded. In N.R. Ellis & N.W. Bray (Eds.), *International review of mental retardation* (Vol. 13, pp. 43–47). New York: Academic Press.

Turnure, J.E., Buium, N., & Thurlow, M. (1976). The effectiveness of interrogatives for promoting verbal elaboration productivity in young children. *Child Development, 47,* 851–855.

Turnure, J.E., & Lane, J.F. (1987). Special educational applications of mnemonics. In M.A. McDaniel & M. Pressley (Eds.), *Imagery and related mnemonic processes: Theories, individual differences, and applications* (pp. 329–357). New York: Springer.

Tversky, B. (1985). Development of taxonomic organization of named and pictured categories. *Developmental Psychology, 21,* 1111–1119.

Uhl, C. (1986). *Zum Zusammenhang zwischen Prognosegenauigkeit, Metagedächtnis, Strategieanwendung und Gedächtnisleistung im Verlauf der Lebensspanne.* Unveröffentlichte Diplomarbeit, Universität Heidelberg.

Uhl, C., & Schneider, W. (1988). *Vergleichende Analysen zum Verhältnis von Metagedächtnis, Strategienutzung und Gedächtnisleistung bei Kindern, Erwachsenen und alten Menschen.* Unveröffentlichtes Manuskript, Max Planck Institut für psychologische Forschung, München.

Underwood, B.J. (1964). Degree of learning and the measurement of forgetting. *Journal of Verbal Learning and Verbal Behavior, 3,* 112–129.

Underwood, B.J., & Schulz, R.W. (1960). *Meaningfulness and verbal learning.* Philadelphia: Lippincott.

Verdonik, F. (in press). Reconsidering the context of remembering: The need for a social description of memory processes and their development. In F.E. Weinert & M. Perlmutter (Eds.), *Memory development: Universal changes and individual differences.* Hillsdale, NJ: Erlbaum & Associates.

Vertes, J.O. (1913). Das Wortgedächtnis im Schulkindesalter. *Zeitschrift für Psychologie, 63,* 19–128.

Vertes, J.O. (1931). Behalten und Vergessen des Kindes. *Zeitschrift für Psychologie und Physiologie der Sinnesorgane, 121,* 241–354.

Vygotsky, L.S. (1978). *Mind in society: The development of higher psychological processes* (M. Cole, V. John-Steiner, S. Scribner, & E. Souberman, Eds. & Trans.), Cambridge, MA: Harvard University Press.

Wagner, D.A. (1974). The development of short-term and incidental memory: A cross-cultural study. *Child Development, 45,* 389–396.

Wagner, D.A. (1978). Memories of Morocco: The influence of age, schooling, and environment on memory. *Cognitive Psychology, 10,* 1–28.

Wagner, D.A. (1981). Culture and memory development. In H.C. Triandis & A. Heron (Eds.), *Handbook of cross-cultural psychology* (Vol. 4, pp. 187–232). Boston: Allyn & Bacon.

Wagner, R.K., & Sternberg, R.J. (1984). Alternative conceptions of intelligence and their implications for education. *Review of Educational Review, 54,* 179–224.

Wagoner, S.A. (1983). Comprehension monitoring: What it is and what we know about it. *Reading Research Quarterly, 18,* 328–346.

Waters, H.S. (1982). Memory development in adolescence: Relationships between metamemory, strategy use, and performance. *Journal of Experimental Child Psychology, 33,* 183–195.

Waters, H.S., & Andreassen, C. (1983). Children's use of memory strategies under instruction. In M. Pressley & J.R. Levin (Eds.), *Cognitive strategy research: Psychological foundations* (pp. 3–24). New York: Springer.

Waters, H.S., & McAlaster, R. (1983). Encoding variability and organization in free recall. *Journal of Experimental Child Psychology, 36,* 380–395.

Waters, H.S., & Waters, E. (1976). Semantic processing in children's free reall: Evidence for the importance of attentional factors and encoding variability. *Journal of Experimental Psychology: Human Learning and Memory, 2,* 370–380.

Waters, H.S., & Waters, E. (1979). Semantic processing in children's free recall: The effects of context and meaningfulness on encoding variability. *Child Development, 45,* 735–746.

Watts, G.H., & Anderson, R.C. (1971). Effects of three types of inserted questions on learning from prose. *Journal of Educational Psychology, 62,* 387–394.

Waugh, N.C, & Norman, D.A. (1965). Primary memory. *Psychological Review, 72,* 89–104.

Weaver, P.A., & Dickinson, D.K. (1984). Scratching below the surface structure: Exploring the usefulness of story grammars. *Discourse Processes, 5,* 225–243.

Weaver, S.L., & Cunningham, J.G. (1985). *Young children's implicit and explicit knowledge of their memory.* Paper presented at the biennial meeting of the Society for Research in Child Development, Toronto.

Weinert, F.E. (1962). Untersuchungen über einige Bedingungen des sprachlichen Lernens bei Kindern und Jugendlichen. *Vita humana, 5,* 185–194.

Weinert, F.E. (1964). Experimentelle Untersuchungen über Formen und Bedingungen des kognitiven Lernens bei Kindern. *Archiv für die gesamte Psychologie, 116,* 126–164.

Weinert, F.E. (1979). Entwicklungspsychologische Lern- under Gedächtnisforschung. Entwicklungsabhängigkeit des Lernens und des Gedächtnisses. In L. Montada (Ed.), *Brennpunkte der Entwicklungspsychologie* (pp. 61–76). Stuttgart: Kohlhammer.

Weinert, F.E. (1984). Metakognition und Motivation als Determinanten der Lerneffektivität: Einführung und Überblick. In F.E. Weinert & R.H. Kluwe (Eds.), *Metakognition, Motivation und Lernen* (pp. 9–21). Stuttgart: Kohlhammer.

Weinert, F.E. (1986). Developmental variations of memory performance and memory related knowledge across the life-span. In A. Sorensen, F.E. Weinert, & L.R. Sherrod (Eds.), *Human development: Multidisciplinary perspectives* (pp. 535–554). Hillsdale, NJ: Erlbaum & Associates.

Weinert, F.E., & Hasselhorn, M. (1986). Memory development: Universal changes and individual differences. In F. Klix & H. Hagendorf (Eds.), *Human memory and cognitive capabilities* (pp. 423–435). Amsterdam: Elsevier (North-Holland).

Weinert, F.E., & Knopf, M. (1983). Gedächtnisentwicklung. In R.K. Silbereisen & L. Montada (Eds.), *Entwicklungspsychologie* (pp. 103–111). München: Urban & Schwarzenberg.

Weinert, F.E., Knopf, M., & Barann, G. (1983). Metakognition und Motivation als Determinanten von Gedächtnisleistungen im höheren Erwachsenenalter. *Sprache und Kognition, 2,* 71–87.

Weinert, F.E., Knopf, M., & Körkel, J. (1983). Zusammenhänge zwischen Metawissen, Verhalten und Leistung bei der Lösung von Gedächtnisaufgaben durch Kinder und ältere Erwachsene. In G. Lüer (Ed.), *Bericht über den 33. Kongreß der Deutschen Gesellschaft für Psychologie in Mainz 1982* (pp. 262–271).

Weinert, F.E., Knopf, M., Körkel, J., Schneider, W., Vogel, K., & Wetzel, M. (1984). Die Entwicklung einiger Gedächtnisleistungen bei Kindern und älteren Erwachsenen in Abhängigkeit von kognitiven, metakognitiven, und motivationalen Merkmalen. In K.E. Grossman & P. Lütkenhaus (Eds.), *Bericht über die sechste Tagung Entwicklungspsychologie* (pp. 313–326). Regensburg: Universitäts-Druckerei.

Weinert, F.E., & Schneider, W. (Eds.) (1986). *First report on the Munich Longitudinal Study on the genesis of individual competencies (LOGIC).* Max Planck Institute for Psychological Research, Munich.

Weinert, F.E., & Schneider, W. (Eds.) (1987a). *The Munich Longitudinal Study on the Genesis of Individual Competencies (LOGIC). Report No. 2: Documentation of assessment procedures used in waves one to three.* Max Planck Institute for Psychological Research, Munich.

Weinert, F.E., & Schneider, W. (Eds.) (1987b). *The Munich Longitudinal Study on the Genesis of Individual Competencies (LOGIC). Report No. 3: Results of wave one.* Max Planck Institute for Psychological Research, Munich.

Weinert, F.E., Schneider, W., & Knopf, M. (in press). Individual differences in memory development across the life-span. In P.B. Baltes, D.L. Featherman, & R.M. Learner (Eds.), *Life-span development and behavior* (Vol. 8). Hillsdale, NJ: Erlbaum & Associates.

Weissberg, J.A., & Paris, S.G. (1986). Young children's remembering in different contexts: A reinterpretation of Istomina's study. *Child Development, 57,* 1123–1129.

Wellman, H.M. (1977a). The early development of intentional memory behavior. *Human Development, 20,* 86–101.

Wellman, H.M. (1977b). Preschooler's understanding of memory-relevant variables. *Child Development, 48,* 1720–1723.

Wellman, H.M. (1977c). Tip of the tongue and feeling of knowing experiences: A developmental study of memory monitoring. *Child Development, 48,* 13–21.

Wellman, H.M. (1978). Knowledge of the interaction of memory variables: A developmental study of metamemory. *Developmental Psychology, 14,* 24–29.

Wellman, H.M. (1979). *The role of metamemory in memory behavior: A developmental demonstration.* Unpublished manuscript, University of Michigan.

Wellman, H.M. (1983). Metamemory revisited. In M.T.H. Chi (Ed.), *Trends in memory development research* (pp. 31–51). Basel: Karger.

Wellman, H.M. (1985a). A child's theory of mind: The development of conceptions of cognition. In S.R. Yussen (Ed.), *The growth of reflection in children* (pp. 169–206). New York: Academic Press.

Wellman, H.M. (1985b). The origins of metacognition. In D.L. Forrest-Pressley, G.E. MacKinnon, & T.G. Waller (Eds.), *Metacognition, cognition, and human performance* (Vol. 1, pp. 1–31). Orlando, San Diego: Academic Press.

Wellman, H.M. (in press). The early development of memory strategies. In F.E. Weinert & M. Perlmutter (Eds.), *Memory development: Universal changes and individual differences.* Hillsdale, NJ: Erlbaum & Associates.

Wellman, H.M., Collins, J., & Glieberman, J. (1981). Understanding the combination of memory variables: Developing conceptions of memory limitations. *Child Development, 52,* 1313–1317.

Wellman, H.M., & Johnson, C.N. (1979). *Children's conception of the mental world.* Paper presented at the biennial meeting of the Society for Research in Child Development, San Francisco.

Wellman, H.M., Ritter, K., & Flavell, J.H. (1975). Deliberate memory behavior in the delayed reactions of very young children. *Developmental Psychology, 11,* 780–787.

Wellman, H.M., & Somerville, S.C. (1982). The development of human search ability. In M.E. Lamb & A.L. Brown (Eds.), *Advances in developmental psychology* (Vol. 2, pp. 41–84). Hillsdale, NJ: Erlbaum & Associates.

Wellman, H.M., Somerville, S.C., & Haake, R.J. (1979). Development of search procedures in real-life spatial environment. *Developmental Psychology, 15,* 530–542.

Werner, H. (1948). *Comparative psychology of the mental development.* New York: International Universities Press, Inc.

Whitely, P.L. (1927). The dependence of learning and recall upon prior intellectual activities. *Journal of Experimental Psychology, 10*, 489–508.

Whittaker, S.J. (1986). Eliminating alternatives: Preschool children's use of indirect memory cues. *British Journal of Developmental Psychologie, 4*, 199–207.

Whittaker, S., McShane, J., & Dunn, D. (1985). The development of cueing strategies in young children. *British Journal of Developmental Psychology, 3*, 153–161.

Wicklund, D.A., Palermo, D.S., & Jenkins, J.J. (1965). Associative clustering in the recall of children as a function of verbal association strength. *Journal of Experimental Child Psychology, 2*, 58–66.

Wilkinson, A.C., De Marinis, M., & Riley, S.J. (1983). Developmental and individual differences in rapid remembering. *Child Development, 54*, 898–911.

Wilkinson, A.C., & Koestler, R. (1983). Repeated recall: A new model and tests of its generality from childhood to old age. *Journal of Experimental Psychology, 112*, 423–451.

Wilkinson, A.C., & Koestler, R. (1984). Generality of a Markov model for repeated recall. *Journal of Mathematical Psychology, 28*, 43–72.

Williams, K.G., & Goulet, L.R. (1975). The effects of cueing and constraint instructions on children's free recall performance. *Journal of Experimental Child Psychology, 19*, 464–475.

Williams, M.D., & Hollan, J.D. (1981). The process of retrieval from very long-term memory. *Cognitive Science, 2*, 87–119.

Wimmer, H. (1976). Aspekte der Gedächtnisentwicklung. *Zeitschrift für Entwicklungspsychologie und Pädagogische Psychologie, 8*, 62–78.

Wimmer, H. (1979). Processing of script deviations by young children. *Discourse Processes, 2*, 301–310.

Wimmer, H. (1980). Children's understanding of stories: Assimilation by a general schema for actions or coordination of temporal relations. In F. Wilkening, J. Becker, & T. Trabasso (Eds.), *Information integration by children* (pp. 267–290). Hillsdale, NJ: Erlbaum & Associates.

Wimmer, H. (1982). *Zur Entwicklung des Verstehens von Erzählungen*. Bern: Huber.

Wimmer, H., & Tornquist, K. (1980). The role of metamemory and metamemory activation in the development of mnemonic performance. *International Journal of Behavioral Development, 3*, 71–81.

Winch, W.H. (1906). Immediate memory in school children. No. II. Auditory. *British Journal of Psychology, 2*, 1906–1908.

Winch, W.H. (1910). The transfer of improvement in memory in school-children. *British Journal of Psychology, 3*, 85–103.

Wine, J. (1971). Test anxiety and direction of attention. *Psychological Bulletin, 76*, 92–104.

Wingard, J.A., Buchanan, J.P., & Burnell, A. (1978). Organizational changes in the memory of young children. *Perceptual and Motor Skills, 46*, 735–742.

Winne, P.H. (1979). Experiments relating teachers' use of higher cognitive questions to student achievement. *Review of Educational Research, 49*, 13–49.

Wippich, W. (1980). Meta-Gedächtnis und Gedächtnis-Erfahrung. *Zeitschrift für Entwicklungspsychologie und Pädagogische Psychologie, 12*, 40–43.

Wippich, W. (1981). Verbessert eine Einkaufssituation die Vorhersage der eigenen Behaltensleistungen im Vorschulalter? *Zeitschrift für Entwicklungspsychologie und Pädagogische Psychologie, 8*, 280–290.

Wippich, W. (1984). *Lehrbuch der angewandten Gedächtnispsychologie (Band 1)*. Stuttgart: Kohlhammer.

Wolff, P., & Levin, J.R. (1972). The role of overt activity in children's imagery production. *Child Development, 43*, 537–547.

Wong, B.Y.L. (1982). Strategic behaviors in selecting retrieval cues in gifted, normal achieving and learning-disabled children. *Journal of Learning Disabilities*, *15*, 33–37.

Wong, B.Y.L. (1985). Self-questioning instructional research: A review. *Review of Educational Research*, *55*, 227–268.

Wood, E., Pressley, M., & Winne, P. (1988). *Children's learning of arbitrary facts in prose as a function of type of elaborative activity*. Presented at the annual meeting of the American Educational Research Association, New Orleans, LA.

Woodworth, R.S., & Schlosberg, H. (1954). *Experimental psychology*, revised edition. New York: Holt & Co.

Worden, P.E. (1974). The development of the category-recall function under three retrieval conditions. *Child Development*, *45*, 1054–1059.

Worden, P.E. (1975). Effects of sorting on subsequent recall of unrelated items: A developmental study. *Child Development*, *46*, 687–695.

Worden, P.E. (1976). The effects of classification structure on organized free recall in children. *Journal of Experimental Child Psychology*, *22*, 519–529.

Worden, P.E., & Sladewski-Awig, L.J. (1982). Children's awareness of memorability. *Journal of Educational Psychology*, *74*, 341–350.

Wozniak, R.H. (1972). Verbal regulation of motor behavior: Soviet research and non-Soviet replications. *Human Development*, *15*, 13–57.

Wozniak, R.H. (1975). Dialecticism and structuralism: The philosophical foundation of Soviet psychology and Piagetian cognitive developmental theory. In K.F. Riegel & G.C. Rosenwald (Eds.), *Structure and transformations: Developmental and historical aspects*. New York: Wiley.

Yates, F.A. (1966). *The art of memory.* London: Routledge & Kegan Paul.

Yendovitskaya, T.V. (1971). Development of memory. In A.V. Zaporozhets & D.B. Elkonin (Eds.), *The psychology of preschool children* (pp. 89–110). Cambridge, MA: MIT Press.

Young, D.R., & Schumacher, G.M. (1983). Context effects in young children's sensitivity to the importance level of prose information. *Child Development*, *54*, 1446–1456.

Yussen, S.R. (1974). Determinants of visual attention and recall in observational learning by preschoolers and second graders. *Developmental Psychology*, *10*, 93–100.

Yussen, S.R. (1985a). Preface. In S.R. Yussen (Ed.), *The growth of reflection in children* (pp. xv–xviii). New York: Academic Press.

Yussen, S.R. (1985b). The role of metacognition in contemporary theories of cognitive development. In D.L. Forrest-Pressley, G.E. MacKinnon, & T.G. Waller (Eds.), *Metacognition, cognition, and human performance* (Vol. 1, pp. 253–283). Orlando, San Diego: Academic Press.

Yussen, S.R., & Berman, L. (1981). Memory predictions for recall and recognition in first-, third-, and fifth-grade children. *Developmental Psychology*, *17*, 224–229.

Yussen, S.R., & Bird, J.E. (1979). The development of metacognitive awareness in memory, communication, and attention. *Journal of Experimental Child Psychology*, *28*, 300–313.

Yussen, S.R., Gagne, E., Gargiulo, R., & Kunen, S. (1974). The distinction between perceiving and memorizing in elementary school children. *Child Development*, *45*, 547–551.

Yussen, S.R., Kunen, S., & Buss, R. (1975). The distinction between perceiving and memorizing in the presence of category cues. *Child Development*, *46*, 763–768.

Yussen, S.R., Levin, J.R., Berman, L., & Palm, J. (1979). Developmental changes in the awareness of memory benefits associated with different types of picture organization. *Developmental Psychology*, *15*, 447–449.

Yussen, S.R., & Levy, V.M. (1975). Developmental changes in predicting one's own span of short-term memory. *Journal of Experimental Child Psychology*, *19*, 502–508.

Yussen, S.R., & Levy, V.M. (1977). Developmental changes in knowledge about different retrieval problems. *Developmental Psychology, 13*, 114–120.

Yussen, S.R., Mathews, S.R., Buss, R.R., & Kane, P.T. (1980). Developmental change in judging important and critical elements of stories. *Developmental Psychology, 16*, 213–219.

Zabrucky, K., & Ratner, H.H. (1986). Children's comprehension monitoring and recall of inconsistent stories. *Child Development, 57*, 1401–1418.

Zelinski, E.M., Gilewski, M.J., & Thompson, L.W. (1980). Do laboratory tests relate to self-assessment of memory ability in the young and old? In L.W. Poon, J. Fozard, L. Cermak, D. Ahrenberg, & L. Thompson (Eds.), *New directions in memory and aging* (pp. 519–544). Hillsdale, NJ: Erlbaum & Associates.

Zembar, M.J., & Naus, M.J. (1985a). *An argument for a more integrative approach to the study of memory development.* Paper presented at the Southwestern Psychological Association, Austin, TX.

Zembar, M.J., & Naus, M.J. (1985b). *The combined effects of knowledge base and mnemonic strategies on children's memory.* Paper presented at the biennial meeting of the Society for Research in Child Development, Toronto.

Zimmerman, B.J., & Pons, M.M. (1986). Development of a structured interview for assessing student use of self-regulated learning strategies. *American Educational Research Journal, 23*, 614–628.

Zinchenko, P.I. (1967). Probleme der Gedächtnispsychologie. In H. Hiebsch (Ed.), *Ergebnisse der sowjetischen Psychologie* (pp. 191–240). Berlin: Akademie Verlag.

Author Index

Abelson, R., 43, *248*
Ach, N., 89, *205*
Ackerman, B.P., 44, 65, 66, 67, 164, *205,*
206, 220, 245
Adams, J.A., 178, *206*
Adams, L.T., 43, *206*
Ahmad, M., 99, 110, 135, 138, 143, 144,
149, 157, 179, 191, *243, 244*
Aivano, S., 48, *237*
Alley, G.R., 181, 184, 187, *219*
Allik, J.P., 47, *206*
Alvermann, D.E., 86, 87, *206, 250*
Anderson, C.W., 87, *206*
Anderson, J.R., 79, 129, 132, 166, 167,
206, 222
Anderson, R.C., 86, *206, 242, 254*
Andreassen, C., 46, 60, 116, 117, 181,
206, 214, 253
Appel, F.L., 45, *206*
Applebee, A.N., 188, *206, 207*
Armbruster, B.B., 38, 122, *214*
Arnold, D.J., 86, *207*
Ashcraft, M.A., 47, *207, 228*

Ashcr, S.R., 83, *207*
Ashmead, D.H., 39, *207*
Atkinson, R.C., 20, 23, 24, 34, 46, 73,
133, 196, *207*
Auble, P.M., 142, *212*
August, D.L., 91, *222*

Baddeley, A., 23, 127, 131, *207*
Baker, L., 91, 96, 124, 131, 166, 167, *207*
Baker-Ward, L., 37, 45, 47, 59, 60, 197,
202, 203, *207, 239*
Baldwin, R.S., 84, *207*
Bandura, A., 161, *207, 208*
Banjeri, R., 178, *246*
Baratz, D., 44, 55, *235*
Barclay, C.R., 51, 109, 163, *208, 212*
Barnett, C., 178, *252*
Barnitz, J., 85, *234*
Baron, J., 122, 126, 127, 128, 131, *208*
Bassiri, D., 125, 189, *219*
Battig, W.F., 53, *208*
Baumeister, A.A., 34, *239*
Beach, D.H., 35, 46, *221*
Beal, C.R., 41, 91, 102, 167, *208*
Bean, J.P., 136, 137, *247*
Begg, I., 153, *208*

Subject Index